ADOLESCENT MEDICINE:
STATE OF THE ART REVIEWS

What's New In Adolescent
Clinical Care?

GUEST EDITORS

Richard B. Heyman, MD
Edward M. Gotlieb, MD

April 2009 • Volume 20 • Number 1

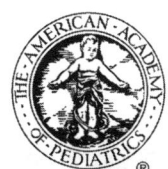

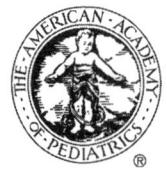

ADOLESCENT MEDICINE CLINICS:
STATE OF THE ART REVIEWS
April 2009
Editor: Diane E. Lundquist
Marketing Manager: Marirose Russo
Production Manager: Shannan Martin

Volume 20, Number 1
ISBN 978-1-58110-333-5
ISSN 1934-4287
MA0478
SUB1006

Copyright © 2009 American Academy of Pediatrics. All rights reserved. No part of this publication may be reproduced or transmitted in any form or by any means, electronic or mechanical, including photocopying, recording, or any information retrieval system, without written permission from the Publisher (fax the permissions editor at 847/434-8780).

Adolescent Medicine: State of the Art Reviews is published three times per year by the American Academy of Pediatrics, 141 Northwest Point Blvd, Elk Grove Village, IL 60007-1098. Periodicals postage paid at Arlington Heights, IL.

POSTMASTER: Send address changes to American Academy of Pediatrics, Department of Marketing and Publications, Attn: AM:STARs, 141 Northwest Point Blvd, Elk Grove Village, IL 60007-1098.

Subscriptions: Subscriptions to *Adolescent Medicine: State of the Art Reviews* (AM:STARs) are provided to members of the American Academy of Pediatrics' Section on Adolescent Health as part of annual section membership dues. All others, please contact the AAP Customer Service Center at 866/843-2271 (7:00 am–5:30 pm Central Time, Monday–Friday) for pricing and information.

Adolescent Medicine: State of the Art Reviews

Official Journal of the American Academy of Pediatrics
Section on Adolescent Health

EDITORS-IN-CHIEF

Victor C. Strasburger, MD
Professor of Pediatrics
Chief, Division of Adolescent Medicine
University of New Mexico School of Medicine
Albuquerque, New Mexico

Donald E. Greydanus, MD
Professor of Pediatrics
Michigan State University and Pediatrics Program Director
Kalamazoo Center for Medical Studies
Kalamazoo, Michigan

ASSOCIATE EDITORS

Robert T. Brown, MD
Upland, Pennsylvania

Cynthia Holland-Hall, MD
Columbus, Ohio

Martin M. Fisher, MD
Manhasset, New York

Paula K. Braverman, MD
Cincinnati, Ohio

Sheryl Ryan
New Haven, Connecticut

Alain Joffe, MD, MPH
Baltimore, Maryland

WHAT'S NEW IN ADOLESCENT CLINICAL CARE?

EDITORS-IN-CHIEF

VICTOR C. STRASBURGER, MD, Professor of Pediatrics, Division of Adolescent Medicine, University of New Mexico, School of Medicine, Albuquerque, New Mexico

DONALD E. GREYDANUS, MD, Professor of Pediatrics, Michigan State University; and Pediatrics Program Director, Kalamazoo Center for Medical Studies, Kalamazoo, Michigan

GUEST EDITORS

RICHARD B. HEYMAN, MD, Suburban Pediatric Associates, Cincinnati, Ohio

EDWARD M. GOTLIEB, MD, The Pediatric Center of Stone Mountain LLC, Stone Mountain, Georgia; Kids Health First Pediatric Alliance, Atlanta, Georgia

CONTRIBUTORS

CHRISTEL A. BILTOFT, MD, FAAP, The Pediatric Center of Stone Mountain, LLC, Stone Mountain, Georgia; Kids Health First Pediatric Alliance, Atlanta, Georgia

JAMIE BRAY, LCSW, Hillside, Inc, Atlanta, Georgia

CHEVON BROOKS, MD, Department of Pediatrics, Morehouse School of Medicine, Atlanta, Georgia

ROBERT L. CERCIELLO, MD, Departments of Neurology and Pediatrics, University of Connecticut School of Medicine, Farmington, Connecticut; Connecticut Children's Medical Center, East Hartford, Connecticut

ROY CHANCEY, LCSW, Hillside, Inc, Atlanta, Georgia

JOSEPH CONGENI, Division of Sports Medicine, Akron Children's Hospital Sports Medicine Center, Akron, Ohio; and Department of Pediatrics, Northeastern Ohio Universities College of Medicine, Rootstown, Ohio

LARAE COPLEY, MD, PHD, Department of Psychiatry, Ohio State University, Columbus, Ohio

KAIYTI DUFFY, MPH, Physicians for Reproductive Choice and Health, New York, New York

PAULA M. DUNCAN, MD, Vermont Child Health Improvement Program, University of Vermont College of Medicine, Burlington, Vermont

BARBARA L. FRANKOWSKI, MD, MPH, Vermont Child Health Improvement Program and Department of Pediatrics, Vermont Children's Hospital, University of Vermont College of Medicine, Burlington, Vermont

GILBERT L. FULD, MD, FAAP, Department of Pediatrics, Dartmouth Medical School, Hanover, New Hampshire; Council on Communications and Media, American Academy of Pediatrics, Elk Grove Village, Illinois

EDWARD M. GOTLIEB, MD, FAAP, FSAM, The Pediatric Center of Stone Mountain LLC, Stone Mountain, Georgia; Kids Health First Pediatric Alliance, Atlanta, Georgia

JAQUELIN S. GOTLIEB, MD, FAAP, The Pediatric Center of Stone Mountain LLC, Stone Mountain, Georgia; Kids Health First Pediatric Alliance, Atlanta, Georgia

RICHARD B. HEYMAN, MD, FAAP, Suburban Pediatric Associates, Cincinnati, Ohio

CHRISTOPHER JONES, PHD, Hillside, Inc, Atlanta, Georgia

LISA J. KOBRYNSKI, MD, MPH, Department of Pediatrics, Allergy/Immunology Section, Emory University School of Medicine, Atlanta, Georgia

ISAAC C. LEADER, University of Vermont College of Medicine, Burlington, Vermont

DAVID A. LEVINE, MD, Department of Pediatrics, Morehouse School of Medicine, Atlanta, Georgia

KATHY LOVE-OSBORNE, MD, Department of Pediatrics, Section of Adolescent Medicine, Denver Health and Hospitals, University of Colorado Denver Health Sciences Center, Denver, Colorado

ANDREW MUIR, MD, Division of Endocrinology, Department of Pediatrics, Emory University School of Medicine, Atlanta, Georgia

EMILY POTTS, LMSW, Hillside, Inc, Atlanta, Georgia

CAROL L. RIZZOLO, RPA-C, MA, Cheshire, Connecticut

PETER D. ROGERS, MD, MPA, FASAM, FSAM, Adolescent Medicine/Addiction Medicine, Nationwide Children's Hospital, Columbus, Ohio; Department of Pediatrics, Ohio State University College of Medicine, Columbus, Ohio

JOHN E. TAYLOR, MA, Child and Youth Mental Health, Ministry of Children and Family Development, British Columbia, Canada

JOAN K. TEACH, PHD, Community Resource Center, Atlanta, Georgia

EAMONN WALSH, LCSW, Hillside, Inc, Atlanta, Georgia

AARON M. WHITE, PHD, Division of Medical Psychology, Department of Psychiatry, Duke University Medical Center, Durham, North Carolina

YOLANDA WIMBERLY, MD, MSC, Department of Pediatrics, Morehouse School of Medicine, Atlanta, Georgia

WHAT'S NEW IN ADOLESCENT CLINICAL CARE?

CONTENTS

Preface xiii

The Nonmedical Use of Prescription Drugs by Adolescents 1
Peter D. Rogers, LaRae Copley

> The abuse of prescription drugs such as opioids, stimulants, tranquilizers, and sleeping pills is the fastest-growing class of drugs being abused by adolescents. Among this class of drugs, prescription opioids are being abused the most, although the abuse of prescription stimulants has been studied the most. There is a paucity of information on the nonmedical use of tranquilizers and sleeping pills. In this article we will discuss the specific prescription drugs that are most commonly abused by adolescents and how physicians need to be cautious when prescribing these drugs. The issue of screening for the abuse of these drugs will be addressed, as will the importance of parents' monitoring the use of these drugs by their own children.

Screening for Substance Abuse in the Office Setting:
A Developmental Approach 9
Richard B. Heyman

> Uptake of the use of alcohol and other drugs is best understood (and, therefore, addressed) as a developmental issue. A variety of risk and protective factors (personal, societal, genetic, etc) play out across the span of childhood, adolescence, and young adulthood, and an understanding of brain and cognitive development may make it easier for the pediatrician to put this into context and address the issue. A simple screening tool that focuses on 6 areas of concern is presented, one that may be used for assessment and educational purposes, as well.

Strength-Based Interviewing 22
Barbara L. Frankowski, Isaac C. Leader, Paula M. Duncan

> Health care for adolescents needs to include both assessment of risk and identification of strengths. Clinicians need practical ways to identify strengths, or assets, by using a proven frame-

work. After eliciting the strengths, clinicians must be ready to help adolescents recognize and build on them. In addition, many will want to go the next step and use this strength-based approach with shared decision-making techniques, including motivational interviewing.

Management of the Adolescent Concussion Victim   41
Joseph Congeni

Increasing awareness and understanding of the implications of concussion have shaped a more proactive management approach to this problem. Although the incidence of brain injuries in adolescent athletes is probably in the range of 1.6 to 3.8 million per year (Centers for Disease Control and Prevention, National Center for Injury Prevention and Control. Facts for physicians about mild traumatic brain injury. Available at: www.cdc.gov/ncipc/pubres/tbi_toolkit/physicians/mtbi/mtbi.pdf), difficulties in recognizing and diagnosing this condition mean that as many as 80% go unrecognized and have led to its being known as "the silent epidemic." Attempts to improve the evaluation on the sidelines, in the outpatient clinic, and in the home are helping to improve management. Better understanding of the prognosis and clinical course of concussion, as well as the importance of physical and mental rest, have also helped healthcare providers to make better decisions about allowing athletes to return to play.

Social Networking and Adolescents   57
Gilbert L. Fuld

Online social networking is a 21st century innovation increasingly embraced by today's young people. It provides new opportunities for communication that expand an adolescent's world. Yet adults, often suspicious of new trends and technologies initially embraced by youth, often see these new environments as perilous places to visit. These fears have been accentuated by media hype, especially about sexual predators. How dangerous are they? Because the rush to go on these sites is a new phenomenon, research is as yet scant. This review explores current beliefs and knowledge about the dangers of social networking sites.

Understanding Adolescent Brain Development and Its Implications for the Clinician   73
Aaron M. White

Contrary to long-held beliefs about brain development, widespread changes occur in the brain during the adolescent years.

These changes involve a shift in control over behavior away from regions geared toward emotional processing, such as the amygdala and reward system, toward the frontal lobes, which are involved in making plans for the future, suppressing impulses, weighing options, and other critical cognitive skills needed to function in the adult world. Experience-dependant sculpting of these developing circuits ensures that each adolescent will be customized to fit the demands of his or her environment, healthy or otherwise. As adolescent brain development unfolds, risk-taking, substance use, and the emergence of psychological pathologies are common. Many recreational and prescription drugs affect adolescents and adults differently, both short-term and long-term. In this review, the changes that take place in the brain during the adolescent years are explored. What happens, how these changes can go awry, and how to help keep adolescent brain development on track will be examined.

An Approach to Obesity Management in Primary Care: Yes, We Can Make a Difference 91
Kathy Love-Osborne

Obesity is a problem encountered in primary care on a daily basis. The author reviews the literature in the area of adolescent obesity and discusses an approach to managing obesity in the office, including screening for comorbidities and motivating teenagers to make lifestyle changes. Medications used for the treatment of comorbidities are reviewed also.

The Metabolic Syndrome in Children and Adolescents: A Clinician's Guide 109
Christel A. Biltoft, Andrew Muir

This article reviews the components of the metabolic syndrome, the theory behind the combined negative effects of insulin resistance and obesity and discusses the clinical utility of this concept in pediatrics. The latest diagnostic criteria for obesity, dyslipidemia and hypertension in children and adolescents as well as management and prevention strategies are also discussed.

Primary Immunodeficiencies Presenting in Adolescence 121
Lisa J. Kobrynski

Recurrent infections are a common problem in pediatrics. For most children the frequency of infection decreases over time, but recurring, severe, or unusual infections may be a sign of a primary immunodeficiency disease. Primary immunodeficiency diseases are a heterogeneous group of more than 120 disorders that affect various parts of the immune system, leading to an increased susceptibility to infection. Many primary immunodeficiency diseases are not diagnosed until late childhood or adolescence. This article will review the diagnosis and treatment of those primary immunodeficiencies that are most likely to present with clinical signs and symptoms during adolescence and young adulthood.

Drop-out Crisis Impacting America: Can We Turn It Around? 149
Joan K. Teach

Increasing numbers of our adolescents are leaving high school before attaining a standard diploma. In today's society, dropping out of high school increases the likelihood of substandard living, lower job potential, and, perhaps, poverty and welfare. As our nation adds more rigorous requirements to graduation, we should develop programs to assist at-risk students to be successful. Without supporting our youth, we will be faced with a nation of undereducated, welfare-level adults, driving down our earning potential, increasing crime, and lowering our community viability. Now is the time for change. This article describes the situation, reviews interventions, and presents a challenge for change.

Adolescent Contraceptive Care for the Practicing Pediatrician 168
Kaiyti Duffy, Yolanda Wimberly, Chevon Brooks

Improved use of contraception has been intrinsic in the decline of teenaged pregnancies in the United States. Recent advances in contraception, including the development of new progestins and longer-acting reversible methods, have greatly increased the options available for adolescents. By frankly discussing adverse effects, offering clear explanations of noncontraceptive benefits, and developing strategies for improving compliance, providers can play a key role in facilitating successful contraceptive use in young patients.

Anxiety and Anxiety-Related Disorders in the Adolescent Population: An Overview of Diagnosis and Treatment 188
Carol L. Rizzolo, John E. Taylor, Robert L. Cerciello

Anxiety is a common component of visits to the doctor's office by adolescents; however, it is often overlooked as a possible causative agent of the presenting complaint. With a high index of suspicion and proper questioning, a clinician can analyze the contribution that anxiety plays in the life of an adolescent patient. Behavioral and pharmacologic interventions exist for this group of disorders, and with proper diagnosis and treatment the symptoms of these disorders can possibly be ameliorated. This article provides a concise guide to the diagnosis and treatment of anxiety and anxiety-related disorders including hyperventilation syndrome, syncope, sleep disorders, panic disorder, and obsessive compulsive disorder.

Helping Adolescents With Attention-Deficit/Hyperactivity Disorder Transition Toward Adulthood 203
Edward M. Gotlieb, Jaquelin S. Gotlieb

Pediatricians can help adolescents with attention-deficit/hyperactivity disorder prepare to enter post–high school training and the workforce. In this article peer-reviewed studies and other resources for informing patients of the issues ahead are identified. We discuss preventive counseling, including long-term monitoring, adherence to treatment, driving, tobacco, alcohol, and other drug usage, career planning, and intimacy. The current status of insurance coverage for young adults and federal programs to assist students with attention-deficit/hyperactivity disorder are reviewed also. Consideration is given for applying for precollege testing and college accommodations and traveling abroad with medications. Pediatricians and young adults are directed to Web-based and other self-management information and tools.

Office-Based Care for Gay, Lesbian, Bisexual, and Questioning Youth 223
David A. Levine

While most gay, lesbian, and bisexual teens are quite resilient, the health disparities in working with this vulnerable population can be significant. This review will define and attempt to quantify the number of our sexual minority youth. The review discusses the unique challenges faced by these young people and suggests some evidence-based interventions that have allowed youth to reduce their risk behaviors. The role of homophobia and heterosexism is discussed and how the two issues impact the developing mind of a gay, lesbian, or bisexual teenager. Finally, issues in providing clinical care and modifying our patient care approaches to providing effective care, is discussed. Essentially, using validated approaches to obtaining a good adolescent psychosocial history, the office-based care for Gay, Lesbian, and Bisexual youth is not different from working with other youth. Many are quite resilient and progress through adolescence without difficulty; others stumble and may fall to mental health issues, substance abuse, and HIV. We must provide excellent care if we are to help this vulnerable population of teenagers.

An Overview of the Use of Dialectical Behavior Therapy With Adolescents for Primary Care Physicians   243
Christopher Jones, Roy Chancey, Eamonn Walsh, Jamie Bray, Emily Potts

Mental health problems among children and adolescents are an area of public health needing increased attention. Children and adolescents whose mental health problems go untreated are at increased risk of suicide, juvenile delinquency, school dropout, and substance abuse. Primary care physicians are often the first point of contact for these youth and left with the task of identifying the most appropriate treatment intervention for these youth and their families. We aim to provide an overview of dialectical behavioral therapy, its effectiveness with adolescents, and its application to work with adolescents.

Index   253

Preface

What's New in Adolescent Clinical Care?

This issue of *AM:STARs* focuses on many apparently disparate concerns of physical and mental health, sexuality, and scientific and sociological issues that have an impact on the primary health care of adolescents. Their commonality is in the attempt by physicians who care for adolescents in the real world to better serve their patients. We are frequently the first, and all too often the only, professionals to whom these patients feel they can turn for help in dealing with their concerns and health care needs. The topics are wide ranging by design. They mean to display the panoply of dilemmas that present themselves on any given day in the clinical office and other primary care settings. Although our concerns may have a somewhat different slant from those of our academic colleagues, the topics we address are broad-based, inquiring, and contemporary. They are frequently enlightened and enlivened by a good story. The authors bring firsthand knowledge and a genuine enthusiasm for their topics, and your editors hope that this energy is projected in their work.

The National Research Council and the Institute of Medicine recently published a workshop report[1] and a text[2] on the problems of providing care in an organized fashion to adolescents in the United States. They place considerable emphasis on the need for a coordinated approach to the delivery of primary health care services for adolescents. Among their recommendations, they make 3 specifically for primary health care:

1. Federal and state agencies, private foundations, and private insurers should support and promote the development and use of a coordinated health care system that strives to improve health services for all adolescents.
2. As part of an enhanced primary care system for adolescents, health care providers and health organizations should focus their attention on the particular needs of specific groups of adolescents who may be particularly vulnerable to risky behavior or poor health because of selected population characteristics or other circumstances.
3. Providers of adolescent primary care services and the payment systems that support them should make disease prevention, health promotion, and behavioral health (including early identification, management, and monitoring of current or emerging health conditions and risky behavior) a major component of routine health services.

The American Academy of Pediatrics Section on Adolescent Health has the task of educating the academy's membership on the health concerns of adolescents. For more than 2 decades the section has presented programs and publications to advance this goal. This journal, and specifically this issue, continues in that tradition. We thank the editors-in-chief of this journal and their associate editors for support and encouragement in bringing primary care physicians and other primary care providers into this discussion.

Richard B. Heyman, MD
Suburban Pediatric Associates
Cincinnati, Ohio

Edward M. Gotlieb, MD
The Pediatric Center of Stone Mountain
Stone Mountain, Georgia

REFERENCES

1. National Research Council; Institute of Medicine. *Challenges in Adolescent Health Care: Workshop Report.* Committee on Adolescent Health Care Services and Models of Care for Treatment, Prevention, and Healthy Development, Board on Children, Youth, and Families, Division of Behavioral and Social Sciences and Education. Washington, DC: National Academies Press; 2007
2. Lawrence RS, Appleton Gootman J, Sim LJ, eds. *Adolescent Health Services: Missing Opportunities.* Committee on Adolescent Health Care Services and Models of Care for Treatment, Prevention, and Healthy Development. Board on Children, Youth, and Families. Division of Behavioral and Social Sciences and Education. Washington, DC: National Academies Press; 2009

The Nonmedical Use of Prescription Drugs by Adolescents

Peter D. Rogers, MD, MPA, FASAM, FSAM[*,a,b], LaRae Copley, MD, PhD[c]

[a]*Adolescent Medicine/Addiction Medicine, Nationwide Children's Hospital, 700 Children's Drive, Columbus, OH 43205, USA*

[b]*Department of Pediatrics, Ohio State University College of Medicine, 700 Children's Drive, Columbus, OH 43205, USA*

[c]*Department of Psychiatry, Ohio State University Department of Psychiatry, 1670 Upham Drive, Columbus, OH 43210, USA*

The abuse of prescription drugs by adolescents has shown an alarming and dramatic increase in the past 2 decades, especially since 2004.[1] Between 1992 and 2002, the US population increased 13% while prescriptions for controlled drugs increased by 154%.[2] The number of people who admitted to abusing controlled prescription drugs increased from 7.8 million in 1992 to 15.1 million in 2003 (an increase of 94%), which is 7 times faster than the increase in the US population. By 2006, 15.8 million people reported abusing controlled prescription drugs, more than the combined number who reported abusing cocaine (6.1 million), hallucinogens (4.0 million), inhalants (2.2 million), and heroin (0.5 million).[3]

The abuse of these controlled prescription drugs by the general population is reflected in the adolescent population. In 2006, 2.2 million teenagers between the ages of 12 and 17 admitted to nonmedical use of a prescription drug in the past year.[4] More adolescents have abused prescription drugs than many illegal drugs including ecstasy, cocaine, crack, and methamphetamine. More than half (56%) of adolescents surveyed believe that prescription drugs are easier to obtain than illicit drugs, and 52% believe that prescription narcotics are "available everywhere."[5]

The abuse of prescription drugs by adolescents has continued to increase since 2005, and there is no reason to believe that the continued increase of the abuse

*Corresponding author.
E-mail address: peter.rogers@nationwidechildrens.org (P. D. Rogers).

Copyright © 2009 American Academy of Pediatrics. All rights reserved. ISSN 1934-4287

of these drugs will abate soon. They now represent the third most widely misused substances among adolescents after alcohol and marijuana.[6]

For adolescents, there is evidence (from our personal experience) to suggest that prescription drugs are not entry-level drugs. Many adolescents who develop a substance abuse disorder and are abusing prescription drugs began their drug use with other drugs, most commonly alcohol and marijuana.[7] Those of us who take care of adolescents have another monster problem of which we need to be aware: the abuse of prescription drugs is dangerous and, if taken with other drugs, can be fatal. There is also mounting evidence to suggest that adolescents and young adults who abuse prescription drugs go on to develop prescription drug abuse and dependence. In this article we discuss the abuse of prescription opioids, stimulants, sleeping pills, and anxiolytic agents.

DEFINITIONS

In referring to prescription drug abuse, terms such as "use," "misuse," and "abuse" are often used interchangeably. In this article, we use the definition used by Boyd et al[1]: prescription drug abuse is defined as the use of prescription medication to create an altered state, to "get high," or for reasons other than those intended by the prescribing clinician. Often the person taking the medication is not the patient for whom the medication was prescribed.

PRESCRIPTION OPIOIDS

An opiate is a drug containing or derived from opium, which is extracted from seeds of the poppy plant and contains morphine or codeine. Heroin is synthesized from the morphine contained in opium.

The term "opioid" refers to compounds that have opioid pharmacologic activity and includes, in addition to codeine and morphine, synthetic and semisynthetic drugs such as hydrocodone, oxycodone (OxyContin [Purdue Pharma, Stamford, CT]), methadone, hydromorphone (Dilaudid [Abbott Laboratories, Abbott Park, IL]), fentanyl, and propoxyphene (Darvon [Xanodyne Pharmaceuticals, Inc, Newport, KY]). The term "narcotics" refers to addictive drugs (eg, opiates and opioids) that reduce pain, induce sleep, and produce euphoria.[8]

The clinician ordering a urine drug screen must understand what specific drugs are included in the test being ordered. Synthetic and semisynthetic opioids, including methadone, are often not identified in urine drug screens that screen for "opiates." Thus, one must understand the implications of the screen and determine if the laboratory method can identify specific compounds.

With the exception of LSD (lysergic acid diethylamide), all substances of abuse, including opioids, cause the release of dopamine in the mesolimbic dopaminergic

Table 1
Source of prescription drugs among those who used them in the past year (12th-graders, 2007)

	Amphetamines, %	Tranquilizers, %	Narcotics Other Than Heroin, %
Bought on Internet	3.1	1.9	1.8
Took from friend/relative without asking	16.5	19.2	26.6
Given for free by friend or relative	56.8	59.1	55.1
Bought from friend or relative	42.5	40.9	38.4
From a prescription I had	15.4	20.6	39.5
Bought from drug dealer/stranger	27.4	21.7	17.9
Other method	19.0	10.3	7.7

Data source: Johnston LD, O'Malley PM, Bachman JG, Schulenberg JE. *Monitoring the Future National Survey Results on Drug Use, 1975–2006.* Vol I: Secondary School Students. Bethesda, MD: National Institute on Drug Abuse; 2007. NIH publication No. 07-6205. Available at: http://monitoringthefuture.org/pubs/monographs/vol1_2007.pdf.

reward system and, for most people, cause euphoria. Opioids have a profound effect on the dopamine receptors and can be highly addictive, with the euphoria being most profound when taking the opioids for a reason other than for treating pain.

Opioids are the most common prescription drugs of abuse among adolescents, and at least 1 author has referred to the misuse of prescription opioids by adolescents as an "epidemic."[7] Use of other, illicit drugs by adolescents is the strongest predictor of nonmedical use of opioids.[9] On the basis of 1 of the author's (Dr Rogers) clinical experiences working with adolescents and young adult opioid users, most adolescents get or steal their prescription opioids from family members and friends or buy the drugs at school or from known drug dealers (see Table 1).

The abuse of opiates by adolescents usually begins by taking the pill(s) by mouth and then may progress to crushing and snorting them. Tolerance for the euphoria-producing effects of opioids builds up quickly, commonly leading the teenager to use the drug more frequently. Many eventually progress to using stronger, longer-lasting, and more potent prescription opioids such as OxyContin, a long-acting preparation of oxycodone.

OxyContin sells for approximately $1 per milligram on the street. When taking this drug becomes a habit, buying enough OxyContin to get high becomes expensive, which often leads to stealing money to buy the drug. Soon the user learns that heroin is cheaper than OxyContin, and when the youth finds where to buy heroin, often in crime-infested areas of the city, addiction often develops. From the authors' experience, it seems that the abuse of prescription opioids is a risk factor for an adolescent developing a heroin addiction.

In a report from the National Center on Addiction and Substance Abuse at Columbia University, the Internet is referred to as a "pharmaceutical candy store," where a youth can purchase controlled prescription drugs, completely lacking in oversight from parents and other family members and frequently hidden from law enforcement.[4] The only published data available for certain opioids used by adolescents has come from the Monitoring the Future Study (2006), which showed that in the past year 9.7% of 12th-grade students had used Vicodin (Abbott Laboratories), 4.3% had used OxyContin, and 9% had used "other narcotics."[6] It seems clear that physicians of all specialties need to be concerned about prescribing opioids (and how much we are prescribing), because so many of the prescription opioids are being diverted.

One suggestion is that if a clinician prescribes an opioid for a minor child, a parent should monitor the use of this drug. Parents should also be cautioned that if there are prescription drugs in the house, such as narcotics, anxiolytic agents, stimulants (including "diet" pills), and sleeping pills, they should be in a safe place, preferably locked, so that others in the family cannot have access to these drugs.

PRESCRIPTION STIMULANTS

The abuse of prescription stimulants among adolescents and college-aged students has been studied longer and more intensely than the abuse of any other prescription drug.[10,11] Attention-deficit/hyperactivity disorder (ADHD) is a prominent neurobehavioral disorder that occurs in 6% to 8% of children and 4% to 5% of adults. Medications including both stimulants and nonstimulants (eg, atomoxetine) are increasingly recognized to contribute to long-term optimal outcome in patients with ADHD.[11] Although useful in the treatment of ADHD, stimulants are controlled, schedule II substances that show a potential for abuse.[12,13]

In recent human studies, the stimulants methylphenidate and amphetamines have been associated with more likeability and euphoria-producing effects than nonscheduled agents such as atomoxetine.[11,14] Although the literature clearly supports the important therapeutic effects of stimulants, human studies have highlighted the abuse liability and, ultimately, dependence on the same stimulants used in the treatment of ADHD.[11,15] One study of 1536 US students in grades 6 to 11 who were using a self-administered Internet-based survey found that 5% reported lifetime prescription stimulant (ADHD medication) misuse.[8,10]

For those of us who prescribe stimulant medications for patients with ADHD and are concerned about the misuse and diversion of these drugs, a recent publication addressed the rates of diversion and misuse of stimulant medications as well as who is at greatest risk for abusing these drugs.[11] The article contains some alarming information, as do other studies on diversion of stimulant medications.

One study reported that 16% of children and adolescents with ADHD were asked to give, sell, or trade their stimulant medications to other students.[16] In another study of a college-aged sample, 23% of students diagnosed with ADHD who had a prescription for stimulant drugs were approached to give, sell, or trade their medications while in college.[11] Two studies of high school students who reported having ADHD prescriptions found that 15% to 24% had given away their stimulant medications,[17] 7% to 19% had sold their medications to other students, and 4% to 6% had their medications stolen.[9,16,18]

Studies on stimulant drug misuse have indicated that females are as likely as males to report stimulant misuse, whites have greater misuse rates than blacks, and adolescents living in metropolitan areas are more likely to abuse stimulant medications than adolescents in rural areas.[11] Those students who misuse stimulant medications often are abusing other substances such as cigarettes, alcohol, and marijuana.[19]

It has also been shown that immediate-release stimulants have a higher rate of misuse than extended-release drugs.[11] Often these immediate-release drugs are crushed and snorted instead of being taken orally.[11,18] The most commonly reported reasons for use of nonprescribed stimulants include studying, staying awake, improved alertness, "getting high and/or partying," and experimentation.[12,14]

It remains unclear whether subjects with neuropsychological deficits or untreated ADHD may be more vulnerable to misuse stimulant medication, but regardless, it is incumbent on those of us who prescribe stimulants to our patients, especially those of high school and college age, to understand that there is a significant potential for abuse of these medications. Our patients and their parents must be told that the unmonitored use of these drugs can have significant effects on the cardiovascular system and that these drugs are often sought by other students with a substance abuse problem and giving away or selling stimulant medications is a felony.

A cautionary note on urine drug screens and the use of stimulant medications: although methylphenidate (Ritalin [Novartis Pharmaceuticals, Basel, Switzerland]) is an amphetamine, because of its unique structure it will not screen positive for "amphetamines" in most urine drug screens. Once again, the clinician ordering a urine drug screen must know what drugs are and are not included in the screening.

It is generally agreed that drugs such as Concerta (Alza Corporation, Mountain View, CA), Vyvanse (Shire Specialty Pharmaceuticals, Wayne, PA), and Strattera (Eli Lilly and Co, Indianapolis, IN) may be "safer" drugs to use for ADHD in adolescents with a substance abuse disorder because of their very low potential for abuse. Concerta (methylphenidate) is manufactured in a slow-release tablet

Table 2
Annual prevalence of sedatives and tranquilizers in 12th grade

	Percent of All Seniors Using These Drugs		
	2002	2005	2008
Sedatives (barbiturates)	6.7	7.2	5.8
Tranquilizers	7.7	6.6	6.2

Data source: Monitoring the Future, National Institutes of Health, News Release. Available at: www.monitoringthefuture.org/pressrelease/08drugs_complete.pdf.

form that is not crushable; Vyvanse (lisdexamfetamine) is an amphetamine/lysine molecule that has rate-limited absorption; and Strattera does not seem to create any euphoria even at high doses (D. Coury, MD, R. Heyman, MD, personal communication, December 15, 2008; R. Heyman, personal communication, December 15, 2008). Although the question has been raised as to whether treating young people with stimulants promotes later substance abuse, research suggests that the use of stimulant medications in children and adolescents with ADHD has a "protective effect" on these children and decreases the likelihood of them developing a substance abuse disorder.[13]

TRANQUILIZERS AND SEDATIVES

Tranquilizers and sedatives, including sleeping pills and barbiturates, are the least studied of prescription drugs abused by adolescents. Although there are data from the Monitoring the Future Study concerning the prevalence of use of these drugs, with the exception of sleeping pills, the specific drugs that are abused in this class remain somewhat hard to define. Tables 2 and 3, from the Monitoring the Future Study, list the prevalence of use of 2 classes of these drugs. There are virtually no data on the misuse of sleeping pills by adolescents.

Although the information on the misuse of tranquilizers is scant, 1 author (Dr Rogers) who works with substance abusing adolescents has found from his

Table 3
Specific tranquilizers: Trends in annual prevalence of use for seniors

	Percent of All Seniors Using These Drugs		
	2002	2004	2007
Valium	2.8	3.1	2.4
Xanax	2.6	2.7	3.3

Data source: Monitoring the Future Study (modified), 2007, Johnston LD. National Institute on Drug Abuse, University of Michigan Institute of Social Research: 112; National Institutes of Health, National Survey on Results of Drug Use 2005–2007.

clinical experience that the immediate-release form of Xanax (Pfizer, New York, New York) is the tranquilizer of choice for adolescents who abuse tranquilizers. Xanax is often referred to as "zanies," and the "holy grail" for these adolescents is "zanibars,"[2] which are 2-mg bar-shaped preparations of Xanax.

CONCLUSIONS

In the most recent Monitoring the Future report, it is stated that for adolescents, "prescription drug abuse is becoming an important part of the nation's drug abuse problem."[13] It seems that prescription drug abuse by adolescents, if rates continue to rise, will be the newest drug epidemic among our youth.

ACKNOWLEDGEMENTS

The authors would like to thank Lisa Blackwell, MLS, Serials/Reference Librarian and Robin Egan, Administrative Assistant, Adolescent Medicine, both at Nationwide Children's Hospital for their help in preparation of this manuscript.

REFERENCES

1. Monitoring the Future: National Survey Results on Drug Use 1975–2007. Johnston, L. National Institute on Drug Abuse, US Department of Health and Human Services. Public Health Service, NIH
2. National Center on Addiction and Substance Abuse at Columbia University. *Under the Counter: The Diversion and Abuse of Controlled Prescription Drugs in the U.S.* New York: Columbia University; National Center on Addiction and substance Abuse. 2005
3. National Center on Addiction and Substance Abuse at Columbia University. *CASA Analysis of the National Survey on Drug Use and Health (HSDUH)*, 2006 [data file]. Rockville, MD: US Department of Health and Human Services, substance Abuse and Mental Health Services Administration; 2005
4. Results from the 2006 National Survey on Drug Use and Health. United States, Substance Abuse and Mental Health Administration; Office of Applied Studies, 2007
5. Results from the 2006 National Survey on Drug Use and Health. United States, Substance Abuse and Mental Health Administration; Office of Applied Studies, 2007
6. Boyd CJ, McCabe SE, Cranford JA, Young A. Adolescents' motivations to abuse prescription medications. Pediatrics. 2006;118(6):2472–2480
7. Sung HE, Richter L, Vaughan R, Johnson PB, Thom B. Nonmedical use of prescription opioids among teenagers in the United States: trends and correlates. *J Adolesc Health*. 2005;37(1):44–51
8. Pharmacology Small, D. in metabolism and interpretation of alcohol and specific drugs (pp205251) in The Medical Officer's Review Manual. Swotinsky R and Smith D. Medical Review Officer Certification Council. Beverly Farms, Ma: EOM Press. 3rd ed. 2006
9. McCabe SE, Boyd CJ, Young A. Medical and nonmedical use of prescription drugs among secondary school students. *J Adolesc Health*. 2007;40(1):76–83
10. Novak SP, Ball JK. Emergency department visits involving ADHD stimulant medications. *The New DAWN Report*. 2006(29). Available at: https://dawninfo.samhsa.gov/files/TNDR09ADHDmedsForHTML.pdf. Accessed Feb. 2, 2009
11. Wilens TE, Adler LA, Adams J, et al. Misuse and diversion of stimulants prescribed for ADHD: a systematic review of the literature. *J Am Acad Child Adolesc Psychiatry*. 2008; 47(1):21–31

12. Teter CJ, McCabe SE, Cranford JA, Boyd CJ, Guthrie SK. Prevalence and motives for illicit use of prescription stimulants in an undergraduate student sample. *J Am Coll Health.* 2005;53(6): 253–262
13. Johnston L. Bachman J and Schulenberg J (2008, Dec.11) National Press Release, "Various stimulant drugs show continuing gradual declines among teens in 2008
14. Musser CJ, Ahmann PA, Theye FW, Mundt P, Broste SK, Mueller-Rizner N. Stimulant use and potential for abuse in Wisconsin as reported by school administrators and longitudinally followed children. *J Dev Behav Pediatr.* 1998;19(3):187–192
15. Kollins SH, MacDonald EK, Cush CR. Assessing the abuse potential of methylphenidate in nonhuman and human subjects: a review. *Pharmacol Biochem Behav.* 2001;68(3):611–627
16. Poulin C. Medical and nonmedical stimulant use among adolescents: from sanctioned to unsanctioned use. *CMAJ.* 201;165(8):1039–1044
17. McCabe SE, Boyd CJ. Sources of prescription drugs for illicit use. *Addict Behav.* 2005;30(7): 1342–1350
18. Poulin C. From attention deficit/hyperactivity disorder to medical stimulant use to the diversion of prescribed stimulants to non-medical stimulant use: connecting the dots. *Addiction.* 2007; 102(5):740–751
19. McCabe SE, Teter CJ, Boyd CJ. Medical use, illicit use and diversion of prescription stimulant medication. *J Psychoactive Drugs.* 2006;38(1):45–56

Screening for Substance Abuse in the Office Setting: A Developmental Approach

Richard B. Heyman, MD, FAAP*

Suburban Pediatric Associates, 752 Waycross Road, Cincinnati, OH 45240

> "Underage alcohol use is not inevitable, and schools, parents and other adults are not powerless to stop it. The latest research demonstrates a compelling need to address alcohol use early, continuously, and in the context of human development using a systematic approach that spans childhood through adolescence into adulthood."

US Department of Health and Human Services[1]

> "[T]he emergence and progression of drinking behavior are influenced by development, ... underage drinking has developmental consequences, alcohol use disorders (AUDs) are developmental in nature, and efforts to prevent or to reduce underage drinking behavior must be developmentally informed to be strategic, sensitive, and effective."

Masten et al[2]

Bright Futures[3] provides an elegant framework to guide those dealing with children and adolescents in providing comprehensive preventive health care. The assessment of alcohol and drug use beginning at the age of 11 is a cornerstone of this series of recommendations.

Countless studies have told us of the role that alcohol and other drug abuse plays in the overall health of America's children. According to the 2007 Monitoring the Future study,[4] nearly half (47%) of high school graduates have tried an illicit drug (and 26% reported having used a drug other than marijuana), and if one includes inhalant abuse, then as many as 28% of our junior and senior high school students have experimented with a brain-altering substance by 8th grade. Alcohol use is even more prevalent, with 72% having reported significant regular alcohol use before the end of high school and 39% by 8th grade. More than half

---

*Corresponding author.
E-mail address: rheyman@aap.org (R. B. Heyman).

Copyright © 2009 American Academy of Pediatrics. All rights reserved. ISSN 1934-4287

of high school seniors have been drunk, as has nearly 1 in 5 8th-graders. Approximately 10% of 9- and 10-year-olds have started drinking, and nearly one third of youth begin before the age of 13.[5]

Although surveys have reflected gradual declines in alcohol and drug use among youth, the problem remains a major public health issue. Alcohol, in fact, is involved in more deaths among adolescents than all other drugs combined, and among the 3 leading causes of death among youth (automobile crashes, homicides, and suicides), alcohol and other drugs are involved in the vast majority of cases.[6] As with other risk behaviors, including the use of personal safety devices such as bike helmets and seatbelts, the choice to become sexually active as well as involvement in gangs and other violent behavior, prevention is clearly a better approach than treatment. As the providers of health care to children and adolescents, pediatricians are in an ideal position to deal with this issue. Yet, although the American Academy of Pediatrics has repeatedly highlighted the role its members should be playing, a 1995 survey suggested that fewer than 50% of those interviewing teenagers raise the topic of alcohol and other drug use.

The article by Frankowski et al[7] in this edition of *AM:STARs* outlines a strength-based approach to interviewing adolescents. This article complements that approach by offering a time-saving and easy-to-remember screening tool for addressing the issue of underage drinking and substance abuse.

ALCOHOL, DRUGS, AND THE DEVELOPING BRAIN

Also in this edition of *AM:STARs*, White[8] discusses the development of the adolescent brain in great detail. His work, as well as that of Giedd[9] and others, shows clearly that the brain undergoes major growth, development, and transformation throughout the second and third decades of life. Alcohol and other drugs can have major effects on that development, and the delay and prevention of use can have long-term health implications.

The work of Hingson et al[10] has shown that delaying the onset of alcohol use decreases the likelihood of subsequent alcohol problems. Those who begin drinking before the age of 14 have as high as a 47% likelihood of developing problems with alcohol later in life, whereas those who wait until the age of 21 have a <10% likelihood. This is significant, suggesting that for each year after age 14 we can prevent the onset of drinking, the risks for alcoholism decrease by ~15%.[11]

There are increasingly clear biological explanations for these behavioral observations. As the brain develops, there are extensive changes that take place as new neural connections develop and unused ones are eliminated (a process referred to as "pruning"). These changes at the neural level help explain how the frontal and prefrontal cortical areas (those involved in planning, decision-making, and executive function) increasingly come to influence the decision-making process compared with areas such as the limbic system, the area that governs emotions.[11] According to Clark et al, "These areas serving cognitive, behavioral, and emotional regulation may be particularly vulnerable to adverse alcohol effects."[12] Animal studies have suggested that alcohol may affect cellular development including myelination and synapse formation in the adolescent brain and almost certainly impairs memory more severely than in the adult brain. The pattern in which adolescents drink (namely, binge drinking) probably exacerbates the neurotoxic effects of the substance and may cause cognitive deficits that persist into adulthood.

It is fascinating to note that the adolescent brain seems to be relatively less sensitive to the negative effects of alcohol, those that might normally serve as clues to cease drinking. These effects include motor and social impairment, sedation, dizziness/lightheadedness, and even the "hangover effects" of nausea and headache. Some of these insensitivities may be genetically predetermined, helping further explain the importance of family history.

Repeated use and early exposure may make the developing brain more susceptible to dependence. Early exposure to alcohol may create increased levels of "craving" and chronic exposure may induce tolerance and, in a sense, "stamp in" this lowered sensitivity to the motor-impairing and mind-altering effects of alcohol,[12] thus perhaps creating increased likelihood of heavy use as an adult.

RISK FOR UNDERAGE DRINKING

The choice to begin using alcohol and other drugs does not occur as a random event. Rather, what has become clear is that it is the result of a complex interplay of genetics, risk and protective factors, community, family and social influences, and, perhaps most importantly, specific individual temperament.

Differences in infant and childhood behavioral patterns are well recognized. It is becoming increasingly clear that the child with poor focus and impulse control and difficulty organizing, planning, and executing was likely to have been an irritable, hyperresponsive, poor-sleeping infant. Many authors have suggested that a "central dysregulatory trait" manifests itself as the "difficult" temperament of infancy, progressing to the deficient development of social, emotional, and intellectual regulation that frequently leads the adolescent to early experimentation with alcohol and other drugs.[13,14] It seems that children demonstrating so-called externalizing behavioral traits (impulsive, aggressive, uninhibited) and, to a lesser degree, internalizing symptoms (depressed, anxious, ruminating) are at greater risk for the development of substance use disorder (SUD) in adolescence.[15]

It is the development of so-called executive function within the frontal lobes that gives rise to the ability to plan, weigh consequences, and make good decisions. Poor development of such function, for whatever reason, may combine with temperament and coping styles and increase the likelihood of alcohol and other drug use.[16] Use of alcohol and drugs during adolescence can have a major long-term impact on the achievement of developmental tasks. Baumrind and Moselle[17] proposed that alcohol and other drugs affect development by distorting reality, changing the way in which teenagers work and play, and creating a situation in which the adolescent is able to coast along with a false sense that he or she lives in a rebellious and isolated world that alcohol and drugs greatly enhance. Jessor's[18] classic research showed clearly that adolescent alcohol and drug use is rarely an isolated phenomenon but, rather, is almost invariably associated with other poor choices such as antisocial behavior, inappropriate sexual exploration, school failure, and trouble with the law. Whether alcohol and drugs serve as a "gateway" to these other behaviors or whether they cluster because of baseline faulty judgment is controversial, but there can be no question that what has been termed "precocious development"[19] is usually associated with multiple antisocial risk behaviors.

The converse, of course, is also true. Children who are calm yet social, have their needs met, and are able to self-soothe seem to be at lower risk for SUDs. Other protective traits among adolescents, including good health and intelligence and a sense of connectedness to family, school, and community, also minimize risk. Adequate executive function seems to serve to motivate young people to achieve, engage, and set goals for themselves.

Rothman et al[20] in the Adverse Clinical Events study cited a number of childhood traumas that predispose to early onset of drinking, presumably to cope with both mental and physical problems. Among the items they identified that achieved statistical significance were physical abuse, sexual abuse, having a mentally ill household member, substance abuse in the home, and parental discord or divorce.

Personal alcohol expectancies represent another predictive factor for subsequent alcohol and other drug use. A number of studies have examined children's perceptions of alcohol use and predictions as to whether they will someday drink. Young children tend to see alcohol as being associated with dangerous, frightening, silly, and inappropriate behavior. Those perceptions tend to change as children grow older such that drinkers are perceived as fun-loving, successful, and part of the "in" crowd. Miller et al[21] have demonstrated that those middle school students who come to perceive significant benefits of drinking were much more likely to drink as adolescents.

There is strong evidence for a genetic basis for these observations. Thus, the fact that alcoholism and drug abuse run in families (1 of every 4 children lives in a family with alcoholism and/or drug abuse) will likely turn out to have more than a social basis. A child exposed to unhealthy drinking patterns and drug use at home may well have inherited 1 of the genes associated with conduct disorder in childhood and drug and alcohol use as an adult. A positive family history of alcoholism makes the likelihood in the offspring some 9 times greater for males and up to 3 times greater for females.[11] The family dysfunction, domestic violence, financial instability, and abuse so characteristic of families with alcoholism certainly serve as additional factors that increase the likelihood of a young person's use.

The home in which a child is raised represents a risk or protective factor. Emotional stability and calmness associated with careful limit setting and the encouragement of self-reliance seem to represent the ideal parenting style. The so-called authoritarian and permissive styles, representing the extremes of harshness and excessive discipline contrasted with submissiveness and inadequate limit setting, seem to be associated with more externalizing behavior during adolescence and, thus, with more SUDs. Parents who do not permit their children to develop decision-making capacity during preadolescence may find that their adolescents are unable to weigh the good things and the not-so-good things about decisions they are called on to make later. Parents who provide little supervision and guidance may find that their adolescents are more subject to outside influences and do not incorporate parental values.

The community in which a young person grows up may represent either a risk or a protective factor. Youth who feel valued and protected, as evidenced, for example, by good schools and recreational facilities and the absence of violence, are less likely to engage in alcohol and drug use. Association with a faith-based organization is an additional protective factor. Vigilance by law enforcement in terms of underage sales and service, as well as monitoring access at festivals and public events, also helps to curtail use. Parental supervising of parties and their children's whereabouts limits access as well, and children who know that their parents explicitly disapprove of underage drinking and drug use are less likely to use them.

A discussion of community standards and influences on adolescent alcohol and drug use would not be complete without mentioning the role of the media and the alcohol industry. The Center on Alcohol Marketing and Youth has extensive data on media exposure, and multiple studies have shown that youth exposed to more media influences (advertisements, product placements, depictions in television, and movies, etc) are substantially more likely to start using at an early age than peers who are not exposed.[22] In 2007 nearly half of youth exposure to alcohol advertising appeared on programs primarily appealing to 12- to 20-year-old audiences. Between 2001 and 2007, youth aged 12 to 20 were exposed to 22 times more ads promoting drinking than to so-called responsibility ads (which pretend to discourage alcohol use while subliminally promoting it). Strasburger[23] pointed out that alcohol advertisements portray use as being fun, ubiquitous, and risk-free. The industry with its billions of dollars is hard to counter, and, sadly, a recent study suggested that between 40% and 60% of its profits come from abusers and underage drinkers.[24]

In most studies that have examined predictors of adolescent alcohol and drug abuse, the peer group is the most important single factor, often accounting for up to 50% of the variance.[12] Adolescents tend to hang out with others with similar interests and values. They take risks in groups, as well, and the fact that most risk-taking behavior takes place in groups suggests that such behaviors have a socializing effect that may overwhelm better judgment. Brown et al[16] noted that the peer group has 3 distinct ways of influencing behavior: through modeling ("Here, try this"), encouragement of affiliation ("Hey, be like us, and we'll like you"), and exaggerated portrayals of normative peer group behavior ("Everyone does it, just look at TV/movies etc"). Cliques are a common phenomenon in middle schools and high schools, but one group that always welcomes new members is the drug-using crowd, for it is always looking for new customers and suppliers. Young people who may have multiple other risk factors or who may have experimented frequently find themselves drawn to like-minded peers, and observations have suggested that those hanging out with users are, in all likelihood, themselves using.

As Johnston et al[4] pointed out, the mere fact that a young person does not frankly condemn underage drinking can be worrisome. The Monitoring the Future study consistently showed a decline in "disapproval" of drinking from 83% in 8th grade to 65% in 12th grade, and a decrease from 57% to 45% that binge drinking is dangerous, in a period of time in which active alcohol use increases from 16% (8th grade) to 44% (12th grade).

PREVENTION, SCREENING, AND EDUCATION

The public health implications of underage drinking and the importance of prevention and identification of those youth who are using alcohol and other drugs are clear. The discussion above suggests that our efforts should focus on patients with the major identified risk factors. These risk factors include family history and perhaps genetic predisposition to alcohol and other drug use; association with peers who use; the sense that alcohol and drugs are acceptable and that they are easy to obtain; personality traits that may include risk taking, impaired executive function, and poor self-monitoring, as well as the judgment that alcohol and drug use is just a normal part of growing up; the opinion that alcohol and drug use is not harmful; and the sense that parents, school, and community will tolerate or even facilitate use without major consequences.

Evaluation of these risk factors can form the basis of a brief, semistructured interview to screen for alcohol and other drug use. Conveniently remembered as "The 6G's," this instrument, although not yet formally evaluated, has face-value validity inasmuch as it screens for these 6 important risk factors.[25] The discussion of substance abuse should include mention of alcohol, tobacco, and other drugs and should be introduced at an early age so that it can serve as a prevention message to children in elementary school. For middle and junior high school students, The 6G's provide an inventory of factors to assess for risk, and it can be used as an educational tool to guide parents in their ongoing childrearing efforts.

THE 6G'S

Content Areas

1. **Genetics**: genetic predisposition to alcoholism; family history of alcoholism; exposure to family drug and alcohol use.
2. **Group**: nature of peer group, including its values, activities, and supervision.
3. **Give**: perception of availability of alcohol and likelihood of someone trying to give alcohol (peer pressure) to the underage patient (at home, friends' houses, illegal sales, adults buying for youth).
4. **Get**: willingness and temptation to seek and get alcohol and other drugs and accept the associated risks; underdeveloped executive function; degree of disapproval of underage drinking.
5. **Great**: recognition of the great dangers associated with underage alcohol and drug use, especially to physical and mental health.
6. **Guidance**: understanding of parental and societal guidance on this issue and understanding of social, family, school, and legal consequences.

For the School-aged Child: A Prevention Message and Conversation Trigger

As mentioned earlier, children as young as 8 or 9 have reported trying alcohol, so raising the issue should be done earlier rather than later. This author uses the following trigger questions with the parent(s) present in the room. Sometimes body language or a nonanswer can tell more than a verbal response, and at times the answers are, quite simply, hilarious.

- Have you learned about alcohol and other drugs in school?
- Do you know anyone who drinks more than he or she should?
- Have you ever seen a person who is drunk?
- What do you think about beer?
- Do you have a favorite beer commercial?
- Do you think you will drink beer when you get older?

With young children, this line of questioning lets them know that this will be a topic of discussion at all visits. It may encourage parents to begin to take the lead in this important discussion and may serve as the impetus for them to begin raising the subject at other appropriate times. Depictions in the media, a family member who drinks too much or uses drugs (especially a sibling), advertisements on television shows, or even family rituals involving small amounts of alcohol are all events that may serve to stimulate discussion. Children form their opinions about alcohol and drugs early (although they evolve, as we have seen), so parents must be pushed to pursue the topic and not leave it up to health class at school.

For the Junior and Senior High School Student: A Screen and a Chance to Talk Alone

By the time children reach early adolescence, it is crucial to conduct a comprehensive psychosocial interview in private. Frankowski et al[7] describe the so-called strength-based interview in their article in this edition of *AM:STARs*, and they reference Ginsburg's SSHADESS mnemonic,[26] which reminds care providers to ask about 8 important areas: strengths, school, home, activities, drugs, emotions, sexuality, and safety. This is an elaboration on the older HEADSS schema of Goldenring and Cohen from the 1970s,[27] which included home, education, activities, drugs, suicidality, and sex. Either way, it is important to interview the adolescent alone and discuss confidentiality with the patient, promising not to reveal topics of discussion unless the care provider feels that the patient is in danger of harm or of harming someone else. Limits on confidentiality vary by state, and each care provider has his or her own comfort limits, but the principle of separating the young teenager from his or her parent is crucial if sensitive topics are to be addressed.

Screening for alcohol and other drug use can become easy and intuitive by using The 6G's mnemonic during this process. A direct approach, favored by this author when other clues suggest that the patient is, in fact, using, might include 1 or more of the following questions:

- "How many beers does it take you to get a buzz?"
- "How many days each week do you drink?"
- "I know a lot of kids at your school drink. Have you ever been caught?"
- "When you party with your friends, where do you get your alcohol?"

Such questions may be met with denial, shock, or resistance, but asking them may pave the way to using The 6G's for a more detailed screen, as follows.

Do you have any **genetic** predisposition to having alcohol problems?
- Do any members of your family drink more than you think they should?
- Do you sometimes feel scared when some of your family members start drinking?

Do any members of the **group** you hang out with drink alcohol or use drugs?
- Where do you and your friends like to hang out?
- What do you do for fun when you are with your friends?

- When you are at a friend's house, is there usually an adult present?
- Have you been to parties where other people were drinking or using drugs?

Has anyone ever offered to **give** you alcohol or encouraged you to try drinking or drugs?
- Has anyone pressured you to try alcohol or drugs?
- Do your friends prefer drinking over other activities?
- Do you ever feel "weird" because you are the only one at a party not drinking or using?

Have you ever been tempted to **get** and try drugs or alcohol, or do you disapprove of drinking by young people?
- Are you the kind who likes to "live on the edge" and take chances?
- Have you ever been in trouble with the law or school officials?
- Do you think people seem to have more fun when they drink or use drugs?
- Have you ever been curious to find out how alcohol or drugs might act on your body?
- Do you just flat-out disapprove of underage drinking and drug use?

Do you understand the **great** dangers associated with underage drinking and drug use?
- Do you understand how alcohol and drugs work differently on a young, growing brain than on a mature one?
- Do you understand how alcohol and drugs affect your judgment and the way you think?
- Do you know someone whose life has been harmed by alcohol or drugs?

Do you feel you receive enough **guidance** about drinking and drug use?
- Do you understand why we grown-ups do not want young people drinking alcohol?
- Do you have a good sense of where your parents stand on the issue?
- Do you recognize the consequences that your parents (not to mention school, law enforcement, and others) are likely to impose if you choose to drink or use drugs?

The Next Step: The Teenager in Need of an Assessment

The confidential interview may raise issues in the alcohol and drug area that warrant further investigation. Any positive answers should concern the care provider, and use of alcohol or other drugs at any level should lead to at least a brief assessment. The 6-item CRAFFT tool of Knight et al[28] is a brief validated office instrument that any provider can administer. Two or more positive answers represent a positive and should be addressed with a more detailed assessment. Depending on the age of the patient, even 1 positive answer may require further investigation.

The CRAFFT Questions

- Have you ever ridden in a **car** driven by someone (including yourself) who was "high" or had been using alcohol or drugs?
- Do you ever use alcohol or drugs to **relax**, feel better about yourself, or fit in?
- Do you ever use alcohol/drugs while you are by yourself, **alone**?
- Do your family or **friends** ever tell you that you should cut down on your drinking or drug use?
- Do you ever **forget** things you did while using alcohol or drugs?
- Have you gotten into **trouble** while you were using alcohol or drugs?

The clinician who is comfortable with the process may want to proceed then with a more thorough assessment. By using a formal instrument or a series of questions, information can be obtained about what drugs are used, in what situations, the pattern and frequency of use, consequences and impact, and level of control. Infrequent, noncompulsive use ("experimentation") can sometimes be addressed through in-office counseling, which might include a contract for nonuse, agreement to urine drug testing, or a motivational intervention. More extensive use on a regular basis or use that involves drugs beyond tobacco, alcohol, or occasional marijuana probably warrants assessment and development of a treatment plan by a certified chemical-dependency counselor. Each clinician should feel comfortable with his or her limits and seek outside consultation when necessary. Levy et al have provided an excellent review of this topic.[29]

For the Parent and Teenager Together

With a negative 6G's inventory, the clinician can have a modicum of confidence that he or she has raised important issues, asked questions in a sensitive and confidential manner, and (assuming the veracity and consent of the patient, of course) can discuss the issue with the parent back in the room. In this setting, The 6G's can serve as an educational tool to help remind parents of the importance of discussing risky behaviors with their children, including not only drug and alcohol use but smoking and perhaps sexual behavior, as well. The parent questions below might serve as the basis for a useful handout.

Genetic: Does Your Child Have Any Genetic Predisposition to Alcohol or Other Drug Use?

- Is there any inappropriate role-modeling to which your child is exposed?
- Do you use alcohol responsibly in your home?

Group: Do Any Members of the Group He or She Hangs Out With Drink Alcohol?

- Know who your child's friends are, and ask if any of them drink alcohol.
- Know where your child hangs out and whether there is adult supervision.
- Ask your child what he or she does with his or her friends when they are together and what it takes for them to have a good time.

Give: Has Your Child Ever Been in a Situation in Which Someone Offered to Give Him or Her Alcohol or Encouraged Him or Her to Try Drinking?

- Ask your child what his or her opinion of drinking is.
- Let your child know that although alcohol may be available (at home, at someone else's home, at school, at a party, etc) you expect him or her not to drink.
- Encourage your child to avoid being with kids who drink and get away from the situation if someone is urging him or her to do so.

Get: Has Your Child Ever Been Tempted to Get and Try Alcohol, or Does He or She Disapprove of Drinking by Young People?

- Find out if your child has ever thought about trying alcohol or has had even a single sip (without your permission) or whether he or she is just totally against it.
- Periodically inquire about other risky behaviors, and let your child know that you expect him or her to make good choices and not to take chances, especially with alcohol.
- Help your child to develop strategies to be able to say "no" without feeling self-conscious.

Great: Does Your Child Understand the Great Dangers Associated With Underage Drinking?

- Remind your child of the great dangers associated with underage drinking, both short-term (accidents, school failure, unwanted pregnancy, etc) and long-term (health, social, economic, legal, etc).
- Understand and talk with your child about how alcohol affects the young developing brain compared with its effects on adults who drink responsibly.
- Use the media to point out examples of alcohol's dangers (eg, car crashes, drug busts, irresponsible behavior, etc).
- Help dispel the media myths that drinking is glamorous and that drinkers are more likeable, attractive, sexy, and fun than nondrinkers.

Guidance: Do You Provide Your Child With Enough Guidance About Drinking?

- Reinforce the fact that underage drinking is dangerous and illegal.
- Regularly remind your child about your hopes and expectations for him or her regarding not drinking.
- Remind your child that, in fact, most kids do not drink and that the behavior is unacceptable and will result in significant consequences.

CONCLUSIONS

The problem of alcohol and drug use by children and adolescents is one that simply is not going away. Although there are certainly other risk behaviors that pediatricians must address, that of alcohol and other drug use is arguably the most important, because it causes such a high percentage of adolescent morbidity and mortality. Addressing the issue in a developmental fashion and recognizing the importance of prevention from childhood through adolescence becomes a major responsibility of pediatric care providers. Understanding the major risk factors and using a simple inventory such as The 6G's may make it easier for those caring for children and adolescents to cover the waterfront in an efficient and comprehensive manner.

REFERENCES

1. US Department of Health and Human Services. *The Surgeon General's Call to Action to Prevent and Reduce Underage Drinking.* Washington, DC: US Department of Health and Human Services, Office of the Surgeon General; 2007
2. Masten AS, Faden VB, Zucker RA, Spear LP. Underage drinking: a developmental framework. *Pediatrics.* 2008;121(suppl 4):S235–S251
3. Hagan JF, Shaw JS, Duncan PM, eds. *Bright Futures: Guidelines for Health Supervision of Infants, Children, and Adolescents.* 3rd ed. Elk Grove Village, IL: American Academy of Pediatrics; 2008
4. Johnston LD, O'Malley PM, Bachman JG, Schulenberg JE. *Monitoring the Future: National Results on Adolescent Drug Use—Overview of Key Findings.* Bethesda, MD: National Institute on Drug Abuse; 2007. NIH publication 08-6418B
5. Donovan JE. Adolescent alcohol initiation: a review of psychosocial risk factors. *J Adolesc Health.* 2004;35(6):529.e7–529.e18
6. Levy DT, Miller TR, Cox KC. *Costs of Underage Drinking.* Washington, DC: US Department of Justice, Office of Justice Programs, Office of Juvenile Justice and Delinquency Prevention; 1999. Available at: www.udetc.org/documents/costunderagedrinking.pdf. Accessed December 11, 2008
7. Frankowski BL, Leader IC, Duncan PM. Strength-based interviewing. *Adolesc Med Clin.* 2009;20(1):22–40
8. White AM. Understanding adolescent brain development and its implications for the clinician. *Adolesc Med Clin.* 2009;20(1):79–90
9. Giedd JN. The teen brain: insights from neuroimaging. *J Adolesc Health.* 2008;42(4):335–343
10. Hingson RW, Heeren T, Winter MR. Age at drinking onset and alcohol dependence. *Arch Pediatr Adolesc Med.* 2006;160(7):739–746
11. White A. *Keeping Adolescence Healthy: Exploring the Issues Facing Today's Kids and Communities.* Charleston, SC: Booksurge Publishing; 2008

12. Windle M, Spear LP, Fuligi AJ, et al. Transitions into underage and problem drinking: developmental processes and mechanisms between 10 and 15 years of age. *Pediatrics*. 2008;121(supple 4):S273–S289
13. Clark DB, Thatcher DL, Tapert SF. Alcohol, psychological dysregulation and adolescent brain development. *Alcohol Clin Exp Res*. 2008;32(3):375–385
14. Clark DB, Cornelius JR, Kirisci L, Tarter RE. Childhood risk categories for adolescent substance involvement: a general liability typology. *Drug Alcohol Depend*. 2005;77(1):13–21
15. Zucker RA, Donoban JE, Masten AS, Mattson ME, Moss HB. Early developmental processes and the continuity of risk for underage drinking and problem drinking. *Pediatrics*. 2008; 121(suppl 4):S252–S272
16. Brown SA, McGue M, Maggs J, et al. A developmental perspective on alcohol and youth 16 to 20 years of age. *Pediatrics*. 2008;121(suppl 4):S290–S310
17. Baumrind D, Moselle KA. A developmental perspective on adolescent drug use. *Adv Alcohol Subst Abuse*. 1985;4(3–4):41–67
18. Jessor R. Risk behavior in adolescence: a psychological framework for understanding and action. *J Adolesc Health*. 1991;12(8):597–605
19. Bachman JG, Schulenberg JE. How part-time work intensity relates to drug use, problem behavior, time use, and satisfaction among high school seniors: are these consequences or merely correlates? *Dev Psychol*. 1993;29(2):220–235
20. Rothman EF, Edwards EM, Heeren T, Hingson RW. Adverse childhood experiences predict earlier age of drinking onset: results from a representative US sample of current or former drinkers. *Pediatrics*. 2008;122(2). Available at: www.pediatrics.org/cgi/content/full/122/2/e298
21. Miller PM, Smith GT, Goldman MS. Emergence of alcohol expectancies in childhood: a possible critical period. *J Stud Alcohol Drugs*. 1990;51(4):343–349
22. Snyder LB, Milici FF, Slater M, Sun H, Strizhakova Y. Effects of alcohol advertising exposure on drinking among youth. *Arch Pediatr Adolesc Med*. 2006;160(1):18–24
23. Strasburger VC. Alcohol advertising and adolescents. *Pediatr Clin North Am*. 2002;49(2):353–376, vii
24. Foster SE, Vaughan RD, Foster WH, Califano JA Jr. Estimate of the commercial value of underage drinking and adult abusive and dependent drinking to the alcohol industry. *Arch Pediatr Adolesc Med*. 2006;160(5):473–478
25. Heyman RB. Combating underage drinking with the 6Gs. *Contemp Pediatr*. 2007;24(6):63–75
26. Ginsburg KR. Engaging adolescents and building on their strengths. *Adolescent Health Update*. 2007;19(2)
27. Goldenring JM, Cohen E. Getting into adolescent heads. *Contemp Pediatr*. 1988;5(7):75–90
28. Knight JR, Sherritt L, Shrier LA, Harris SK, Chang G. Validity of the CRAFFT substance abuse screening test among adolescent clinic patients. *Arch Pediatr Adolesc Med*. 2002;156(6):607–614
29. Levy S, Vaughan BL, Knight JR. Office-based intervention for adolescent substance abuse. *Pediatr Clin North Am*. 2002;49:329–343

Strength-Based Interviewing

Barbara L. Frankowski, MD, MPH[*,a], Isaac C. Leader, BA[b], Paula M. Duncan, MD[c]

[a]*Vermont Child Health Improvement Program and Department of Pediatrics, Vermont Children's Hospital, University of Vermont College of Medicine, 1 South Prospect Street, Burlington, VT 05401, USA*

[b]*University of Vermont College of Medicine, 89 Beaumont Avenue, Burlington, VT 05401, USA*

[c]*Vermont Child Health Improvement Program, University of Vermont College of Medicine, 1 South Prospect Street, Burlington, VT 05401, USA*

Bright Futures,[1] in its 2007 guidelines, called for an assessment of adolescent development and the use of strength-based approaches in the adolescent health supervision visit. The 7 developmental tasks of adolescence noted in the developmental surveillance at each yearly visit include:

- healthy behaviors;
- caring and supportive relationships;
- physical, cognitive, emotional, social, and moral competencies;
- self-confidence, hopefulness, and well-being;
- resiliency, when confronted with life stressors;
- responsible and independent decision-making; and
- positive engagement in the life of the community.[2]

Using strength-based approaches in the clinical setting requires that clinicians have the following skills and knowledge:

- understanding what constitutes strengths;
- knowing how to ask about and elicit strengths by using a framework;
- improving youth confidence by reflecting strengths back to youth and their parents;
- providing guidance about adding strengths in domains where they may be lacking; and
- using shared decision-making strategies when behavior change is needed.

The rationale for using a strength-based approach and building developmental assets has been reviewed by us previously.[3] Risk assessment is still mandatory,

*Corresponding author.
E-mail address: barbara.frankowski@vtmednet.org (B. L. Frankowski).

Copyright © 2009 American Academy of Pediatrics. All rights reserved. ISSN 1934-4287

especially for the health behaviors that contribute the most to adolescent and adult morbidity and mortality. These risk behaviors include inadequate physical activity and nutrition, sexual behavior that may lead to unintended pregnancy or infection, substance use and abuse, and behaviors that contribute to unintentional injuries and violence (ie, homicide/suicide).[4] Much of our literature review focused on finding a lower number of these risky behaviors in youth who had a greater number of developmental assets.[1,5-8]

A list of approaches that the medical home can use to support healthy adolescent development (eg, physical and psychological safety, supportive relationships, and opportunities for skill building) was provided in our previous article (see Table 3 in ref[3]). This list was adopted from a report on community approaches prepared by Eccles for the National Research Council and Institute of Medicine Committee on Community- Level Programs.[9]

The advocacy for strength-based approaches in the medical home is supported by the field of positive psychology, which builds on Bandura's social cognitive theory.[10] Both emphasize self-efficacy. A list of strengths that enable human thriving[11] can also inform this work. In addition to facilitation of self-management and behavior change, strength-based approaches can also result in more positive engagement with youth and their parents.

The work described here, which has been developed over the past 8 years, was inspired by the work of Brendtro, Van Bockem, and Brokenleg,[12] Benson,[13] and Pittman et al[14] and initiatives of the Vermont Agency of Human Services and Vermont Regional Partnerships, which have focused on community and school-level interventions.

To participate in this strength-based model, health care practitioners needed clinically workable models for integrating these services into their busy practices. Design of the practice-level implementation involved input from adolescents, parents, and professionals from schools, community groups, and youth-serving agencies as well as health care and mental health professionals. Actual implementation relied on the expertise and suggestions of Vermont pediatricians, family physicians, nurse practitioners, physician assistants and nurses, in the settings of practices, clinics, and school-based health centers.

The Search Institute work identifies 40 assets arranged in the following categories: support, empowerment, boundaries and expectations, constructive use of time, commitment to learning, positive values, social competencies, and positive identity.[5] Pittman has focused on 5 C's (competence, connection, contribution, character, and confidence)[14]; Brendtro et al, in the Circle of Courage, identified the importance of generosity, independence, mastery, and belonging.[12] Our practices were given an opportunity to choose 1 of these frameworks, and almost all chose the Circle of Courage model. Many practices have implemented strength-based approaches and have allowed chart audits to measure their use as part of a quality improvement effort.[15] Many health care professionals, parents, and advocates in various settings outside Vermont have participated in workshops on strength-based approaches and have shared their ideas and experiences.

Several other pediatricians have devoted significant effort to similar issues, and their contributions have provided additional examples and tools for the incorporation of strengths into preventive services. Ginsberg has recommended the use of the SSHADESS (strengths, school, home, activities, drugs, emotions/depression, sexuality, safety) interview format[16] and the 7 C's, adding coping and control to Pittman's 5 C's.[17] Sege served as the project director and co-editor with Spivak, Flanigan, and Licenziato for the American Academy of Pediatrics *Connected Kids: Safe, Strong, Secure Clinical Guide* (2007).[18] *Connected Kids*, which includes parent handouts and a practitioner guide, outlines a strength-based approach to violence prevention.

IDENTIFYING STRENGTHS: A PRACTICAL APPROACH

Most pediatricians are already asking a lot of questions about strengths, although not necessarily in a systematic way. We commonly ask questions related to mastery and belonging, but adolescents need to develop all the strengths to be successful adults. Incorporating strengths in your adolescent interviews is not an "add-on" to the clinical visit but, rather, a rethinking of the way you work with adolescents, a way to efficiently reorganize and prioritize the content of anticipatory guidance.[19] The goals of a strength-based approach are to raise adolescents' awareness of their developing strengths and to motivate them to take responsibility for the role they can play in their own health and well-being. Discussing strengths orients youth toward actively seeking out and acquiring the personal, environmental, and social assets that are the "building blocks" of future success.

If you are already using a HEADSSS (home, education, activities, drugs, sexual activity/sexual identity, suicide/depression, and safety) type of interview strategy,[20] you would just need to add a few more questions (Table 1). Ginsburg has suggested using the SSHADESS format[16] as a way to remember to ask about strengths. He comments that "we risk losing the opportunity to inspire (adolescents) when they quietly become defensive and close themselves off."[16] Respectful, reflective listening, rather than teaching or preaching, allows adolescents to reveal their strengths.

If you choose to use the Brendtro et al Circle of Courage as your framework, you will be asking about strengths in 4 essential areas (Table 2). You would not use all the questions, and you would probably want to ask slightly different questions on the basis of the age of the adolescent and what you already know about his or her strengths and challenges.

Table 1
Using HEEADSSS with a strength-based approach

HEEADSSS Risk Areas	Questions to Help Identify Strengths	Example Responses Indicating the Presence of Strengths	Strengths
Home	Who lives at home with you?	Close family relationships (as opposed to living alone)	Belonging
	What responsibilities do you have at home?	Care-taking responsibilities	Generosity
Education/employment	What's going well at school?	Working with a tutor	Independence
	Are you working?	Working for college money	Mastery
Eating	How do you stay healthy?	Choosing healthy foods	Independence
	What do you think about your diet?	Making healthy meals	Mastery
Peer-related activities	What do you do for fun?	Volunteer/civic activities	Generosity
	Do you have friends you socialize with?	Hanging out with friends	Belonging
Drugs	Do you have friends who use drugs? Do you?	Pledge to abstain	Independence
		Friendships with people who do not use drugs	Belonging
Sexuality	Have you ever had sex?	Consistently responsible behavior	Independence
	Has anyone ever made you do something you didn't want to?	Supportive or understanding relationships	Mastery; belonging
Suicide/depression	What do you do when you feel sad?	Access to a confidant	Belonging
	Do you have someone you talk to about your problems?	Successful coping skills	Mastery; independence
Safety from injury and violence	Do you wear a seatbelt? Do you wear a helmet when riding bikes?	Seatbelt and helmet use	Independence
	Do you feel safe at home?	Feelings of safety or security at home and school	Belonging

Adapted from Goldenring JM, Rosen DS. Getting into adolescents heads: on essential update. *Contemporary Pediatrics.* 2007. Reprinted with permission from Duncan PM, Garcia AC, Frankowski BL, et al. Inspiring healthy adolescent choices: a rationale for and guide to strength promotion in primary care. *J Adolesc Health.* 2007;41(6):531

Some may want to use a different framework with older adolescents. The "READY for Life" framework[21] can work well with older adolescents:

Am I READY for life as an adult[21]?

- Relationships with friends, other students, co-workers, and family

Table 2
Identifying Strengths

Belonging (connection)	How do you get along with the different people in your household?
	What do you like to do together as a family? Do you eat meals together?
	Do you feel you have at least 1 friend or a group of friends with whom you are comfortable?
	What do you and your friends like to do together after school? On weekends?
	How do you feel you "fit in" at school? In your neighborhood?
	Do you feel like you matter in your community?
	Do you have at least 1 adult in your life who cares about you and to whom you can go if you need help?
	When you're stressed out, who do you go to?
Mastery (competence)	What do you do to stay healthy?
	What are you good at?
	How are you doing in school?
	What do you like to do after school with your free time?
	Do you feel you are particularly good at doing a certain thing like math, soccer, theater, cooking, hunting, or anything else?
	What are your responsibilities at home? At school?
Independence (confidence)	Do you feel that you have been allowed to become more independent or make more of your own decisions as you have become older?
	Do you feel you have a say in family rules and decisions?
	Are you able to take responsibility for your actions even when things don't work out perfectly or as you planned?
	Have you figured out a way to control your actions when you're angry or upset?
	Everyone has stress in their lives. Have you figured out how to handle stress?
	How confident are you that you can make a needed change in your life?
Generosity (contribution, character)	What makes your parents proud of you?
	What do your friends like about you the most?
	What do you like about yourself?
	What do you do to help others (at home, or by working with a group at school, church, or community)?
	What do you do to show your parents or siblings that you care about them?
	How do you support your friends when they are trying to do the right thing, like quitting smoking or avoiding alcohol and other substances?

- Energy to give to the things you enjoy
- Awareness of the world around you, your place in the world, and your contribution
- Decision-maker (you know how to get things done and control your behavior)
- Yes—you should say yes to healthy behavior: eat well, play hard, work hard

This can be used to help adolescents take stock of what strengths they already have, on what strengths they need to work, and how they can use strengths to make needed changes. The READY brochure, written for the parents of adolescents, outlines these concepts further.[21]

TEACHING STRENGTHS TO PARENTS

Pediatricians may find it helpful to explain strengths to parents of adolescents. Just as we use anticipatory guidance in early childhood to help parents watch for expected milestones, the strengths are expected and necessary milestones for adolescents. Parents can play a needed role in encouraging strengths in areas that are lagging. In addition, pediatricians should be committed to recognizing and reinforcing parents' strengths by using a similar framework. Pointing out a parent's strengths can be particularly helpful when he or she is going through a difficult time with an adolescent son or daughter.

Parents are often worried about the risks of adolescence and are sometimes so put off by their own child's behavior that they tend to worry about and focus on the negative aspects of adolescence rather than seeing it as a growth experience for them and their child. Adolescence takes many parents by surprise. By teaching them to "watch out" not only for risky behavior, we can help them see their own child's strengths and help them figure out ways to build strengths that may need boosting. All parents want their children to experience joy, success, love, and hope, and adolescents need to develop all the strengths to end up as happy, productive adults.

strengths = assets = protective factors = developmental milestones for adolescents

Using the Circle of Courage framework is 1 way to explain the strength-based approach to parents.

Mastery

"What am I good at?" Parents need to help their adolescent figure this out, especially if he or she is not a great student. Encourage your adolescent to try sports, clubs, a musical instrument, etc. Make him or her an expert on something in the family (research driving directions on-line before a family trip). Model problem-solving behaviors when something does not go well. Help the adolescent to be persistent when he or she does not succeed at something the first time around (or second). Make him or her feel competent in more than 1 area.

Belonging

"Who do I fit in with? Who do I feel connected to?" Parents are often disappointed as friends become more important, but peer relations are vital to adolescents. Keeping your adolescent attached to your family as he or she develops friendly and romantic relationships is tricky. Get to know your adolescent's friends and make your home a welcome place for them. Encourage appropriate relationships with other adults you trust. Be sure your child knows to whom he or she can go if there is a problem that he or she does not feel can be shared with you (his or her doctor could be one of these people). Help your adolescent figure out how he or she "fits in" with your extended family ("Your little cousins sure look up to you and love to play soccer with you!"), your neighbors ("If I wasn't home and you had a problem, you could get help from Mrs X or Y." "Let's help Mr Z shovel his driveway/mow his lawn."), his or her school ("Who are the teachers/students you get along with the best?"), and his or her community (attend neighborhood events together, or encourage your adolescent to go with his or her friends), including faith-based organizations.

Independence

This is scary for parents of early adolescents, but we all want our children to grow up and be able to function independently (yet remain attached). For many adolescents, this means starting to make healthy independent decisions for themselves, especially decisions to avoid unhealthy risks. Guide your adolescent in healthy decision-making; let him or her work out the solution to a problem and then run it by you for final approval. Independence also means being responsible; as time goes by, this should happen more and more with less and less reminding from you. Some adolescents have a harder time gaining independent control of their behavior and showing self-discipline. Point out to your adolescent that every time he or she makes a healthy decision and controls his or her behavior without reminders from you, he or she is exercising independence. Encourage confidence in your adolescent by putting your trust in him or her when you assign a task to do. Good teachers will try to do the same thing. Let your adolescent take a leadership role in something he or she is good at.

Generosity

This can be the most difficult strength for some adolescents to develop, because most of them go through a stage when they are naturally self-centered as they try to figure out who they are. Point out and name qualities such as caring, sharing, loyalty, and empathy when you see your adolescent displaying them with his or her friends. Encourage the adolescent to practice these qualities when it is more difficult (eg, with a younger brother or an unpopular classmate). The broadest definition of this strength is the sense of giving back to one's community. This can start with parents involving adolescents in volunteering in their neighborhood, school, or faith-based community. Many older adolescents who have not developed this strength feel like they do not "matter" in their family, school, or community. The ability to feel like what you do matters—that the world (or at least your family, school, or community) is a little better because you are there—is very empowering, gives adolescents confidence and hope, and keeps them engaged.

Armed with these strengths, adolescents can be encouraged to take "healthy" risks. As youth advocate Matt Morton has noted, "If you don't give us healthy risks to take, we'll take unhealthy ones."[22] Remember, it is the taking of risks and failing, then having the strength, confidence, and hope to try again, that helps adolescents become resilient adults.

GOING TO THE NEXT LEVEL: USING STRENGTHS

After eliciting strengths in an adolescent, there are several things a clinician can do with the information. First, you can identify or reflect back the adolescent's strengths as a teaching tool about strengths and youth development (much as we encourage parents to identify or put into words a younger child's emotions). Many talented youth do not recognize their own strengths until they are pointed out to them. Second, you can make suggestions to boost strength areas that may be lacking or deficient, because adolescents need strengths in all areas to become healthy, happy, productive adults. Third, you can use strengths as an engagement strategy to lead into a discussion about a needed behavior change. Fourth, you can bring strengths into a structured discussion about behavior change, such as shared decision-making or motivational interviewing.[23]

Some examples of using the Circle of Courage as a teaching tool for adolescents are as follows:

- For a younger adolescent: "Some kids struggle in middle school or high school and get involved in unhealthy, risky behaviors. Others have an easier time becoming a healthy adult. Young people who develop strengths in these 4 areas seem to be 'protected' from a lot of these risks. I can't help but notice that you have developed strengths in these areas [point out strengths that you have elicited]. Are there any areas you think you could work on getting better at?"
- For an adolescent with special health needs (eg, spina bifida): "Have you heard of the Circle of Courage? It represents strengths I look for in adolescents that can help them mature into healthy adults. I can't help but notice how many strengths you have developed over the past 2 years. You struggled, especially with friendships and independence in middle school, but you're doing well in those areas now. And you've really developed your talent for art, and you are thinking of becoming an art teacher. Generosity, making a contribution in your community, is also important. Have you ever done any volunteer work? Would you consider working with children at the homeless shelter? They have program called 'Art From the Heart,' and I think the kids would really enjoy working with you."

Sometimes we notice that a particular strength is lacking in some adolescents. See Table 3 for some examples of how you and parents can boost needed strengths.

Table 3
Promoting strengths that are lacking

Generosity
- Ask "What are you doing to help out at home?" "How can you contribute to your community?" Suggest a volunteering commitment that takes advantage of something the youth is good at or interested in. Parents can help steer towards a volunteer experience.

Independence
- Ask "How do you make a decision about something important?" "How do you control your feelings when you are angry?" Suggest writing down pros and cons the next time they are struggling with a decision, or point out ways to alleviate stress with deep breathing, etc. Parents can help by discussing how they make decisions (about saving money for a needed item, for whom to vote in an election).

Mastery
- Ask "What are you getting good at?" "What are you interested in outside of school?" Suggest joining a club or sport. Parents can help by providing transportation to or from after-school or weekend meetings or events.

Belonging
- Ask "Who do you go to for help?" "Who are the adults you trust?" Suggest getting involved in a mentoring program. Parents can help by pointing out relatives or neighbors who can be trusted to go to for help and advice.

What if your patient has a particular problem or challenge? Here are some examples:

- Obesity (strengthen mastery): "Become an expert and take control of your exercise and eating."
- Attention-deficit/hyperactivity disorder (strengthen independence): "You and I have discussed how your attention problems have a biological basis, but you can learn to develop inner control and self-discipline. Learn a way to stop and think before you make an impulsive decision, and practice this skill. The goal is not to get off all your meds, but your appropriate decision-making will make you more independent and get your parents and teachers off your back!"
- Special health needs (developmentally delayed) (strengthen belonging): "Who are your friends, and what do you like to do with them? How are you a good friend? Who are the adults you can go to if you have a problem?"
- "Smart but selfish" (strengthen generosity): "Be aware of the world around you, and see how you can contribute to it. Think about how you could volunteer in the community; maybe you can help set up a Web site for the local teen center. Think about ways you can help out at home or in your extended family."

MAKING STRENGTHS WORK IN DIFFICULT SITUATIONS

Adolescents in difficult situations (eg, those living in foster care or who have dropped out of high school) often have trouble seeing their own strengths and can benefit greatly from having their strengths pointed out to them. For adolescents who have many challenges, you can use strengths as an "engagement strategy" to enhance communication, help establish trust, promote self-efficacy, and increase patient satisfaction.[16] You can use strengths to work on a needed behavior change by using an established model.

There are several models, from relatively straightforward (the "helping skill"[23]) to more complex (motivational interviewing[24]), that pediatricians can use with adolescents. The "helping skill" involves the following steps: identify the issue; explore the options; consider the consequences; make a plan; and follow-up. Motivational interviewing is a structured set of interviewing skills that help patients move along the stages of change from precontemplation to contemplation, to preparation, and to action. Strategies for motivational interviewing involve expressing empathy, developing discrepancy, avoiding argumentation, rolling with resistance, and supporting self-efficacy. Using strengths can enhance these techniques. The following cases provide a few examples.

Case 1

Tiffaney is a 16-year-old girl who is living in her fifth foster home and fourth school district and comes in for a health supervision visit. She has been in her current foster home for ~9 months and is able to keep the rules pretty well. She has her own room and feels safe. She does some chores but mostly is out of the house. She eats breakfast with both foster parents most mornings. She is a vegetarian and walks 2 or 3 miles per day "getting around" because none of her friends have a car.

She attends public school, is in the 10th grade, and is passing all her courses except one with mostly Cs and Ds. She is failing algebra at the moment, but she loves her art class and gets along well with her teacher. She thinks she may be able to graduate on time in 2 years if she really tries, but it is "a little iffy." She is not sure what she wants to do after high school, but she would like to figure out a way to help kids who are like her.

She had a social worker in a different county whom she still calls and sees occasionally. She feels that this woman helped her a lot with encouragement and choices. She is not currently smoking or drinking, although she has in the past. She now hangs out with a "straight-edge" crowd that does not do drugs of any kind. She is artistic and can draw well. She is interested in body art and has 2 piercings. She keeps a journal and feels that she can express her emotions and thoughts pretty well.

She has had a boyfriend for 6 months, and she spends much of her time with him at his friend's apartment. He works and plays music and enjoys spending time with her and their friends. He tries to support her in her decision to finish high school, although he did not. She has been sexually active with him (her third sexual partner in her life) for 5 months. They use a condom "sometimes," but he does not really like them. When she is in a car she wears her seatbelt. She describes her mood now as happy and positive. Although she has felt very depressed in the past, she never considered hurting herself.

Her examination is normal. She is in the 50th percentile for height and the 30th percentile for weight; her BMI is in the 25th to 50th percentile.

Tiffaney's risk is unprotected sexual intercourse. Her strengths are:

- generosity (wants to help other kids in foster care);
- independence (expresses herself well, gets around town, makes healthy decisions about substance use, manages her health care);
- mastery (keeping on track at school, art, "survival skills"); and
- belonging (foster parents, art teacher, former social worker, friends, boyfriend).

Use the helping skill:

- Identify the issue: "I just met you and I can't help but notice how many strengths you have . . . . But, I am concerned that you are having sex without using a condom. Can we talk about that?"
- Explore the options with Tiffaney: "What could you do? What else could you do?"
- Consider the consequences of each option that Tiffaney comes up with: "What could happen if you did that? How would that work with your life now?"
- Make a Plan: "It sounds like you are thinking about hormonal birth control, probably the patch. Can I give you a prescription for that today, along with some condoms?" (Tiffaney indicates that she would like to talk it over with her boyfriend first.)
- Follow-up: "That's great! Why don't you make an appointment to come in next Tuesday with your boyfriend and we can talk about it together. Because your pregnancy test today is negative, do you think you two could abstain from sexual intercourse until then?"

Case 2

Carlos, a 17-year-old boy, comes in for a physical for his job.

He lives with his dad, who has a history of involvement with the law for driving while intoxicated. His dad used to hit him but does not really bother with him too much now. He loves his mom, but he thinks that she should take more responsibility for his 3 younger brothers.

He dropped out of school this year in his junior year. He was never good in school, but he did well in weightlifting, and he felt that the coach gave him encouragement. Because his dad does not give him any financial support beyond a place to live, he decided to drop out of school and work. He thinks he will get a GED (general equivalency diploma) someday, but not right now. He works at a gas station 30 hours/week. Because he likes to talk about car engines, and he likes the money, he is pretty reliable at work. His boss thinks that he is basically a good kid and thinks of him as an apprentice. He is pretty good with his hands and works on 4-wheelers. His dad has one that he rides a lot.

His friends think he is reliable. They like having him around, and they describe him as funny. He always spends 1 evening and 1 weekend afternoon with his brothers, because he wants his brothers to have a guy to look up to because he never did. He is teaching them to shoot hoops and lift weights. He goes to church with them some Sundays.

He eats a lot of "fast food" for breakfast and lunch but often has dinner at his boss' house. He binges on the weekend but usually does not drink more than 1 beer per day after work. He has been in trouble with the law for possession of malt beverage and was picked up for "doing doughnuts" with his car in the school parking lot. He does not use any other substances.

He is sexually active once a month with different partners, and he always uses a condom. He is not depressed or suicidal. He is basically content and deals with what his life has to offer. He wears a helmet whenever he rides his 4-wheeler.

He is proud to be self-reliant. He knows a few things in depth (engines, nature [hunting, fishing]) and almost nothing about many life skills (bank accounts, college applications). He says he would never expect help from outsiders or an "agency."

Carlos' risks are alcohol use and sexual activity with multiple partners. For the alcohol use, use the CRAFFT screening tool[25] with him:

- Have you ever ridden in a car driven by someone (including yourself) who was "high" or had been using alcohol or drugs?
- Do you ever use alcohol or drugs to relax, feel better about yourself, or fit in?
- Do you ever use alcohol/drugs while you are by yourself, alone?
- Do you ever forget things you did while using alcohol or drugs?
- Do your family or friends ever tell you that you should cut down on your drinking or drug use?
- Have you ever gotten into trouble while you were using alcohol or drugs?

Carlos has 2 positive responses on the screen (he has driven while using and has gotten in trouble).

Carlos' strengths are:

- generosity (really cares about his younger brothers);
- independence (has a job, earns his own money, makes some healthy decisions);
- mastery (has a job he is getting good at [but did not finish high school], likes outdoor sports [hunting, fishing] and weight lifting); and
- belonging (family [brothers], friends, boss, church).

Try motivational interviewing:

- "Carlos, I haven't seen you in a couple of years, and I'm impressed with your maturity and sense of independence, and there are so many things you are getting good at. Sounds like your job is going well, although it would be great for you to get your GED sometime soon. Your younger brothers really look up to you, and you are very generous with your time that you spend with them. However, I'm really concerned about how your drinking could affect your health and your plans for the future. Could we talk about that some more?" (Carlos might indicate that, sure, he can talk about it, but he does not see any problem with his drinking, because he is not an alcoholic like his dad. He only got in trouble once, and he will not let that happen again. He is in the precontemplative stage.)
- Develop discrepancy: "Carlos, what do you like about your drinking? What else?" Keep asking until there are no more "good things." (Carlos may indicate that he likes how it makes him feel relaxed, he feels more like a part of the gang at work, he feels his sense of humor is better when he's had a few beers, etc.) "Carlos, what are the 'not-so-good' things about your drinking? What else?" (Keep asking until there are no more not-so-good things. Carlos may indicate that he does not like the way he feels the next morning after he has been drinking, he hates the way his dad tells him he is 'just like him' when he drinks, he disappointed his boss by not showing up for work a couple of times when he felt too 'hung over,' he was really ashamed that his mother and little brothers found out when he got in trouble with the police.)
- "So, it sounds like you enjoy drinking, but it may be starting to interfere with some things that are really important to you, like your job and your relationship with your brothers. What do you make of that?" (Carlos may indicate that he never really thought about it that way.)
- "Would you be willing to start cutting down on your drinking? When would be the easiest time of the week to not use? Could I meet with you next week during your lunch break at work to see how it went?"
- "You have many strengths in your life now, especially your generosity and your sense of independence. I know you can use that independence to help you make the healthiest decision for yourself right now."

Case 3

Rochelle, who is 12½ years old, comes in with her mother for her checkup.

She continues to live at home with both parents and her younger brother. Rochelle gets along "fine" with everyone in the house, although her mother comments that they "clash" over things more than they have in the past. When asked what they disagree on, Rochelle shrugs, and her mother expresses concern about Rochelle's weight. She does mention that Rochelle continues to get along with her younger brother, aged 10, and has a lot of patience with him and helps him with his math homework.

Rochelle just started the 6th grade 2 months ago; this is her first year in middle school. She expresses disappointment that most of her friends from last year are not in her classes, and she occasionally eats lunch by herself. She continues to do well in her classes and got all A's in her first-quarter report card. She did not join the soccer team this year, because she wanted to focus on her schoolwork. In addition, her mother had been finding it difficult to drive Rochelle to practice with her new job. Rochelle now has to baby-sit her brother after school. She does not mind, because they watch television together. Her father has a demanding job in sales that requires him to work 10-hour days and travel a lot, but the family manages to eat dinner together 4 nights per week.

Her diet is "okay," with fruits and vegetables, 2% milk, lots of cheese, and mostly chicken and fish. She usually buys soda at school; there is a new vending machine in the cafeteria. She admits to snacking a lot after school with her brother. She denies the use of tobacco, alcohol, marijuana, and other drugs. Her parents do not smoke, and neither do her friends. She is not interested in any "romantic relationships" at this time, although she does have some friends who are boys, mostly ones with whom she played soccer last year. She has never had sex. She always wears a seatbelt in the car and a helmet on her bike. She used to ride her bike more often but now stays home after school.

Rochelle says that things are "fine," but she is disappointed that school is not as fun as it was in the 5th grade. Her mom has been "getting on her" about her weight, but she thinks it is not her fault, because both her parents are overweight. She says she feels "kind of down" a lot of days but not really bad, and she would never consider harming herself.

On physical examination, Rochelle has sexual maturation ratings (SMRs) of 4 (breasts) and 4 (pubic hair). She is 61 in tall (75th percentile) and 135 lb (95th percentile); her BMI is 25.5 (just below the 95th percentile). The rest of examination is unremarkable. She started her period ~6 months ago and has had it ~3 times; she has had no problems with heavy bleeding or cramps.

Rochelle's risks are:

- poor nutrition (more snacking, soda at school);
- inadequate physical activity (not playing soccer this year, more television time); and
- sadness or depressed mood (misses friends from soccer, school not as fun).

Her strengths are:

- generosity (takes care of her brother after school, helps him with his homework);
- independence (knows how to keep herself and brother safe when parents are not home);
- mastery (good at school, all A's); and
- belonging (family, but not as much with friends now).

Use a written change plan[26]:

- "Rochelle, you are showing a lot of strengths in your life now. You've successfully transitioned to middle school and are keeping up your excellent grades. You are demonstrating independence and maturity by watching your brother after school, and you are very generous to be spending the time helping him with his homework. But, it seems that you are not as active and not eating as well as you were last year, and you seem not as happy with things. Can we talk about that today?" (Rochelle indicates that she really wanted to talk about her weight, because she does not like the way she is looking these days. She wants some help deciding what to do.)
- "Rochelle, on a scale of 1 to 10, with 1 being not ready and 10 being very ready, how ready are you to start making a change?" (Rochelle says 10!)
- "Some people find it helpful to write down their ideas about change. Would you like to fill out this change plan with me today while you are here?"

Fill out the change plan together (see Fig 1), and give her a copy to take home.

TOOLS

If you are just getting started with strengths, pick a framework or model that works well for you (Circle of Courage, 5 C's, READY, etc). Think about what questions you want to ask to identify strengths in each major developmental area. The following are some ideas that have helped other clinicians incorporate strengths in their practice:

- Consider a previsit questionnaire that asks about risks and strengths. Although most practitioners cannot extend the time they spend with patients, the use of tools can help optimize this precious time we do have

How important is it to make a change? How ready am I to make a change now?	
__1 __2 __3 __4 __5 __6 __7 __8 __9 __10	
Nutrition	**Physical Activity**
Change:	Change:
How will I make this happen?	How will I make this happen?
Who or what can help me? My strengths: My family's strengths:	Who or what can help me? My strengths: My family's strengths:
What can get in the way?	What can get in the way?
How confident am I that I can make this change? __1 __2 __3 __4 __5 __6 __7 __8 __9 __10	

Return visit: _____

_____

Patient Signature   Parent Signature_____Clinician Signature

Fig 1. Fit & healthy change plan. Data source: http://healthvermont.gov/family/fit/documents/Promoting-Healthier-Weight_pediatric_toolkit.pdf.

face-to-face with youth and parents. Instead of asking questions about strengths, this information can be collected by questionnaire, on paper or electronically on a computer or handheld device. Olsen et al[27] have piloted the use of a personal digital assistant (PDA) with an expanded GAPS (Guidelines for Adolescent Preventive Services) questionnaire for use by teenagers in the waiting room. The questionnaire does not substitute for the conversation to elicit strengths, but it gets the youth (and parents if they are going to be involved) thinking in this direction. You can use ones that have been developed or construct your own with your

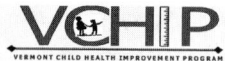

Date of Screening:_____
- ❏ Nutrition
- ❏ Generosity

- ❏ Physical Activity
- ❏ Independence

- ❏ Substance Abuse
- ❏ Mastery

- ❏ Sexual Activity/Development
- ❏ Belonging

- ❏ Safety

CRAFFT? Yes No
2+ or   -

- ❏ Emotional Health/Suicide
Office Intervention
Referral

Check Indicates a Preventive Screening   ©

Fig 2. Vermont Child Health Improvement Program (VCHIP) reminder sticker. The sticker is attached to patient charts to remind primary care practitioners to track a set of 6 risk behaviors and 4 wellness-promoting assets during patient screening visits.

favorite questions to elicit strengths. You could also choose questions suggested in Table 2. Consider asking different questions for different age groups. Consider asking parents to describe their adolescent's strengths.
- Use prompts: If you have paper records, you can add a sticker on your encounter form that cues you to ask questions about risks and strengths. The example in Fig 2 was developed by the Vermont Child Health Improvement Program and encourages practitioners to try new interviewing skills before they make changes to their encounter forms.
- You can use a Circle of Courage poster in your examination rooms as your prompt,[28] or the 5 C's or READY brochure. If you are not facile with motivational interviewing, consider using a worksheet such as SMART (Specific, Measurable, Achieveable, Realistic, Time-framed)[29] or a Fit & Healthy change plan worksheet.[26]
- Have educational materials or resources available for parents and/or patients. Some examples could include the READY pamphlet,[21] Gins-

berg's book,[17] *Connected Kids* brochures,[18] parent books, and handouts from the Search Institute.[13]

CONCLUSIONS

In our experience, the implementation of strength-based approaches in the medical home setting requires only a modest restructuring of the visit. A conscious focus on protective factors and strengths does not take the place of the essential risks assessment but, rather, reinforces the commitment of our practitioners and their staff to wellness and health promotion in addition to disease prevention.

REFERENCES

1. Hagan JF, Shaw JS, Duncan P. *Bright Futures: Guidelines for Health Supervision of Infants, Children, and Adolescents*. 3rd ed. Elk Grove Village, IL: American Academy of Pediatrics; 2008
2. Fine A, Large R. *A Conceptual Framework for Adolescent Health: A Collaborative Project of the Association of Maternal and Child Health Programs and the State Adolescent Health Coordinators Network*. Washington, DC: Association of Maternal and Child Health Programs; 2005
3. Duncan PM, Garcia AC, Frankowski BL, et al. Inspiring healthy adolescent choices: a rationale for and guide to strength promotion in primary care. *J Adolesc Health*. 2007;41(6):525–535
4. Centers for Disease Control and Prevention. *Healthy People 2010: Leading Health Indicators*. Atlanta, GA: Centers for Disease Control and Prevention; 2004
5. Leffert N, Benson PL, Scales PC, Sharma AR, Drake DR, Blyth DA. Developmental assets: measurement and prediction of risk behaviors among adolescents. *Appl Dev Sci*. 1998;2(4):209–230
6. Murphey DA, Lamonda KH, Carney JK, Duncan P. Relationships of a brief measure of youth assets to health-promoting and risk behaviors. *J Adolesc Health*. 2004;34(3):184–191
7. Vesely SK, Wyatt VH, Oman RF, et al. The potential protective effects of youth assets from adolescent sexual risk behaviors. *J Adolesc Health*. 2004;34(5):356–365
8. Borowsky IW, Ireland M, Resnick MD. Violence risk and protective factors among youth held back in school. *Ambul Pediatr*. 2002;2(6):475–484
9. National Research Council; Institute of Medicine. *Community Programs to Promote Youth Development*. Washington, DC: National Academy of Press; 2002
10. Bandura A. Self-efficacy mechanism in human agency. *Am Psychol*. 1982;37(2):122–147
11. Seligman ME, Steen TA, Park N, Peterson C. Positive psychology progress: Empirical validation of interventions. *Am Psychol*. 2005;60(5):410–421
12. Brendtro LK, Brokenleg M, Van Bockern S. *Reclaiming Youth at Risk: Our Hope for the Future*. Bloomington, IN: National Education Service; 2002
13. Benson P. 40 Developmental Assets. Available at: www.search-institute.org/system/files/40Assetts.pdf. Accessed February 20, 2009
14. Pittman KJ, Irby M, Tolman J, Yohalem N, Ferber T. *Preventing Problems, Promoting Development, Encouraging Engagement: Competing Priorities or Inseparable Goals?* Washington, DC: Forum for Youth Investment; 2003. Available at: www.forumfyi.org/files/Preventing%20Problems,%20Promoting%20Development,%20Encouraging%20Engagement.pdf. Accessed February 3, 2009
15. Duncan P, Kullock E, Frankowski B, et al. Will primary care providers incorporate a strengths assessment into preventive service visits for the 11–18 year old? Poster presented at: meeting of the Pediatric Academic Society; May 2, 2006; Washington, DC
16. Ginsburg KR. Engaging adolescents and building on their strengths. *Adolesc Health Update*. 2007;19(2)

17. Ginsberg KR, Jablow MM. *A Parent's Guide to Building Resilience in Children and Teens: Giving Your Child Roots and Wings*. Elk Grove Village, IL: American Academy of Pediatrics; 2006
18. Spivak H, Sege R, Hatmaker-Flanigan E, Kozial B, Licenziako V, Bardy K. *Connected Kids: Safe, Strong, Secure Clinical Guide*. Elk Grove Village, IL: American Academy of Pediatrics; 2006
19. Ozer EM, Adams SH, Lustig JL, et al. Can it be done? Implementing adolescent clinical preventive services. *Health Serv Res*. 2001;36(6 pt 2):150–165
20. Goldenring JM, Rosen DS. Getting into adolescent heads: an essential update. *Contemp Pediatr*. 2004;21(1):64–80
21. Duncan P. *READY for Life: Building Adolescent Strengths* [brochure]. Burlington, VT: Vermont Department of Health; 2004. Available at: www.med.uvm.edu/vchip/downloads/READYbrochure.pdf. Accessed February 3, 2009
22. Morton M. Lunch key note speech. Presented at: the 2nd Annual Vermont Working With Youth Conference; May 18, 2007; Burlington, VT
23. Comprehensive Health Education Foundation. The Helping Skill. Natural Helpers. Available at: http://web1.msve.edu/4h/cls/documents/NH-buscard.pdf. Accessed February 20, 2009
24. Miller WR, Rolnick S. *Motivational Interviewing: Preparing People to Change Addictive Behaviour*. New York, NY: Guilford; 1991
25. Knight JR, Sherritt L, Shrier LA, Harris SK, Chang G. Validity of the CRAFFT substance abuse screening test among adolescent clinic patients. *Arch Pediatr Adolesc Med*. 2002;156(6):607–614
26. Vermont Department of Health, Vermont Area Health Education Center. Promoting healthier weight in pediatrics. Available at: http://healthvermont.gov/family/fit/documents/Promoting-Healthier-Weight_pediatric_toolkit.pdf. Accessed February 20, 2009
27. Olson AL, Gaffney CA, Hedberg VA, et al. The Healthy Teen Project: tools to enhance adolescent health screening. *Ann Fam Med*. 2005;3(suppl 2):S63–S65
28. Reclaiming Youth Network. The Circle of Courage philosophy. Available at: www.reclaiming.com/about/index.php?page=philosophy. Accessed February 20, 2009
29. Gold M, Kokotailo P. Motivational interviewing strategies to facilitate adolescent behavior change. *Adolesc Health Update*. 2007;20(1). Available at: www.hcet.org/resource/postconf/08/MI4FPpros/GOLD/AHUOct07GoldKokotailo.pdf. Accessed February 3, 2009

Management of the Adolescent Concussion Victim

Joseph Congeni, MD, FAAP*

Division of Sports Medicine, Akron Children's Hospital Sports Medicine Center, 215 West Bowery Street, Suite 7300, Akron, OH 44308-1062; Department of Pediatrics, Northeastern Ohio Universities College of Medicine, 4209 Street Rt. 44, P.O. Box 95, Rootstown, OH 44272

The evaluation, treatment, and long-term prognosis of concussion have traditionally been among the most poorly understood medical problems in the adolescent age group. An increase in the number of studies over the past decade has helped medical practitioners better understand this confusing condition, and the more we understand the constellation of medical symptoms, the more we recognize the inadequacy of our previous approach to its management.

A study by the Centers for Disease Control and Prevention in 1999 estimated that some 300 000 sports and recreational traumatic brain injuries occur per year.[1] However, this study took into account only those concussions resulting in loss of consciousness. More recent studies have shown that concussions resulting in loss of consciousness account for only 8% to 19% of concussive injuries,[2,3] suggesting that, in fact, ~1.6 to 3.8 million sports-related concussions occur each year.[4]

A majority of head injuries in children between the ages of 2 and 10 years are caused by falls. A majority of brain injuries that occur over age 20 are caused by motor vehicle crashes. A significant number of brain injuries that occur in the adolescent years from age 13 to 20 occur in the sports or athletic arena. Those athletes most at risk for concussion include high school football players, with hockey players close behind.[5] Approximately 20% of high school football players who played through a 4-year career admit to sustaining a concussion, and that number jumps to 40% for those who played college football. The incidence for high school soccer and soccer goalies was estimated to be ~10% and 15%, respectively. There continues to be an increased incidence in nonhelmeted sports as well, including soccer, basketball, martial arts, and gymnastics.

---

*Corresponding author.
E-mail address: jcongeni@chmca.org (J. Congeni).

One of the major problems with addressing the issue of concussion is that because it is so poorly understood, there has been significant underreporting. A study from the University of Akron (Kaut et al[6]) confirmed that only 19% of athletes suffering symptoms that would fit the description of concussion were diagnosed accurately. Several other studies had similar findings,[7–10] leading some to refer to the condition as the "silent epidemic."

One of the other noteworthy concerns regarding concussion is the recurrence rate, with a four- to fivefold increased risk for a second injury after the first concussion. Recent studies seem to indicate that the major reason for this problem is the premature return of brain-injured athletes to sporting activity,[7,10] a decision that can have long-term complications of major concern. Learning disabilities and cognitive deterioration have been associated with multiple concussions,[10] and there is a suggestive relationship to concentration issues and attention-deficit/hyperactivity disorder as well. The use of medication to treat these issues is currently being studied in patients with previous concussion. Recent studies in Medicine and Science in Sports and Exercise showed a threefold increase in the diagnosis of clinical depression and the need for psychotherapy and antidepressants in patients with more than 3 concussions.[11] Studies also have shown an increased incidence of chronic headache[12] in this group. Finally, the rare but deadly condition know as "second-impact syndrome" (an apparently trivial head injury after a recent concussion) still leads to death and permanent brain damage in a small number of patients with concussions per year.[13,14]

DEFINITION/LOCATION OF CONCUSSION

The definition of concussion has evolved over time, and the challenge most recently has been to define the clinical syndrome. In 1966 the Congress of Neurologic Surgeons wrote that concussion was "a clinical syndrome characterized by the immediate and transient posttraumatic impairment of neural functions, such as alteration of consciousness, disturbance of vision, or equilibrium, etc."[15] The evolution of this definition into the 1990s included the American Academy of Neurology's description of "any trauma-induced alteration in mental status that may or may not include a loss of consciousness."[16] It further noted that the effects are typically "transient."

Many of these initial definitions were used to develop concussion guidelines and grading scales that guided return-to-play decisions. There are at least 19 different scales described in the literature, contributing greatly to the confusion for the medical practitioner because of the tremendous variability between grading scales and the fact that guidelines are not based on scientific research or outcome studies of any kind.

At the first international symposium on concussion in sport, held in Vienna, Austria, in 2001, the definition was refined further: "Concussion can be caused either by a direct blow to the head, face, or neck, or elsewhere on the body with

Table 1
Concussion criteria

Complex concussion criteria
At point of injury, athlete has concussive convulsion; or
At point of injury loss of consciousness for >1 min; or
Athlete has history of multiple previous concussions; or
Retrospectively, athlete has not recovered within 10 d
Simple concussion criteria
Concussion that does not include complex criteria and recovery occurs in <10 d

an impulsive force transmitted to the head."[17] The important distinction is that "brain injury" can occur without a direct blow to the head. Findings went on to suggest that "concussion is typically associated with grossly normal structural neuroimaging studies" and "concussion may result in neuropathological changes but the acute clinical symptoms largely reflect the functional disturbance, rather than a structural injury." This definition clearly emphasizes symptoms and neurocognitive functioning and calls for abandoning the grading-scale approach. The second international symposium on concussion held in Prague, Czech Republic, in 2004 maintained the emphasis on symptoms rather than on guidelines.[18] The report went a step further to describe concussion retrospectively as either simple or complex (see Table 1).

This functional and metabolic model of brain injury, as opposed to structural change such as brain bleed, also contributes to the difficulty in recognizing this medical condition. Current imaging studies, such as MRI and computed tomography, do not show structural changes in athletes with concussion.[10,17] Studies have been performed, however, on the metabolic cascade after cerebral concussion.[19] These studies from the UCLA Brain Injury Research Center are summarized in Fig 1. CMR indicates cerebral metabolic rate. With the use of animal studies, Giza and Hovda[19] identified several chemical markers that are abnormal

Table 2
Signs and symptoms of concussions

Signs Observed	Symptoms Reported by Athlete
Appears to be dazed or stunned	Headache
Is confused about assignment	Nausea
Forgets plays	Balance problems or dizziness
Is unsure of game, score, or opponent	Double or fuzzy/blurry vision
Moves clumsily	Sensitivity to light or noise
Answers questions slowly	Feeling sluggish or slowed down
Loses consciousness	Feeling "foggy" or groggy
Shows behavior or personality change	Concentration or memory problems
Forgets events prior to play (retrograde)	Change in sleep pattern
Forgets events after hit (posttraumatic)	Feeling fatigued

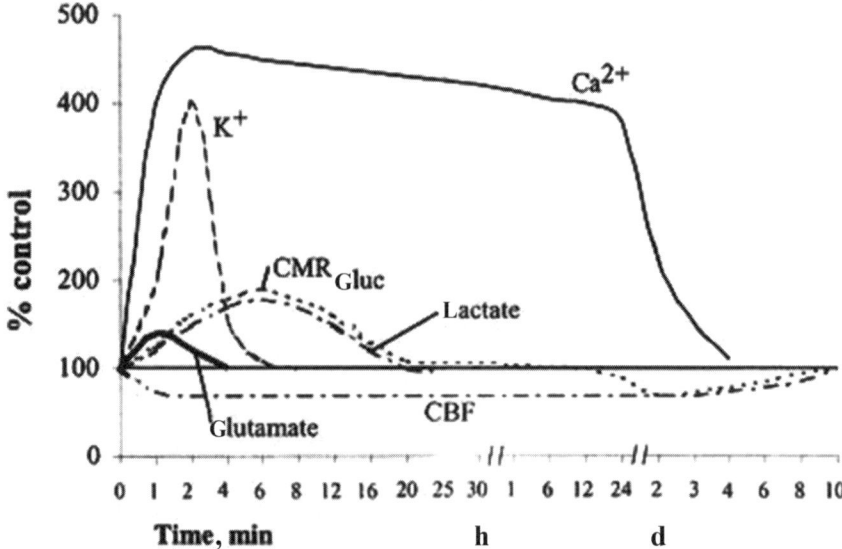

Fig 1. Reprinted with permission from Giza CC, Hovda DA. The neurometabolic cascade of concussion. *J Athl Train.* 2001;36(3):228–235; CMR, cerebral metabolic rate, CBF, cerebral blood flow.

after brain trauma. Most notable is the drop in cerebral blood flow during the period of time that the brain is recovering from this trauma. These chemical markers someday may be useful in tracking the progress of cerebral concussion.

The location of the brain injury can provide a better understanding of the symptoms that occur in concussion. The cerebellum, the balance center of the brain, is involved in some but not all brain injuries, as is the visual center in the occipital lobe. Symptoms referable to the parietal lobe (responsible for arithmetic, spelling) and temporal lobe (involved in memory and language) are affected in many concussions. Injuries to the frontal lobe may lead to emotional and behavioral symptoms such as extreme irritability, anger, or crying. It is felt that concussion that involves loss of consciousness may involve injury to the reticular-activating system or the "central command post" of the brain. Clinicians hoping to see a consistent injury profile are often frustrated by the clinical variability associated with concussive brain injuries. Medical personnel who assess such injuries may expect to see most or all of the symptoms of concussion in each athlete, although it is clear that many victims manifest only 1 or 2 symptoms.

EVALUATION/ASSESSMENT OF CONCUSSION

Evaluation and assessment of concussion are difficult for the many reasons described above. Further complicating the matter is the fact that concussion evolves over time, and the implications of the assessment can be different depending on the setting in which the adolescent patient is first encountered. On the sideline or on the field of play, the presentation is not always obvious. This is especially true in settings where there are multiple players, and the coaching staff and medical staff may be a distance away from those players on the court or the field. Although most medical people are looking for the obvious loss of consciousness, as stated earlier, only 8% to 19% display this symptom.[2,3] Athletes may also appear dazed, move clumsily, appear confused about play, or show signs of confusion, memory loss, or loss of awareness of their surroundings, symptoms that may initially be recognized by another teammate or a coach. The athletes themselves may be reluctant to report these symptoms for a variety of reasons.[8] They may feel this is just "a part of the game" and that the symptoms will go away quickly, or they may be concerned about being removed from the game and attempt to "tough it out." This is another reason for this condition being known as the silent epidemic, because without the athlete's reporting these symptoms, it is very difficult for medical people, most commonly the athletic trainer, to even recognize that an injury has occurred.

Sideline evaluation relating to this condition has been discussed for many years, and researchers recently developed tools that can be useful to medical personnel attempting to conduct on-the-spot assessments. The first of the standardized tools was the Standardized Assessment of Concussion, which has been well studied by McCrea et al[20] (Fig 2). It includes specific items to assess orientation, immediate memory, neurologic screening, concentration, exertional maneuvers, and delayed recall. There is a summary of total scores, and baseline scores for college or high school athletes are generally in the range of 26 of 30 points. Athletes suffering from a concussion often score well below that number. There are 4 versions of this test so that there is not a learning effect by athletes. This tool has been expanded with a Sport Concussion Assessment Tool (SCAT) card (a SCAT evaluation being recommended in the guidelines from Prague)[18] (see Fig 3).

Evaluating athletes with brain injury at home is equally difficult. Parents and caregivers may see only subtle degrees of the symptoms shown in Fig 4.

Physicians who see these adolescents in their office also struggle to find objective tests that help them make an easy assessment. Traditionally, athletes and their parents are much more likely to seek evaluation of musculoskeletal injuries than they are of what may seem to be insignificant brain injuries. Nevertheless, a complete office evaluation is necessary to avoid the risk of sending these athletes back onto the field of play in contact and/or collision sports. The risk of reinjury and the complications discussed here make that a high-stakes decision for the medical caregiver.

A comprehensive clinical examination should include 6 components:

1. Neurologic evaluation: The results of this examination are most likely to be normal. The findings of focal neurologic abnormalities in the sensory-motor or cranial nerve evaluation are most likely to be seen in structural

SAC Card

1) ORIENTATION:

Month: _____	0	1
Date: _____	0	1
Day of week: _____	0	1
Year: _____	0	1
Time (within 1 hr.): _____	0	1

Orientation Total Score _____ / 5

2) IMMEDIATE MEMORY: (all 3 trials are completed regardless of score on trial 1 & 2; total score equals sum across all 3 trials)

List	Trial 1	Trial 2	Trial 3
Word 1	0 1	0 1	0 1
Word 2	0 1	0 1	0 1
Word 3	0 1	0 1	0 1
Word 4	0 1	0 1	0 1
Word 5	0 1	0 1	0 1
Total			

Immediate Memory Total Score _____ / 15

(Note: Subject is not informed of Delayed Recall testing of memory)

NEUROLOGICAL SCREENING:

Loss of Consciousness: (occurrence, duration)

Retrograde & Posttraumatic Amnesia: (recall of events pre- and post-injury)

Strength:

Sensation:

Coordination:

3) CONCENTRATION:

Digits Backward (If correct, go to next string length. If incorrect, read trial 2. Stop after incorrect on both trials)

4-9-3	6-2-9	0 1
3-8-1-4	3-2-7-9	0 1
6-2-9-7-1	1-5-2-8-6	0 1
7-1-8-4-6-2	5-3-9-1-4-8	0 1

Months in reverse order: (entire sequence correct for 1 point)
Dec-Nov-Oct-Sep-Aug-Jul
Jun-May-Apr-Mar-Feb-Jan _____ 0 1

Concentration Total Score _____ / 5

EXERTIONAL MANEUVERS
(when appropriate):
5 jumping jacks   5 push-ups
5 sit-ups   5 knee-bends

4) DELAYED RECALL

Word 1	0	1
Word 2	0	1
Word 3	0	1
Word 4	0	1
Word 5	0	1

Delayed Recall Total Score _____ / 5

SUMMARY OF TOTAL SCORES:

Orientation	_____	/ 5
Immediate Memory	_____	/ 15
Concentration	_____	/ 5
Delayed Recall	_____	/ 5

Overall Total Score _____ / 30

Fig 2. SAC Card.

brain injuries such as bleeds. Neurologic examination is an important part of the assessment, but it is not especially sensitive.
2. Subjective scale: The Post-concussion Scale (Fig 5) can be useful and can be given separately or as a part of computerized neurocognitive testing. This scale is most useful if it is given at the time of or shortly after the diagnosis of the concussion and then serially as the athlete recovers. This component has limitations, however, in that it is subject to self-reporting,

Fig 3. Sport Concussion Assessment Tool (SCAT).

1. **HEADACHE**—Especially with reading, using computers, increased physical activity, or during concentration.
   - Athletes frequently will ask for medicines like Acetaminophen, or Ibuprofen.

2. **FEELING SLOWED DOWN OR MENTALLY FOGGY**
   - Talking to your child after a concussion could be like changing from a high-speed cable modem connection to a slow moving dial up connection.

3. **SENSITIVITY TO LIGHT OR NOISE**
   - Throbbing, pounding and uncomfortable being in noisy areas, in the sun, or under bright light.

4. **DIZZYNESS OR BALANCE PROBLEMS**
   - This doesn't have to be dramatic; they just don't feel right after standing up from sitting.

5. **MEMORY**
   - Trouble finding the right words in a sentence.

6. **TIRED or EASILY FATIGUED**
   - Just wants to sit down or lay down.
   - Does not sleep well even though tired.

7. **MORE EMOTIONAL or IRRITABLE**
   - Easily cries, excessive laughing, arguing

8. **DOUBLE VISION OR BLURRY VISION**

9. **NAUSEA OR VOMITING**

Fig 4. Parent's checklist for concussion (developed by Akron Children's Hospital, Sports Medicine Center).

and its usefulness seems to decrease as the athlete improves. Athletes tend to be more realistic early on in the process.

3. Cervical evaluation: There is clearly much overlap between cervical spine injuries and brain injury. The full cervical evaluation and aggressive treatment of cervical injury is crucial in the care of patients with concussion.
4. Balance assessment: At our clinic we use head injury and postural stability testing based on the Balanced Error Scoring System popularized by Guskiewicz at the University of North Carolina (Fig 6).[21] This 6-step test is performed in different positions on a firm and foam surface, and the numbers of errors are recorded and the information used in assessing the concussed athlete. Far more advanced computerized balance systems are available in some tertiary clinical settings.
5. Neuropsychological and cognitive testing: Neuropsychological evaluations were initially administered to the injured athlete as part of concussion evaluation by a neurophysiologist. These tests have evolved in recent years to

POST-CONCUSSION SCALE-REVISED
Mark Lovell, Ph.D., Joseph Maroon, M.D., John Norwig, ATC, Julian Bailes, M.D.

Patient/Athlete: _____ Team: _____

SYMPTOM	RATING None Mod. Severe	BASELINE Date:	TESTING 2 Date:	TESTING 3 Date:	TESTING 4 Date:	TESTING 5 Date:
Headache	0 1 2 3 4 5 6					
Nausea	0 1 2 3 4 5 6					
Vomiting	0 1 2 3 4 5 6					
Balance problems	0 1 2 3 4 5 6					
Dizziness	0 1 2 3 4 5 6					
Fatigue	0 1 2 3 4 5 6					
Trouble falling asleep	0 1 2 3 4 5 6					
Sleeping more than usual	0 1 2 3 4 5 6					
Sleeping less than usual	0 1 2 3 4 5 6					
Drowsiness	0 1 2 3 4 5 6					
Sensitivity to light	0 1 2 3 4 5 6					
Sensitivity to noise	0 1 2 3 4 5 6					
Irritability	0 1 2 3 4 5 6					
Sadness	0 1 2 3 4 5 6					
Nervousness	0 1 2 3 4 5 6					
Feeling more emotional	0 1 2 3 4 5 6					
Numbness or tingling	0 1 2 3 4 5 6					
Feeling slowed down	0 1 2 3 4 5 6					
Feeling mentally "foggy"	0 1 2 3 4 5 6					
Difficulty concentrating	0 1 2 3 4 5 6					
Difficulty remembering	0 1 2 3 4 5 6					
TOTAL SCORE						

Fig 5. Post-concussion Scale-Revised.

computerized versions that can be used in a more standardized and accessible system. One such system, used at Akron Children's Hospital in the past 6 years, is known as ImPACT (immediate post-concussion assessment and cognitive testing). This system has a demographic and concussion history questionnaire, which can be useful for clinical evaluation and research purposes, and a concussion symptom scale. There are several neurocognitive measures within this testing, including memory, attention, reaction time, and mental speed. The program comes with a detailed clinical report, and the evaluation is automatically scored by computer, which allows comparison to national norms. In the ideal situation, the test is also compared with the athlete's baseline, although most high school athletes have not had a baseline test performed. Nevertheless, these tests have become a readily available and clinically useful objective tool for clinicians to assess an athlete's recovery from a concussion.

6. Exertional testing: When athletes have improved and passed the first 5 components of the examination, they may be subjected to exercise on a bike, treadmill, or step test in the office. Progressive exertional testing can be administered by the athletic trainer at the high school as well. If athletes do not have a recurrence of symptoms, the discussion about return to play may begin.

PROGNOSIS/CLINICAL COURSE OF CONCUSSION

Every athlete who is assessed for concussion is anxious to return to the playing field or court and wants to know how long it will take to recover. Recent studies have shown that fewer than 50% of concussion victims recover within 1 week.[22] At the 2-week mark, the number increases to nearly 60%, and by 3 weeks nearly 80% have returned to normal status (Fig 7).

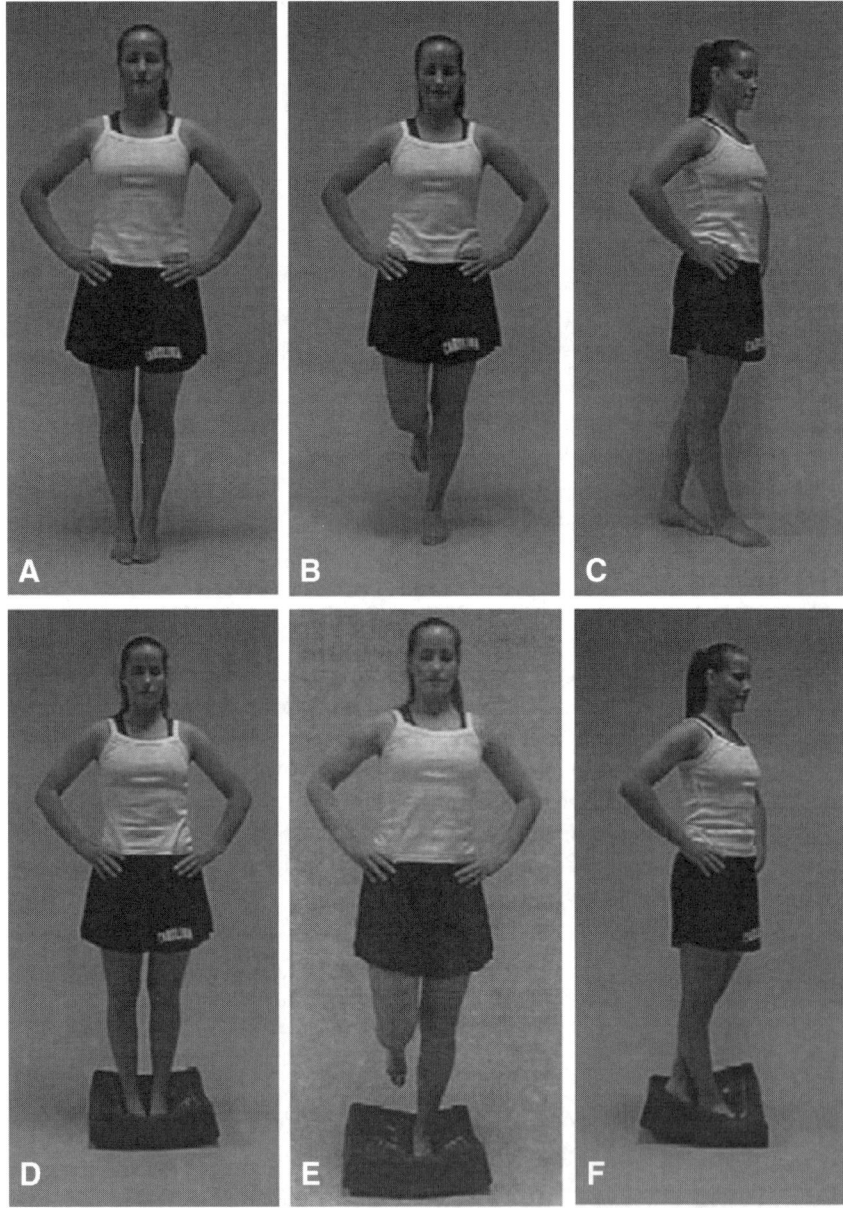

Fig 6. Balanced Error Scoring System. Reprinted with permission from Guskiewicz KM. Postural stability following concussion: one piece of the puzzle. *Clin J Sport Med.* 2001;11(3):182–189.

We also have come to better understand the factors that slow recovery from sports concussion. The most important of these factors is age. Younger athletes, in whom the brain is still maturing, are known to recover at a slower rate.[5,7,10,19,20,23,24]

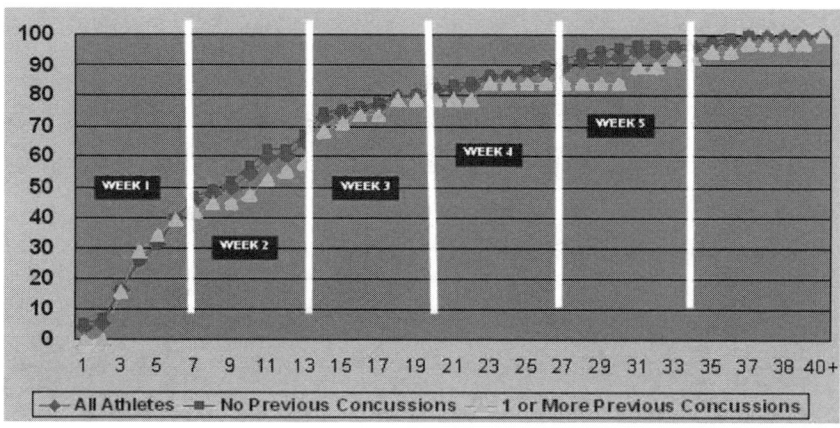

Fig 7. Recovery from concussion: how long does it take?

Athletes who have had repetitive concussion are notoriously slower healers.[10,19] The presence of personal or family history of migraine headache seems to have an association with protracted recovery from this injury as well.[10,25] Finally, those athletes who return to exertion too soon frequently complete recovery more slowly.

INITIAL MANAGEMENT OF TRAUMATIC BRAIN INJURY: FIRST WEEK

Initial management of traumatic brain injury includes physical rest, because athletes need to avoid physical exertion until the brain begins to recover. More recently, we have become aware of the role of mental rest. Mental rest includes specifics such as withholding students from school in the initial stages (full day or partial day), restriction of driving, reduction of work load and homework, and restriction or postponement of standardized testing, especially achievement tests and final examinations. Mental rest at home includes avoiding activities associated with loud noise such as parties, dances, concerts, and sporting events and avoiding the use of headphones. These athletes should also be instructed to avoid bright sunlight, computer games, carnival rides, and, of course, alcohol and drugs. The restriction of brain stimulation is related to speed of brain recovery (see Fig 8).

Ideally, those athletes (10%) who have not recovered by 1 month may need a more detailed, specific individualized educational plan put together by a neurophysiologist with input from the school.

This student has sustained a concussion (mild traumatic brain injury). Post-concussive symptoms may last for several days to several weeks depending on the severity of the injury. These symptoms include headache, vision problems, inability to concentrate, fatigue, and irritability which could affect school performance. Healing requires both mental and physical rest, therefore we recommend the restrictions listed below:

☐ Restricted from school until ____/____/____   ____ until cleared by physician.

☐ Restricted from sports/phys. ed. until ____/____/____   ____ until cleared by physician.

☐ Return to school for: ____ period (s) until ____/____/____   ____ until cleared by physician.

☐ Full return to school on ____/____/____ .

☐ Academic accommodations as specified below:

    _____ NO tests for _____ week (s)   _____ un-timed tests

    _____ reduced work load when possible   _____ pre-printed class notes

    _____ tutoring Other: _____

☐ Restricted from work until ____/____/____   ____ until cleared by physician

☐ Restricted from driving until ____/____/____   ____ until cleared by physician

☐ Restricted from loud noises (parties, concerts, MP3 players, headphones, loud sporting events).

☐ Restricted from bright lights (strobe lights, computer screens, video games). Wear sunglasses in bright daylight as needed.

☐ Restricted from spinning rides, and any activities that include excessive head motion.

☐ Alcohol or any other mind-altering substance should be strictly avoided.

The next physician appointment will be in ____ week(s).

Additional Recommendations / Instructions: _____

Fig 8. Physical and mental rest guidelines.

RETURN TO PLAY AFTER A TRAUMATIC CONCUSSION

When athletes recover from a concussion and become asymptomatic, they may begin gradual return to sporting activity in a graded fashion. An example of this is the 5-day functional progression guidelines for traumatic brain injury included in the summary and agreement statement of the second international conference on concussion in sports[18] (Fig 9).

Perhaps the most difficult decision in the care of a brain-injured athlete is when to suggest or insist on retirement. This is best answered by a medical care team, which may include an athletic trainer, primary care doctor, sports medicine physician, neurologist, neurosurgeon, and neuropsychologist. Factors that might point toward such a recommendation include the athlete's having increased length of postconcussion symptoms, milder degrees of trauma causing concus-

The athlete named above has suffered a concussion, and may not return to ANY contact sport activity (practice, games, contact drills, physical education class) unless listed on this form and cleared by the Sport Medicine Physician. Activity is permitted as tolerated only - that means that symptoms should not return or worsen during or after the activity.

Step 1: No activity, complete rest. Once asymptomatic, proceed to level.2

Step 2: Light aerobic exercise such as walking or stationary cycling, no resistance training.

Step 3: Sport specific exercise (eg, skating in hockey, running in soccer), progressive addition of resistance training at steps 3 or 4.

Step 4: Non-contact training drills.

Step 5: Full contact training after medical clearance.

Step 6: Game play.

Do not move on to the next step if symptoms develop. If any post-concussion symptoms develop, drop back to the previous step. You must remain symptom free for 24 hours before you can progress to the next higher step.

Fig 9. Return to physical activity guidelines.

sion, and decreasing time between concussions. There are no hard-and-fast rules for when to retire. However, it is important to remember that the competitive years are few (for most participants, high school only), and life is increasingly long. You cannot ice your brain like your quads and hope that it works next week.

PREVENTION OF TRAUMATIC BRAIN INJURY

There are many suggestions in the medical literature for the prevention of traumatic brain injury, some with strong research support and others with somewhat anecdotal evidence. Medical personnel involved in sports medicine need to advocate for rules changes and enforcement that can help prevent brain injury in young athletes. These changes include banning spearing and head-to-head contact (football), rough goal play (soccer), avoiding backward head flick (soccer), requiring padded goal posts in soccer, and enforcement of the rules against elbowing in basketball. Helmets should be a part of standard equipment for biking, snow sports, skateboarding, and inline skating as well.

There has been a long discussion in the literature regarding use of mouth pieces to help prevent traumatic brain injury.[26] Controversy also surrounds the use of head gear for nonhelmeted sports[27,28] such as soccer and basketball, which happen to be 2 sports that are seeing continued increase in the incidence of concussions. Finally, athletes need to be instructed on proper neck and shoulder girdle strengthening for contact and collision sports during the off season. The most effective way to prevent traumatic brain trauma, however, is awareness of the problem and awareness of the guidelines to protect athletes from brain injury. Coaches and parents need to be made aware of the standing knockout, and coaches and trainers must be taught never to return a symptomatic athlete to play. Other prevention tools include education kits such as the ones distributed by the Centers for Disease Control and Prevention.[4,29] It also may be useful to think of baseline neurophysiologic testing at the time of the preparticipation examination in contact and collision sports.

WHAT IS THE FUTURE OF OUR UNDERSTANDING OF CONCUSSION?

Several imaging techniques are being studied that may help to add clinical understanding to concussion and may ultimately help in making the decision about return to play as well. Imaging techniques that hold the most promise include functional MRI[10,30] and positron emission tomography (PET)[30] scanning. Studies are currently going on to better understand the clinical utility of these techniques.

There is also much study going on to examine genetics and traumatic brain injury. The gene locus ApoE4 is being evaluated, especially in boxers. The presence of ApoE4 is a known risk factor for Alzheimer disease.[25] Questions in this area may be answered that would allow us to use genetic testing as future modifiers and predictors of athletes' risk for traumatic brain injury.

SUMMARY OF TRAUMATIC BRAIN INJURY

1. The medical team has been charged with a major educational effort to improve the awareness and identification of traumatic brain injury, particularly in sports. Parents, coaches, athletes, and medical personnel need to reduce the silent epidemic of concussion by improving the timely and appropriate diagnosis of the injury.
2. The medical community needs to reduce the confusion in the clinical and radiographic diagnosis of concussion.
3. The medical community needs to highlight the management principles as an important part of the treatment of concussion. The concept of physical and mental rest is important in the recovery period for the brain.
4. Medical personnel need to eliminate long-standing myths in the care and treatment of brain-injured athletes, including the notion that all concussions are associated with loss of consciousness. Coaches, parents, athletes, and medical personnel need to be aware of the fact that only 10% to 20% of concussions include loss of consciousness.
5. Medical personnel need to understand that concussion is a functional and symptomatic injury rather than a structural injury to the brain. Therefore, "normal" MRI or computed tomography scan results do not rule out a concussion.
6. The medical community needs to increase awareness among coaches, parents, and athletes that all concussions are not brief transient injuries

with full recovery. The short and long-term consequences of concussion need to be explained well to nonmedical personnel.
7. The medical community must continue to push for further research and grant funding to improve our knowledge and understanding of traumatic brain injury. Much good work has been done in the past 10 years, but much work still remains to be done.
8. The medical community needs to ensure that coaches, parents, and athletes understand that no symptomatic athlete can ever be allowed to return to play.

REFERENCES

1. Thurman D, Alverson C, Dunn K, Guerrero J, Sniezek J. Traumatic brain injury in the united states: a public health perspective. *J Head Trauma Rehabil.* 1999;14(6):602–615
2. Centers for Disease Control and Prevention, National Center for Injury Prevention and Control. Facts for physicians about mild traumatic brain injury. Available at: www.cdc.gov/ncipc/pub-res/tbi_toolkit/physicians/index.htm. Accessed September 17, 2008
3. Collins M, Field M, Lovell M, et al. Relationship between post-concussion headache and neuropsychological test performance in high school athletes. *Am J Sports Med.* 2003;31(2):168–173
4. Schulz M, Marshall S, Mueller F, et al. Incidence and risk factors for concussion in high school athletes, North Carolina, 1996–1999. *Am J Epidemiol.* 2004;160(10):937–944
5. Gerberich SG, Priest JD, Boen JR, Straub CP, Maxwell RE. Concussion incidences and severity in secondary school varsity football players. *Am J Public Health.* 1983;73(12):1370–1375
6. Kaut KP, Depompei R, Kerr J, Congeni J. Reports of head injury and symptom knowledge among college athletes: implications for assessment and educational intervention. *Clin J Sport Med.* 2003;13(4):213–221
7. Grant L, Iverson G, Gaetz M, Lovell M, Collins M. Cumulative effects of concussion in amateur athletes. *Brain Injury.* 2004;18(5):433–443
8. LaBotz M, Martin MR, Kimura IF, Hetzler RK, Nochols AW. A comparison of a preparticipation evaluation history form and a symptom-based concussion survey in the identification of previous head injury in collegiate athletes. *Clin J Sport Med.* 2005;15(2):73–78
9. Valovich-McLeod TC, Bay RC, Heil J, McVeigh SD. Identification of sport and recreational activity concussion survey in the identification of previous head injury in collegiate athletes. *Clin J Sport Med.* 2008;18(3):221–226
10. Lovell M, Collins M, Bradley J. Return to play following sports-related concussion. *Clin Sports Med.* 2004;23(3):421–441, ix
11. Guskiewicz KM, Marshall SW, Bailes J, et al. Recurrent concussion and risk of depression in retired professional football players. *Med Sci Sports Exerc.* 2007;39(6):903–909
12. Packard RC. Chronic post-traumatic headache: associations with mild traumatic brain injury, concussion, and post-concussive disorder. *Curr Pain Headache Rep.* 2008;12(1):67–73
13. Kelly JP, Rosenberg JH. Diagnosis and management of concussion in sports. *Neurology.* 1997;48(3):575–580
14. Schmidt MS, Caldwell D. Brain injury puts player in critical condition. *The New York Times.* October 18, 2008. Available at: www.nytimes.com/2008/10/16/sports/16prep.html?_r=2&fta=y&pagewanted=print Accessed December 4, 2008
15. Committee on Head Injury Nomenclature of the Congress of Neurological Surgeons. Glossary of head injury, including some definitions of injury to the cervical spine. *Clin Neurosurg.* 1966;12:386–394
16. American Academy of Neurology. Practice parameter: the management of concussion in sports (summary statement). Report of the Quality Standards Subcommittee. *Neurology.* 1997;48(3):581–585

17. Aubry M, Cantu R, Dvorak J, Graf-Baumann T, et al. Summary and agreement statement of the 1st international symposium on concussion in sport, Vienna 2001. Clin J Sport Med. 2002;12(1): 6–11
18. McCrory P, Johnston K, Meeuwisse W, et al. Summary and agreement statement of the 2nd international conference on concussion in sport, Prague 2004. Clin J Sport Med. 2005;15(2): 48–55
19. Giza CC, Hovda DA. The neurometabolic cascade of concussion. J Athl Train. 2001;36(3):228–235
20. McCrea M, Kelly JP, Randolph C, et al. Standardized assessment of concussion (SAC): on-site mental status evaluation of the athlete. J Head Trauma Rehabil. 1998;13(2):27–35
21. Guskiewicz KM. Postural stability following concussion: one piece of the puzzle. Clin J Sport Med. 2001;11(3):182–189
22. Collins MW. Management of sports concussion: research and clinical application. Presented at: Akron Children's Hospital's Sports Medicine Update; March 2, 2007; Akron, OH 44308
23. Lovell MR. Recovery from mild concussion in high school athletes. J Neurosurg. 2003;98(2): 296–301
24. Field M, Collins MW, Lovell MR, Maroon J. Does age play a role in recovery from sports-related concussion? A comparison of high school and collegiate athletes. J Pediatr. 2003;142(5):546–553
25. Jordan BD. Genetic influences on outcome following traumatic brain injury. Neurochem Res. 2007;2(4–5):905–915
26. Knapik JJ, Marshall SW, Lee RB, et al. Mouth guards in sports activities: history, physical properties, and injury prevention effectiveness. Sports Med. 2007;37(2):117–144
27. McIntosh AS, McCrory P. Impact energy attenuation performance of football headgear. Br J Sports Med. 2000;34(5):337–341
28. Delaney JS, Al-Kashmiri A, Drummond R, Correa JA. The effect of protective headgear on head injuries and concussions in adolescent football (soccer) players. Br J Sports Med. 2008;42(2): 110–115
29. Centers for Disease Control and Prevention. Heads Up: Concussion in High School Sports. Atlanta, GA: Centers for Disease Control and Prevention; 2005. Available at: www.cdc.gov/ncipc/tbi/Coaches_Tool_Kit.htm. Accessed November 19, 2008
30. Johnston KM, Ptito A, Chankowsky J, Chen JK. New frontiers in diagnostic imaging in concussive head injury. Clin J Sport Med. 2001;11(3):166–175

Social Networking and Adolescents

Gilbert L. Fuld, MD, FAAP*

Department of Pediatrics, Dartmouth Medical School, 1 Rope Ferry Road, Hanover, NH 03755 and Council on Communications and Media, American Academy of Pediatrics, 141 Northwest Point Boulevard, Elk Grove Village, IL 60007

Adolescents have been networking on the Internet for years on sites such as AOL and Yahoo, entering chat rooms, using instant and text messaging, and revealing personal and identifying information about themselves. However, the advent of the social networking sites MySpace and Facebook has markedly increased the popularity and ease of communicating on the Internet, both with people known offline and those known only online.

Adolescents are knowledgeable about computers but too comfortable about disclosing private information and posting provocative photographs. This places them in danger according to law enforcement authorities, school and church officials, and worried parents.[1]

Although concerns about mushrooming worldwide networks of child pornographers, pedophiles, and sexual predators predate the inception and rapid acceptance by young people of social networking sites,[2] these new services are the current lightning rods for parental and societal concern. But, do social networking sites increase the risks or merely change the direction from which dangers to adolescents appear? And, what are those perils? This review will highlight some of the dangers that the 21st century presents to our youth, especially those related to the Internet and the World Wide Web.

SOCIAL NETWORKING SITES: WHAT ARE THEY?

Social networking sites combine the attributes of several already-existing ways to communicate: e-mail, instant messaging, Web logs, chat rooms, and message boards. Web logs (blogs for short) are unedited online journals generally written by a single person. The sites allow users to create profiles of themselves and form a network of online friends. Teens and young adults are among the most enthusiastic users of these Web sites.[3]

---

*Corresponding author.
E-mail address: glfuld@ne.rr.com (G. L. Fuld).

Copyright © 2009 American Academy of Pediatrics. All rights reserved. ISSN 1934-4287

A profile is a Web page within the social networking site and generated online by a Web-based questionnaire. Programming skill is not required to set up or maintain a profile. It may include information as basic as an individual's name, age, and hometown but with options to add detailed contact information, academic and work affiliations, interests, Web journals, hyperlinks, and more. Text-based personal information can be augmented by other user-generated content such as photographs, video, or music. A profile is a user's description of himself or herself and represents how the user wants to be presented to the online universe.

Once a profile is created, a user is then able to join a "community," which is simply a linkage of his or her profile with someone else's. A community is developed member by member and can be as large as the individual wants it to be. Facebook also automatically creates communities by linking users if they are related in other ways, such as students or alumni of an academic institution. Thus, users can belong to many different communities.[4]

Profiles can be private (requiring that anyone sending a message to the site know the individual's user name and limiting access by unknown people), or they can be public (allowing anyone to send a message to the individual, view the profile, or identify someone by searching for his or her name or other key identifying information).

Interactive communication can occur concurrently, as with instant messaging or chat rooms, but can also be posted for later perusal, as with e-mail or message boards. The gravitation of young people to social networking sites is not surprising, given the great number of options for communication. In communicating with friends, talking on the telephone (even the cell phone) has become supplanted by other technology, and the medium of choice for many young people is instant (or text) messaging. Blogs, which function as online journals, allow people to express themselves as in a diary while also receiving responses from anybody who has access to the personal site.[5,6]

Thus, social networking sites allow adolescents to experiment with and develop a personal identity that can be changed at any time. Young people "can represent themselves in a creative way and keep in touch with (and involved in) each others' lives."[7]

SPECIFIC SOCIAL NETWORKING SITES

At present, the most popular social networking sites in the United States are MySpace and Facebook. Although other sites exist and may supplant one or both of these in future popularity, most of the articles in the media and the scant data about such sites are about these two.

MySpace was launched in August 2003 and has grown rapidly since. Estimates of its membership vary, although it may have more than 200 million users.[8] It is the most visited US-based Web site. Facebook began in February 2004 and counts more than 60 million members.

Although on the surface they seem similar, they are, in fact, different in many ways. Right from the start, MySpace embraced openness and inclusiveness. Currently anyone can join who has an e-mail address and claims to be 13 years of age or older. After creating their profiles, users can connect with other users and create communities. The default setting for users 18 and older is to leave their profiles open to anyone including nonmembers, although the user does have the option of limiting access to his or her friends. MySpace users originally needed to choose whether to share their entire profiles. There was no way to limit access to private information to friends while exposing other parts of the profile to all viewers.[4] A profile currently can be customized so that parts of it are visible to specific groups of friends. For users 13 to 17 years old (previously only for users younger than 16), the profiles are supposed to be automatically limited to identified friends, restricting the ability of users older than 18 to become friends with younger users.[6] However, I easily found the profile of a boy who signed onto MySpace as a 32-year-old but gleefully states in the text of his public profile that he is really 11.

Facebook was started at Harvard University and, at first, limited access to college students. It subsequently opened the site to high school students, professional and regional networks, and the general public ≥13 years of age. Similar to MySpace, Facebook's Web-based questionnaires allow easy development of profiles plus the addition of multimedia and Internet links. However, in contrast to MySpace, it uses a "confirmed friendship" model to emphasize interaction with users' "real friends based on real relationships and the real world around them."[4] Facebook networks depend on a user's affiliations with institutions or employers, geographic location, or individual relationships.

Facebook restricts profile views to users within the same community or to identified friends. Given the self-contained nature of the networks, most users can view fewer than 1% of the profiles on the site. Furthermore, members are able to decide what information they want to expose to geographic or institutional networks and what more (such as contact information) to expose to real friends. Users can easily block particular people from seeing their profile or any part of it.[4] Indeed, the site is set up to encourage that activity. People younger than 18 must join the communities of their educational institutions, and Facebook does, in fact, authenticate its members.

HOW DO YOUNG PEOPLE USE SOCIAL NETWORKING SITES?

In a survey conducted by the Pew Internet and American Life Project 2006, 93% of teenagers used the Internet, and 55% of 12- to 17-year-old Internet users created a profile on a social networking site.[9]

- Forty-eight percent of teenagers said that social networking sites help them manage their friendships.
- Ninety-one percent of all social networking teenagers said that they use the sites to stay in touch with friends they see frequently, whereas 82% used the sites to stay in touch with friends they rarely see in person.
- Seventy-two percent of all social networking teenagers used the sites to make plans with friends.
- Forty-nine percent used the sites to make new friends. Older boys (aged 15–17) who use social networking sites are more likely than girls of the same age to say that they use the sites to make new friends (60% vs 46%, respectively).[10]

A survey for the National School Boards Association revealed that 9- to 17-year-old respondents spent ~9 hours/week on social networking activities (not all on social networking sites). Almost 60% of the students using social networking talked about education topics online, and >50% talked specifically about homework.[11]

What information do users post on their profiles?

- Eighty-two percent included their first name, and 29% disclosed their last names.
- Seventy-nine percent included photographs of themselves, and 66% included photographs of friends (girls were more likely to post photographs than boys).
- Sixty-one percent named their hometown, and 49% identified their school.
- Two percent listed their cell phone numbers (boys were more likely to include this information), and 29% gave out their e-mail address.
- Although two thirds of the teenagers with an online profile limited access to their profiles in some way, a small but not insignificant number (11%) gave their first and last names on publicly accessible profiles, and 5% disclosed full names, photographs of themselves, and the name of their hometown on publicly accessible sites.

Posting information on social networking sites opens the electronic door to the millions of people using the Internet and may expose youth to having blind contact with strangers. More than 30% of social networking teenagers have "friends" on their social network they have never personally met. Some 43% have reported being contacted online by complete strangers. Of those contacted, 21% have responded to find out more information about that person, whereas 65% have simply ignored and deleted the unwanted messages. Yet, 23% of teenagers contacted by a stranger online felt scared or uncomfortable because of the online contact.[3] Girls are approximately twice as likely to be frightened by an online experience than boys.[12]

This is similar to the findings of the National School Boards survey,[11] in which 7% of 9- to 17-year-old students said that someone on a social network has asked for identifying information, 4% have had conversations on social network sites that made them uncomfortable, and 2% said that a stranger they met online tried to meet them in person. Only 1 (0.08%) of the 1277 students surveyed admitted to meeting someone that they had first met online in person without their parents' permission. According to the Pew Internet and American Life Project report, many, but not all, teenagers realize the hazards of disclosing identifying information on a publicly viewed site, and many, but not all, of them make thoughtful choices about what and where to share it.[9]

In a 2000 review, Hinduja and Patchin[7] examined teenagers' MySpace profiles before the Web site's automatic restriction of access to identified friends only, for those younger than 18. They reported that only 38% listed a first name, 9% listed their full name, 28% listed their school, 81% listed their hometown, and 1% listed their e-mail address. Virtually no one revealed a telephone number (<0.5%), although 57% included a photograph. Almost 40% of the sites were listed as private. Presumably all sites of users younger than 18 would be private at present, but the study found evidence of age inflation, both to avoid the restriction of public posting and the age restriction of developing a profile at all.

DANGERS TO YOUTH OF SOCIAL NETWORKING SITES

Is there something inherently dangerous and different about social networking sites, or is it simply that sexual predators and others who would take advantage of our children go there because that's where the kids are? With the popularity of MySpace (85% of social networking teenagers use MySpace) and the declining use of chat rooms, concerns have been expressed that social networking sites are a new and dangerous place for youngsters to visit.

Media reports, peaking to the point of hysteria in early 2006, warned about this new method of group communication.[13]

- A February 2006 NBC news report detailed the arrest of a 21-year-old man for allegedly raping a 14-year-old girl he met on MySpace.[14]
- Three days later on the CBS Evening News, the mother of a daughter who was sexually assaulted by a 26-year-old man said: "Please don't allow your children to go onto MySpace. It's a very unsafe environment for them to be in."[15]
- In April 2006, *Wired News* ran the names of randomly selected registered sex offenders in San Francisco, California, and neighboring Sonoma County through MySpace's user search engine. The search turned up the profiles of 5 men whose self-reported names and

descriptions matched those of profiles on the state's online sex offender registry.[16]

An article in *AM:STARs* by Wolak et al[17] in 2007 summarized then-current knowledge about the Internet and adolescent victimization as it related to Internet-associated sex crimes and online sexual solicitation, Internet harassment, risky online behavior, and exposure to online pornography. Much of the research in this area has been performed at the Crimes Against Children Research Center at the University of New Hampshire. Published works include the first[18] and second[19] Youth Internet Safety Surveys (YISS-1 and YISS-2), both of which were telephone interviews of separate youth Internet users, and the National Juvenile Online Victimization (N-JOV) study,[20] which interviewed law enforcement investigators to determine the characteristics of Internet-related sex crimes.

Most of the adult offenders were up front in their online communications about their interest in a sexual encounter. Only 5% passed themselves off as adolescents, although many shaved some years off their actual age. Therefore, most of the teenage victims who met the molesters offline expected to engage in sexual activity. The major deceptions were promises of love and romance to a vulnerable adolescent from an individual who was interested only in sex. Violent confrontations were rare: 5% of the offenders committed violent crimes, mostly rape or attempted rape. However, most of the sexual encounters, although nonforcible and developed through seduction, represented statutory rape, because many of the victims were too young (usually younger than 16) to consent to sexual intercourse.[21]

In 2000 there were 6594 arrests nationwide for statutory rape. During a similar time period covered by the N-JOV study (July 1, 2000, to June 30, 2001), an estimated 500 arrests for Internet-initiated sex crimes were made by federal, state, and local law enforcement agencies.[22] Wolak et al[22] conceded that the increase in Internet use and the greater ability to respond to Internet-related crimes developed by law enforcement personnel since 2000 would probably increase the proportion of arrests from 7%. Nevertheless, they argued that Internet-related sex crimes account for a small proportion of statutory rape offenses and relatively few of the sex crimes that involve underaged victims.

In the 2005 YISS-2,[19] 1 in 7 youth Internet users received an unwanted sexual solicitation during the year before the interview. Only 1 in 7 of these solicitations came from offline friends and acquaintances; the others were from individuals known only online. Within the previous year, 4% of those surveyed received an aggressive solicitation, one in which the solicitor attempted or actually made an offline contact such as asking to meet the youth in person, calling on the telephone, or sending offline money, mail, or gifts. Another 4% of users reported themselves to be very or extremely upset or afraid because of the online solicitation. Approaches that were both aggressive and disturbing were reported by some 2% of the respondents.

WHICH YOUNGSTERS ARE VULNERABLE TO ONLINE SEXUAL PREDATORS?

According to Wolak et al,[22] young people are neither naive about the Internet nor innocent about sex. "The factors that make youth vulnerable to seduction by online molesters are complex and related to immaturity, inexperience, and the impulsiveness with which some youths respond to and explore normal sexual urges."[22]

Youth Internet users with histories of offline sexual or physical abuse are more likely to receive online sexual solicitations. Sending personal information and talking about sex with unknown people is more likely to attract individuals who make online sexual advances and then try to move on to face-to-face encounters. Users who engaged in such high-risk online interactive behavior had high rates of offline problems such as rule-breaking behavior, depression, and social interaction problems, adding online risky behavior to the list of risk behaviors that cluster. One study suggested that a combination of behaviors is related to online interpersonal victimization, but merely sharing information is not.[23] Aggressive behaviors in the form of making rude or nasty comments or frequently embarrassing others, meeting people in multiple ways, and talking about sex online with unknown people were significantly related to online sexual solicitation. Someone engaging in those 4 types of online behaviors magnified their chances of receiving unwanted overtures by a factor of 11. This seems to indicate that adolescents are not putting themselves at great risk just because they post identifying information about themselves but, rather, because of other behaviors not unique to the Internet experience.

Girls who become sexually active during early adolescence may be more likely to be involved with older partners and engage in risky behavior, thus putting themselves at increased risk. Although girls are more at risk for Internet-related sexual victimization, boys who question their sexual orientation or identify themselves as gay constitute up to 25% of such victims. These are youngsters who may turn to the Internet to find answers to questions about their sexuality or to meet potential romantic partners and thereby put themselves at risk for sexual exploitation.

PROTECTING OUR CHILDREN

Parry Aftab, an Internet privacy and security lawyer and executive director of WiredSafety.org, a children's Internet safety group, characterized MySpace on an NBC Dateline program as "one stop shopping for predators, and they can shop by catalog."[24] Not surprisingly, public fears spawned an industry dedicated to warning and protecting children, including a book that describes MySpace as "a dangerous gateway to a completely different world."[25] Various Web sites provide information,[26,27] as well as parental control software[28–30] and products that also allow parents to spy on what their children are doing online.[31]

However, with time comes familiarity and acceptance. For example, a recent MSNBC advice column recently offered calm advice on cyberspying, older "friends," and whether parents should forbid access to social networking sites,[32] and a young adult book series, which explores issues with opposing views, presents a discussion of the risks and benefits of social networking sites.[33] Because of the recent rapid growth of social networking sites, data specific to this mode of communication are scant. The only available study indicated that unwanted sexual solicitations are received more commonly through instant messaging and in chat rooms than on social networking sites.[5] Although only 4% of the respondents received solicitations on a social networking site, what is not clear is how much time was spent on such a site in comparison to other online activities. There is much more research to be done to delineate the true extent of danger to young people from using a social networking site and to determine if such activity is inherently more or less dangerous than other Internet activities that were popular (and are still used by some) before the sites became available.

Notwithstanding the lack of data, bills have been introduced on the federal and state levels to limit access to social networking. The Deleting Online Predators Act was passed overwhelmingly by the House of Representatives in 2006 but died in the Senate. Reintroduced in 2007, it would effectively ban access to social networking sites and blogs in libraries and schools.[4]

Political pressure eventually drove MySpace and Facebook to agree to voluntary measures designed to improve the safety for its users. After years of criticism for inaction in blocking sex offenders from the sites, MySpace in coordination with 49 state attorneys general announced new ways to increase the safety for users. This followed a voluntary agreement that Facebook made in October 2007 with Attorney General Andrew Cuomo of New York.

MySpace committed to creating an Internet Safety Technical Task Force to find ways to verify ages and identities online.[34] The task force will include Internet businesses and nonprofit organizations interested in children's safety. It will operate out of the Berkman Center for Internet and Society at Harvard Law School and will be chaired by Berkman Center Executive Director John Palfrey.[35]

Specific steps agreed to by MySpace include:

- installing safeguards that require an adult user to prove that he or she knows a child user by, for instance, typing in an address or telephone number before being permitted contact;

- automatically setting profiles of users younger to 18 to "private," preventing casual browsers from seeing them;
- improving technology to prohibit underaged children from creating profiles;
- allowing parents who do not want their children using the site to be able to submit their children's e-mail addresses to MySpace, thereby preventing users of those addresses from creating profiles; and
- hiring a contractor to identify and remove pornographic images and links to pornographic sites from its Web site.

In May 2008, Facebook followed suit with a similar voluntary agreement with a few new stipulations[36]:

- prevent older users from trying to masquerade as youngsters (when users try to change their ages, a customer service agent reviews their profiles);
- ensure that companies offering services on its site comply with its safety and privacy guidelines;
- remove groups whose comments or images suggest incest, pedophilia, bullying, or other inappropriate content; and
- send warning messages when a child is in danger of giving personal information to an adult.

The expectation was that once the 2 leaders agreed to these measures, competing sites would follow suit.[36] Criticism was immediate. An obvious problem was that, without their parents' knowledge, many kids obtain multiple e-mail addresses available for free through AOL, Yahoo, and other sites or otherwise find their way around the barriers. Texas attorney general Greg Abbott opted out of both agreements over concerns about the lack of a reliable age-verification system that allows an adult to "go on there right now and establish a profile as a 15-year-old. That poses a great danger."[37] (However, this is an uncommon event; the N-JOV study indicated that 95% of the time, sexual predators do not pass themselves off as adolescents[20]).

Parry Aftab of WiredSafety.org, who said the agreement was a good first step, warned about unforeseen consequences. "There's no system that will work for age verification without putting kids at risk," she said. "Age verification requires that you have a database of kids, and if you do, that database is available to hackers and anyone who can get into it."[38] Other controls may be equally ineffective. Ryan Hupfer, owner of the social networking site www.indymojo.com and author of "MySpace for Dummies," believes that most parents are not savvy enough to monitor their kids online. He also believes that tools such as age-verification software or setting profiles to private for a certain age group do not really work in the long run.[39]

A new federal law, Keeping the Internet Devoid of Sexual Predators (KIDS) Act, signed in October 2008, will require registered sex offenders to submit their e-mail addresses, instant message addresses, or other identifying information they use on the Internet. The information will be placed on the National Sex Offender Registry, which already keeps track of the home addresses of convicted offenders. The law also will allow qualifying social networking Web sites to check user information against the registry,[40] but it attracted immediate criticism as well. One critic maintained that it does nothing to stop first-time offenders, asks known criminals to be honest, and lets the social networking sites off the hook by having them match e-mail addresses to a registry instead of doing the hard wok of policing their sites.[41]

Public education campaigns may play a role in improving Internet safety. From 1999/2000 to 2005 the proportion of youth Internet users communicating online with people they did not know in person declined from 40% to 34%, the proportion of users who admitted to forming close online relationships with people they met online declined from 16% to 11%, and use of chat rooms (felt by many youth to be "unpleasant places attracting unsavory people") declined from 56% to 30%.[19] Another report[9] documented a drop in teenagers visiting chat rooms from 55% in 2000 to 18% in 2006 and attributes it to prominent media campaigns alerting teens and parents about the dangers of chat rooms. In addition, chat rooms now represent old technology, and teens may be finding instant messaging and social network sites to be safer and more attractive.

OTHER INTERNET HAZARDS

Despite an increase in use of filtering, blocking, and monitoring software on home computers between the first (1999–2000) and second (2005) YISS, there was also an increase in exposure to unwanted sexual material from 25% to 34% of youth Internet users. Three reasons for this have been suggested: an increase in youth Internet access and use; technologic change resulting in greater ease of access to visual images and increased capacity of computers to transmit and receive visual images; and aggressive marketing of sexual images on the Internet. Exposure to pornographic sites or sites that lead teenagers to gamble (an illegal activity in every state),[42] promote racism and hate, or encourage adolescents to engage in self-destructive behaviors such as anorexia ("pro-ana" sites), bulimia ("pro-mia" sites), self-cutting, or even suicide also alarm adults.[25] The increasing power of search engines such as Google makes finding such sites quick, efficient, and easy. Links from one kind of site to those promoting other dangerous activities increase the exposure to and, thus, encourage the clustering of such risky behaviors.

Perhaps the most insidious threat for young people is lack of privacy.[8] The large number of adolescents who have public profiles with personal and identifying information available to all viewers suggests not that they are unaware of a lack of privacy but that they may not care about the loss of their privacy. Once something is posted publicly online, the poster no longer controls it, and anyone can distribute it worldwide with a few clicks. (This is even worse if someone is the subject of a malicious post, true or not, because that someone may not even be aware of the posting). The full impact of social networking on all of these issues has yet to be understood.

CYBERBULLYING

Receiving unwanted sexual material is not the only potential problematic area for adolescents. Cyberbullying occurs when any digital medium is used to harm others.[8] Social networking sites have joined the older communication techniques (e-mail, instant messaging, and text messaging [often via cell phones]) to enable bullying to extend beyond the schoolyard. Such harassing activities range from benign to annoying to truly alarming and include threatening messages, forwarding private e-mails or text messages without consent, posting embarrassing pictures, or spreading rumors.

Girls are victimized more than boys; they are the subjects of more rumors and the unauthorized posting of embarrassing pictures, and they are recipients of more online threats. Twice as many users of social network sites report that they are targets of these actions than those who do not use the sites. Teenagers who create content for the Internet (produce blogs, post photographs, share artwork, or help others create Web sites) are more likely to report being harassed or cyberbullied.

Among social network users in one study, 39% reported personal experience of being an object of cyberbullying, although the report did not state through which medium the e-mail, instant message, or text message was received.[43] Other studies have stated that 9% of youth report being harassed,[5] and 7% say they have experienced cyberbullying[11] while specifically on a social network site. These were the earliest attempts to quantify the problem, but the rapidly increasing popularity of social network sites may quickly make these figures obsolete.

Although the impulses for bullying probably remain the same as they always have been, the anonymity of the Internet allows adolescent cruelty to move "from the school yard, the locker room, the bathroom wall, and the phone onto the Internet."[43] Anonymity further isolates bullies from the results of their actions. The new technology allows bullying actions, which have often been private or known to only a few persons, to be transmitted to thousands of people through a social network. Public concern about how far cyberbullying can go was heightened by a teenager's suicide after a false MySpace identity was created to deceive and attack her.[44]

WHAT CAN AND CANNOT BE DONE TO PROTECT KIDS?

Media publicity about Internet-related sex crimes was previously mentioned. In April 2006, a 14-year-old girl (13 when she established a MySpace profile) was sexually assaulted by a 19-year-old man she met on MySpace. Citing 11 cases between December 2005 and June 2006 in which criminal charges were pending for adults who had contact with underaged MySpace users, suit was filed in federal court against MySpace claiming that the site had a duty to protect underaged users from sexual predators. The suit was dismissed in 2007 by the trial judge, who rejected the family's claim and also ruled that interactive computer services are immune from such lawsuits under the 1996 Communications Decency Act, which shields online publishers from online content. The judge further wrote that if anyone had the duty to protect the girl, it was her parents, not MySpace.[45] The ruling was upheld on appeal in 2008.

Much of the proposed and enacted legislation, and the agreements between attorneys general and social networking sites designed to forestall suits or legislation, deal with technology aimed at restricting access to social network sites or making them safer. Yet, as one attorney general notes, technologic improvements can be bypassed. "Children can create new e-mail addresses that their parents do not know about; adult strangers could obtain enough information about children to get past the site's safeguards; pornographic links spring up as quickly as they can be removed."[34] Furthermore, restrictions may run afoul of First Amendment guarantees of free speech.

One researcher argued that the money spent on legislation and legal action would be better spent on prevention: "online youth outreach programs, school anti-bullying programs, and online mental health services."[5] A recent Virginia law, for example, mandates Internet safety lessons in public schools at all grade levels.[46]

Most parents are aware of their responsibility to deal with potential Internet threats to their children. In a survey of adolescents aged 12 to 17 and their parents, many parents stated that they had rules about computer use.

- Eighty-five percent of parents of online teenagers claim to have rules about Internet sites that the teenager can and cannot visit.
- Eighty-five percent have rules about what kind of personal information can be disclosed online.
- Seventy percent limit their teenager's Internet time.
- Fifty percent of both parents and teenagers say that filtering software for preventing access to certain Web sites is installed on the computer used by the youngster.
- Forty-five percent of parents use software that monitors what users do online, although only 35% of the teenagers were aware that it was being used.

- Seventy-five percent of the teenagers said that the computer they use at home is in a public area.[3]

Law enforcement personnel encourage parental monitoring and emphasize that parents must prevent teenagers from posting descriptive information about themselves and stop them from talking online with strangers.[47]

Others have warned that parental tracking of online activities will undermine mutual trust.[8] Wolak et al[21,22] from the Crimes Against Children Research Center called for a reorientation of prevention materials, which currently focus on the technology or emphasize avoiding deception, not trusting people met online, not meeting strangers, and not giving out identifying information. They maintain that this does little to decrease the number of young teenagers knowingly and voluntarily meeting with adult men to have sex. Rather, increased emphasis must be placed on educating teenagers about the dangers of seduction and that, although it is normal to have strong sexual feelings, it is wrong for adults to exploit them. They should be told directly why such liaisons are a bad idea for both parties and that any risqué pictures sent online may end up all over the Internet or in a courtroom as evidence.

Physicians working with adolescents are encouraged to educate parents and children about what does and does not increase the risk of sexual victimization. A social networking site is not intrinsically dangerous, but parents can be educated about the adolescent "personal fable" of invincibility and alerted to the internal and external factors that make teenagers vulnerable. Girls who are alienated from their parents, are victims of family abuse, or are lonely or depressed and boys who are gay or conflicted about their sexual orientation are most at risk for abuse. These young people and their parents deserve special counseling about the attractiveness and dangers associated with Internet activities. Furthermore, the interactive behaviors some children pursue online make them more likely to attract online sexual attention.[21,22] Mention should also be made of other risk behaviors that may be promoted on Web sites, including sexual promiscuity, disordered eating, weapon use and procurement, drug and alcohol use, gang affiliation, violence, and a host of other behaviors to which our youth fall prey. Comprehensive, candid discussions beginning at an early age are arguably the best hope for prevention.

Parents should know with whom, when, and about what topics their teenagers are talking online. One way to do that is to keep the computer in a public area of the home. The best time for parents to talk to their children about online activity is before they first begin to explore the Internet. That way limits on use are something that the youngster grows up with, rather than being something suddenly imposed by frightened parents.

Palfrey and Gasser[8] see not only a technologic gap between parents and teachers on one side and children on the other but also too much media fear-mongering.

Adults have better digital-literacy skills than adolescents, but young people understand the technology better. Rather than banning technology, Palfrey and Gasser have called for parents to pay increased attention to the online disinhibition effect (people do and say things online they wouldn't do face-to-face) and to help children and adolescents understand the difference between healthy experimentation and truly risky behavior.

CONCLUSIONS

According to Fred Turner, a communications professor at Stanford, excessive parental concern is fueled by a generation gap. He stated that "[e]very time that a new communications technology becomes popular there's usually a moral panic. When the telephone was introduced in the 19th century, there was widespread fear that it would decrease the authority of parents over their daughters, that men would be entering the house through the telephone line. That's something we are going through right now. . . ."[48] Yet, parents do play a role in helping protect their children from the potential dangers of this new medium. As pediatricians, we know that brief interventions are effective in dealing with other risky behaviors including smoking, bicycle helmet use, and sexual behavior. There is every reason to believe that incorporating the discussion of Internet safety into our regular routine may help to raise awareness and be an effective prevention tool.

REFERENCES

1. Marvel M, Churnin N. Parents fear MySpace is playground for pedophiles. *Dallas Morning News*. March 5, 2006. Available at: www.dallasnews.com/sharedcontent/dws/dn/latestnews/stories/030506dnlivmyspace.2976283.html. Accessed December 18, 2008
2. Nordland R, Bartholet J, Johnson S, et al. The Web's dark secret. *Newsweek*. March 19, 2001;137:44
3. Lenhart A, Madden M. Pew Internet and American Life Project: teens, privacy & online social networks. Available at: http://pewinternet.org/pdfs/PIP_Teens_Privacy_SNS_Report_Final.pdf. Accessed December 18, 2008
4. Guo R. Stranger danger and the online social network. *Berkeley Technol Law J*. 2008;23(1):617–644
5. Ybarra ML, Mitchell KJ. How risky are social networking sites? A comparison of places online where youth sexual solicitation and harassment occurs. *Pediatrics*. 2008;121(2). Available at: www.pediatrics.org/cgi/content/full/121/2/e350
6. Subrahmanyam K, Greenfield P. Online communication and adolescent relationships. *Future Child*. 2008;18(1):119–146. Available at: www.futureofchildren.org/usr_doc/18_06_Subrahmanyam.pdf. Accessed December 18, 2008
7. Hinduja S, Patchin J. Personal information of adolescents on the Internet: a quantitative content analysis of MySpace. *J Adolesc*. 2008;31(1):125–146
8. Palfrey J, Gasser U. *Born Digital*. New York, NY: Basic Books; 2008
9. Lenhart A, Madden M, Macgill A, Smith A. Pew Internet and American Life Project: teens and social media. Available at: http://pewinternet.org/pdfs/PIP_Teens_Social_Media_Final.pdf. Accessed December 18, 2008
10. Lenhart A, Madden M. Pew Internet and American Life Project: Pew Internet Project data memo. Available at: www.pewinternet.org/pdfs/PIP_SNS_Data_Memo_Jan_2007.pdf. Accessed December 18, 2008

11. De Boor T, Kramer-Halpern L. Creating and connecting/research and guidelines on online social—and educational—networking. Available at: www.nsba.org/SecondaryMenu/TLN/CreatingandConnecting.aspx. Accessed December 18, 2008
12. Smith A. Pew Internet and American Life Project: data memo. Available at: www.pewinternet.org/pdfs/PIP_Stranger_Contact_Data_Memo.pdf. Accessed December 18, 2008
13. Bahney A. Don't talk to invisible strangers. *The New York Times.* March 9, 2006:G1
14. Williams P. MySpace, Facebook attract online predators. Available at: www.msnbc.msn.com/id/11165576. Accessed December 18, 2008
15. Hughes S. MySpace.com responds to Web risks. Available at: www.cbsnews.com/stories/2006/02/06/eveningnews/main1286130.shtml. Accessed December 18, 2008
16. Shreve J. MySpace faces a perp problem. Available at: www.wired.com/culture/lifestyle/news/2006/04/70675. Accessed December 18, 2008
17. Wolak J, Ybarra M, Mitchell K, Finkelhor D. Current research knowledge about adolescent victimization via the Internet. *Adolesc Med State Art Rev.* 2007;18(2):325–341, xi
18. Finkelhor D, Mitchell K, Wolak J. *Online Victimization: A Report on the Nation's Youth.* Alexandria, VA: National Center for Missing & Exploited Children: 2000. Available at: www.unh.edu/ccrc/pdf/jvq/CV38.pdf. Accessed December 18, 2008
19. Wolak J, Mitchell K, Finkelhor D. *Online Victimization of Youth: 5 Years Later.* Alexandria, VA: National Center for Missing & Exploited Children; 2006. Available at: www.missingkids.com/en_US/publications/NC167.pdf. Accessed December 18, 2008
20. Wolak J, Mitchell KJ, Finkelhor D. *Internet Sex Crimes Against Minors: The Response of Law Enforcement.* Alexandria VA: National Center for Missing & Exploited Children; 2003. Available at: www.unh.edu/ccrc/pdf/jvq/CV70.pdf. Accessed December 18, 2008
21. Wolak J, Finkelhor D, Mitchell K. Internet-initiated sex crimes against minors: implications for prevention based on findings from a national study. *J Adolesc Health.* 2004;35(5):424.e11–424.e20
22. Wolak J, Finkelhor D, Mitchell K, Ybarra M. Online "predators" and their victims: myths, realities, and implications for prevention and treatment. *Am Psychol.* 2008;63(2):111–128
23. Ybarra ML, Mitchell KJ, Finkelhor D, Wolak J. Internet prevention messages: targeting the right online behaviors. *Arch Pediatr Adolesc Med.* 2007;161(2):138–145
24. Stafford R. Why parents must mind MySpace. Available at: www.msnbc.msn.com/id/11064451. Accessed December 18, 2008
25. Edmiston WD. *Why Parents Should Fear MySpace.* Longwood, FL: Xulon Press; 1997
26. Wired Safety [an Internet safety, help, and education resource]. Available at: www.wiredsafety.org. Accessed December 18, 2008
27. NetSmartz.org [educational resource from the National Center for Missing & Exploited Children]. Available at: www.netsmartz.org. Accessed December 18, 2008
28. Net Nanny News. Net Nanny Internet filter software for your home. Available at: www.netnanny.com. Accessed December 18, 2008
29. InternetSafety.com [internet safety solutions]. Available at: www.internetsafety.com. Accessed December 18, 2008
30. CyberPatrol [powerful Internet filtering software to protect your kids online]. Available at: www.cyberpatrol.com. Accessed December 18, 2008
31. SpyBuddy [Internet monitoring software]. Available at: www.buy-spybuddy.com. Accessed December 18, 2008
32. Persch JA. Answering parents' MySpace questions. Available at: www.msnbc.msn.com/id/24507454. Accessed December 18, 2008
33. Espejo R, ed. *Should Social Networking Sites Be Banned? At Issue Series: Mass Media.* Farmington Hills, MI: Greenhaven Press; 2008
34. Barnard A. MySpace agrees to lead fight to stop sex predators. *New York Times.* January 15, 2008:B03
35. The Berkman Center announces formation of Internet safety task force to identify and develop online safety tools. Available at: http://cyber.law.harvard.edu/newsroom/Internet_Safety_Task_Force. Accessed December 18, 2008

36. Worden A. Facebook reaches agreement on sex predators. *The Philadelphia Inquirer*. May 9, 2008:B1
37. King L. My not so safe space, still? Experts say new pact won't faze predators. *The Philadelphia Inquirer*. February 10, 2008:A1
38. Texas AG. MySpace agreement offers "false sense of security." Available at: www.dallasnews.com/sharedcontent/dws/dn/latestnews/stories/011508dnnatmyspace.2d6c721.html. Accessed December 18, 2008
39. Bora M, Raghunathan A. MySpace plan to shield kids won't work, experts say. *St Petersburg Times*. January 16, 2008:4A. Available at: www.sptimes.com/2008/01/16/Worldandnation/MySpace_plan_to_shiel.shtml. Accessed December 18, 2008
40. Weiner M. Sen. Charles Schumer's crackdown on sex offenders is signed by President Bush. Available at: www.syracuse.com/news/index.ssf/2008/10/sen_charles_schumers_crackdown.html. Accessed December 18, 2008
41. Windish J. McCain's sex offender e-mail registry signed into law. Available at: http://themoderatevoice.com/society/children/23483/mccains-sex-offender-e-mail-registry-signed-into-law. Accessed December 18, 2008
42. Federal Trade Commission. Online gambling and kids: a bad bet. Available at: www.ftc.gov/bcp/edu/pubs/consumer/alerts/alt116.shtm. Accessed December 18, 2008
43. Lenhart A. Pew Internet and American Life Project: cyberbullying and online teens—data memo. Available at: www.pewinternet.org/PPF/r/216/report_display.asp. Accessed December 18, 2008
44. Steinhauer J. Woman indicted in MySpace suicide case. Available at: www.nytimes.com/2008/05/16/us/16myspace.html. Accessed December 18, 2008
45. Puzzanghera J, Chmielewski DC. Judge says MySpace isn't liable for alleged sexual assault on girl. *Los Angeles Times*. February 15, 2007:C1. Available at: http://articles.latimes.com/2007/feb/15/business/fi-myspace15. Accessed December 18. 2008
46. Vargas T. New focus in the classroom: Internet safety for children [reprint]. *New Hampshire Sunday News*. May 4, 2008:A6
47. Shoichet CE. MySpace pal called a predator. *St Petersburg Times*. December 3, 2007:1B. Available at: www.sptimes.com/2007/12/03/State/MySpace_pal_called_a_.shtml. Accessed December 18, 2008
48. Minaya Z. Pedophiles trolling in MySpace raise alarm. *Houston Chronicle*. March 3, 2006:A1

Understanding Adolescent Brain Development and Its Implications for the Clinician

Aaron M. White, PhD*

Division of Medical Psychology, Department of Psychiatry, Duke University Medical Center, Box 3374, Durham, NC 27710, USA

Adolescence is the stage of human development during which we make the transition from childhood dependence to adult autonomy. Soon after our bodies begin the physical metamorphosis of puberty, the brain undergoes a fascinating array of gene- and experience-driven modifications that prepare us to survive in the current cultural context. In essence, puberty reflects the physical changes that allow us to survive in the adult world, whereas adolescence embodies the psychological/neurologic changes that allow us to survive in the adult world as it is now. In this article, adolescent brain development will be explored, and the implications of such development for both normal and abnormal behavior during the teenage years will be discussed. As we will see, the neurologic changes that take place during adolescence provide incredible opportunities for personal growth but also enhanced vulnerabilities to consequences ranging from psychological disorders to substance abuse.

THE MALLEABLE DEVELOPING BRAIN

The brain is a remarkably complex, still poorly understood organ. Hundreds of billions of neurons, 1 of the 2 key types of cells in the brain, bathe one another in chemical messengers that influence moment-to-moment changes in brain processing, behavior, and experience. Glial cells, the other main category of brain cells, nurture and sustain neurons by holding them in place, feeding them partially metabolized glucose, fighting immune battles, cleaning up debris, and forming a key part of the blood-brain barrier that regulates the flow of molecules in and out of the brain. The basic layout of the brain is encoded by genes, but the specifics of the wiring are dependent on experience. The malleability of the developing brain allows each individual to be customized to fit the demands of the environments in which he or she is raised.

---

*Corresponding author.
E-mail address: aaron.white@duke.edu (A. M. White).

Copyright © 2009 American Academy of Pediatrics. All rights reserved. ISSN 1934-4287

Until quite recently, it was generally believed that the majority of brain development is finished by the age of 10. Learning languages becomes much harder after this age, and the brain reaches its adult size at about this time. Indeed, the brain is 90% of its adult size by the age of 7.[1] The moodiness, risk-taking, rule-breaking, and general tumult of the adolescent years were long assumed to stem from the hormone changes of puberty. We now know that, although hormones certainly do contribute to the roller-coaster ride of adolescence, hormone changes are just part of the puzzle. Thanks in large part to research by Jay Giedd and colleagues at the National Institute of Mental Health, it has become clear that, during the adolescent years, the organization and functioning of the brain go through complex changes. Importantly, these changes seem to be unique to the adolescent years and not simply the trailing remnants of childhood brain development.

CHANGES IN THE FRONTAL LOBES DURING ADOLESCENCE

Some of the most intriguing changes in the brain during adolescence take place in the frontal lobes. These brain areas, located just behind the forehead, play critical roles in memory, intentional movement, controlling emotional urges, making decisions, planning for the future, and other higher-order cognitive functions on which adults rely for survival. Frontal lobe gray-matter volumes, which represent dense concentrations of neurons and their parts, increase throughout childhood and do not reach their peak until approximately the age of 11 (girls) or 12 (boys), at which point they decline throughout the second decade of life and into young adulthood.[1]

Why might frontal lobe gray-matter volumes go up during childhood and down during adolescence? Recent data suggested that, during childhood, neurons in the frontal lobes are allowed to overgrow and form far too many points of communication, or synapses, with other neurons. As a result, gray-matter volumes increase. As childhood draws to a close and adolescence begins, the brain switches from overproduction mode to selection mode. Early in the second decade of life, the brain stops overproducing synapses in the frontal lobes and puts the synapses that exist on the chopping block. Hundreds of billions of points of communication will be sacrificed through the teenage years. Only those that form meaningful, useful points of contact will be kept. Guided by a teenager's experiences, the frontal lobes are shaped and molded into a configuration that will carry the individual, for better or worse, through the adult years. As this pruning process unfolds, gray-matter volumes decrease.[2]

The activity of neurons requires energy. As frontal lobe gray-matter volumes rise during childhood and fall during adolescence, a parallel increase in overall metabolism occurs in the frontal lobes during the first decade of life and then decreases during early adolescence, reaching adult levels by the age of 16 to 18.[3] Importantly, declines in gray-matter volumes and energy usage during adoles-

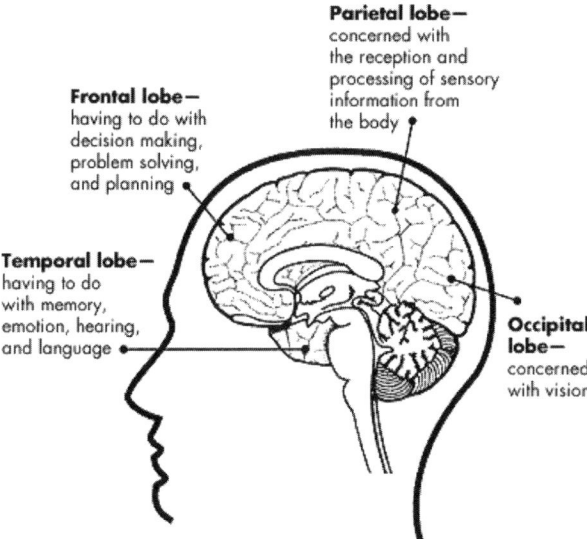

Fig 1. The human brain. (Reproduced with permission from National Institute on Drug Abuse. *Mind Over Matter: The Brain's Response to Drugs.* Teacher's Guide. Bethesda, MD: National Institute on Drug Abuse; 2002:10. Available at: http://teens.drugabuse.gov/mom/teachguide/MOMTeacherGuide.pdf).

cence do not reflect a diminution of frontal lobe function. Quite the opposite. As gray-matter volumes and metabolism decrease, neural activity during the performance of frontal lobe–dependent tasks becomes more focused and efficient, and the accuracy of performance improves.[2] The changes taking place in the frontal lobes during adolescence reflect a fine-tuning of circuitry that allows for enhanced efficiency and accuracy of functioning.[4] Indeed, there seems to be a general increase in reliance on the frontal lobes to organize and control behavior as we progress through the teenage years toward young adulthood. This developmental transition of power to the frontal lobes has become known as frontalization.[5] Concurrent molding of circuitry as frontalization unfolds means that each individual will learn to control impulses, make plans, and regulate emotions in ways consistent with the contingencies of the current culture. Such cultural-specific molding of behavior manifests in the generation gap that frustrates so many parents.

The frontal lobes do not function in isolation (see Fig 1). That is, they gather information and exert their influences by interacting with other brain areas. In addition to revealing that changes take place within the frontal lobes during adolescence, recent science has begun to shed light on how circuits formed between the frontal lobes and other structures develop during the second decade of life. The overall picture is one of increasing specialization of function within specific subregions of the frontal lobes and increasing cohesion between these subregions and the brain areas with which they interact. For instance, in the

Stroop interference task, in which subjects are shown words in different colors and must inhibit the tendency to read the words to name the colors, coordinated activity between the lateral prefrontal cortex and the basal ganglia, the lenticular nucleus of the striatum in particular, comes online during adolescence. Both the accuracy of performance on the task and the magnitude of activation of circuits involving the frontal lobes and basal ganglia increase throughout the adolescent years and into adulthood.[6] Similar age-related increases in activity within circuits involving the frontal lobes and basal ganglia have been observed in the tracking stop task, a response-inhibition task in which subjects must inhibit a response to a go signal if it is followed by a stop signal.[7]

CHANGES IN OTHER PARTS OF THE CORTEX

The frontal lobes are not the only cortical areas that undergo construction during the adolescent years.[8,9] As with the frontal lobes, the amount of gray matter in the parietal lobes peaks at approximately age 11 and decreases throughout adolescence. Located on the sides and toward the back of the brain, the parietal lobes are primarily involved in processing sensations from the body and understanding spatial relationships such as where the body is relative to other objects in the world. They are also very important for interpreting and creating music, solving math problems, and other higher-order abstract cognitive functions.

In the occipital lobes, located at the back of the brain and entirely dedicated to processing visual information, gray-matter volumes increase throughout adolescence and into the early 20s.

The temporal lobes, which are critical for memory formation as well as processing auditory information and seeing detailed patterns and shapes, do not reach their maximum levels of gray matter until the age of 16 to 17, at which point they plateau. The temporal lobes contain the hippocampus, a structure that is central to creating an autobiographical record of what one does and what one learns.

Clearly, much of the cortex undergoes changes during adolescence, each area with its own unique progression.[1,2]

STRUCTURES INVOLVED IN EMOTIONAL REACTIVITY AND RISKY BEHAVIORS

On the surface, changes in the frontal lobes and other cortical structures seem capable of explaining a wide range of typical adolescent behaviors, including difficulties inhibiting impulses and the tendency to measure the future in hours and minutes rather than weeks and days. However, Casey et al[10] were quick to point out that changes in the frontal lobes and other cortical areas cannot explain the whole of adolescent behavior, particularly when it comes to risk-taking and strong emotional reactions. The authors argued that, similar to adolescents, children have immature frontal lobes, too, but do not exhibit the degree of risky behavior exhibited by many teenagers. According to the authors, "[a]dolescence is a developmental period characterized by suboptimal decisions and actions that are associated with an increased incidence of unintentional injuries, violence, substance abuse, unintended pregnancy, and sexually transmitted diseases." Indeed, the National Center of Health Statistics has estimated that there are 13 000 adolescent deaths per year, 70% of which are caused by motor vehicle crashes, unintentional injuries, homicide, and suicide[11] and all of which are activities suggestive of problems with impulse control and the presence of strong and often maladaptive impulses.

Casey et al concurred that immature frontal lobes certainly help explain problems regulating impulses. Maturation of the frontal lobes leads to the ability to suppress inappropriate thoughts and actions and to forego short-term satisfaction in exchange for reaching long-term goals. Immature cognitive control centers make it easier for emotional impulses to break through to the surface and influence behavior, but what about the strong emotional impulses themselves? From where do they originate, and why are they so strong during adolescence? The authors suggested that several important emotional areas of the brain reach full operating power by midadolescence at a time when the frontal lobes are still in flux. Adolescents are driven by strong emotions arising from these areas and do not yet have the cognitive control necessary to stifle, consistently, these strong emotional urges. The fact that the frontal lobes are not yet working at their full potential simply makes it easier for these deep emotions to influence moment-to-moment changes in behavior.

In support of their position, neuroimaging studies suggested that, when making risky choices and processing emotional information, adolescents exhibit larger increases in activity in the amygdala and nucleus accumbens relative to the activity seen in children and adults.[2] The amygdala, a small almond-shaped structure located just in front of the hippocampus in the temporal lobes on each side of the brain, plays a prominent role in learning and evoking emotional responses, particularly negative emotional responses, to stimuli.

The nucleus accumbens, deep within the center of the brain, is the heart of the reward system. The nucleus accumbens receives signals in the form of the neurotransmitter, dopamine, from another deep-seated structure called the ventral tegmental area. This system is strongly activated both in anticipation of reward and on the delivery of reward. In essence, activation of this circuitry leads to pleasure, and pleasure increases the odds that the rewarded behavior will be repeated. Animal studies[2] have suggested that the density of dopamine receptors is highest in the nucleus accumbens during adolescence, perhaps making this region particularly responsive to the rewarding signals that dopamine provides. As will be discussed in a subsequent section, these poorly understood changes in the reward system are thought to contribute to the heightened risk of abuse and dependence people face when substance use begins during the adolescent years.

In addition to exhibiting differences in responsiveness to both fear-inducing and rewarding stimuli, adolescents exhibit an exaggerated stress response relative to children and adults.[12] This exaggerated stress response seems to contribute to the periodic difficulties that many teenagers have regulating their emotional reactions. At the core of the stress response is the hypothalamic-pituitary-adrenal (HPA) axis. In response to stressful stimuli or environments, the hypothalamus releases corticotropin-releasing hormone, which causes the pituitary to release adrenocorticotropin, which in turn triggers the adrenals, located just above the kidneys, to release cortisol. Puberty brings increased activity in the HPA axis. Sharp increases in urine and salivary cortisol levels happen at approximately the age of 13 and remain elevated into adulthood. A little cortisol goes a long way and helps the body prepare itself to deal with stressors and form memories of stressful events. Too much cortisol is associated with the onset of depression, the death of brain cells in the hippocampus, the memory center of the brain, and with weakened immune activity and cardiovascular problems down the road. Cortisol triggers anxiety via receptors on neurons in the amygdala, and high cortisol levels are commonly seen in adolescents, as well as children and adults, with anxiety disorders.[13] A stronger association exists between adverse life events and depression during adolescence than during adulthood, perhaps reflecting heightened reactivity in the HPA axis during the adolescent period.[14]

Additional evidence that adolescents are particularly reactive to stress comes from evidence that stressful stimuli cause greater skin-conductance changes in adolescents than in adults. In adolescents, these changes in skin conductance also take longer to habituate. In other words, the stress response is not only larger in adolescents than adults but also stays activated longer once initiated.

Collectively, heightened activity in the amygdala, reward system, and HPA axis, combined with the still-developing frontal lobe circuits, could explain the presence of particularly strong emotional impulses and reactions during adolescence and the trouble many adolescents have regulating them.

WHITE-MATTER VOLUMES AND PSYCHOLOGICAL DEVELOPMENT DURING ADOLESCENCE

Most research on adolescent brain development has focused on changes in gray-matter volumes during the teenage years. As discussed above, gray-matter volumes reflect the density of neurons and parts of neurons. Understanding the changes that occur in neurons and the circuits they form during adolescence is critical if we are to understand adolescence as a neurodevelopmental stage. However, we also must understand the changes taking place in the other major category of brain matter, white matter.

White matter reflects the density of glial cells, which help protect and nurture neurons and the circuits they form. This diverse group of cells contains micro-

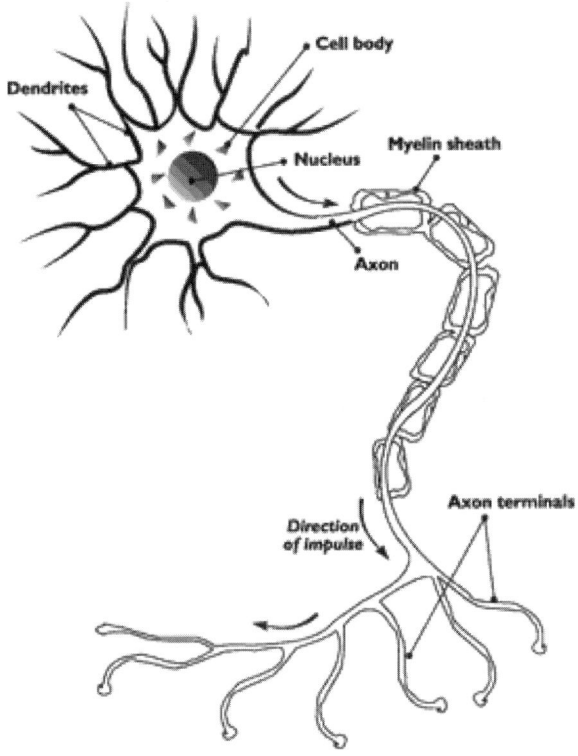

Fig 2. Depiction of a neuron. (Reproduced with permission from National Institute on Drug Abuse. *Mind Over Matter: The Brain's Response to Drugs*. Teacher's Guide. Bethesda, MD: National Institute on Drug Abuse; 2002:11. Available at: http://teens.drugabuse.gov/mom/teachguide/MOMTeacherGuide.pdf).

glia, which help fight brain infections, and astroglia, which form a critical component of the blood-brain barrier by surrounding blood vessels. Oligodendroglia, another type of glial cell, perform one of the most important acts performed by glia in the brain, namely, myelination of neuronal axons. Myelination will be discussed briefly, and then its role in adolescent brain development will be explored.

Neurons are capable of harnessing the electrical charges of ions (such as sodium, potassium, and chloride) located around their cell membranes to generate tiny electrochemical impulses called action potentials (see Fig 2). Action potentials begin near the cell bodies of neurons and travel down long arms called axons, which reach away from the cell bodies, branch out, and form synapses with other neurons. In essence, the axon is like a gun barrel down which the electrical impulse travels. Once the electrical signal reaches the distal tips of the axon, which could be several inches away from the cell body and number in the thousands by the time the axon stops branching, neurotransmitters are released onto the neuron's targets.

Myelination is a process by which oligodendroglia grab onto the axons of neurons and wrap around them. This increases the resistance across neuronal membranes relative to the resistance of the cytoplasm contained in the axons and allows action potentials to travel down the axon farther and faster. As such, myelination speeds processing times in the brain and reduces the amount of energy that neurons need to exert to send signals to one another. Myelination essentially supercharges circuits in the brain and allows them to function quicker and more efficiently.

As has been discussed, gray-matter volumes in the frontal lobes increase during childhood, peak early in adolescence, and then decrease as a result of experience-driven molding throughout the adolescent years. Although gray-matter volumes in the frontal lobes follow an inverted U-shaped function, white-matter volumes seem to increase linearly throughout development into young adulthood. In a general sense, myelination progresses in a posterior-to-anterior fashion, with myelination being completed in cortical areas toward the back of the brain before the completion of myelination in the frontal lobes. Increased myelination leads to increased efficacy of the brain circuits formed within the frontal lobes and between the frontal lobes and the structures with which they communicate.

Several studies have suggested that changes in white-matter volumes are associated with cognitive and emotional development during the adolescent years. An MRI-based technique called diffusion tensor imaging allows researchers to use the patterns of movement of water molecules to infer not just the volumes of white matter in various areas of the brain but also the coherence or maturation of myelinated circuits. Several studies have suggested that cognitive abilities improve as myelinated circuits mature. For instance, Nagy et al[15] observed an association between working-memory performance and maturation of fiber tracts connecting the frontal and parietal lobes. The thickness of the corpus callosum, a bundle of myelinated axons traveling between the left and right hemispheres of the brain, increases during adolescence, eventually reaching a larger size in females than in males. Increased thickness here reflects increased myelination of axons in the corpus callosum, which presumably allows the 2 sides of the brain to communicate faster and more efficiently.

The importance of the corpus callosum in organizing behavior is revealed in cases in which the tract is intentionally severed to prevent seizure activity in one side of the brain from spreading to the other side. When the corpus callosum is cut, signals cannot get from one side of the brain to the other. Although most people automatically integrate the activity arising on both sides of the brain into their experiences and behaviors from moment to moment, a person with a severed corpus callosum cannot. In fact, the 2 sides of the brain can actually end up competing with each other for control of the person's actions.

Several recent studies suggested that increases in white-matter volumes in the corpus callosum during adolescence are associated with improvements in cognitive abilities. Using diffusion tensor imaging, Fryer et al[16] observed that, during adolescence, the maturation of white matter in the corpus callosum is associated with improvements in vocabulary and reading abilities, visuospatial skills (such as copying complex line drawings), and psychomotor performance (such as reacting quickly and in a coordinated manner in response to stimuli). This was particularly true with regard to maturation of the splenium, which is located in the posterior portion of the corpus callosum and seems to reach full maturity later in adolescence than other regions of the corpus callosum. This is an exciting new area of research, and future studies should yield useful insight into the role of myelination in the corpus callosum and elsewhere in improved cognitive skills during the adolescent years.

ADOLESCENT BRAIN DEVELOPMENT AND TYPICAL TEENAGE BEHAVIORS

Time-lapse recordings during the adolescent years would capture a true metamorphosis. The second decade of life brings a multitude of changes on psychological, physiologic, and neurologic levels. If life were a white-water rafting trip, adolescence would be the rapids. We enter adolescence as kids who tag along with adults and have our needs met for us. We exit as semiautonomous young adults responsible for meeting most of our own needs and perhaps the needs of our own children. Without the normal upheaval in behavior that adolescence brings, the transition to adult autonomy could not occur.

The changes taking place in the adolescent brain explain many of the behavioral quirks that make adolescence successful as a stage of development. Highly reactive emotional centers imbue adolescents with impulses to explore and take risks while simultaneously providing both a mild paranoia of adults in general and a desire to spend copious amounts of time with their peers. As such, these changes serve as biological wedges that insert themselves between developing adolescents and the adults around them, primarily their immediate caregivers. Development of sex-specific brain structures leads to increased motivation to attract members of the opposite, and sometimes the same, sex and to work hard to gain their attention and acceptance.[17] Although not reviewed in this brief article, these changes serve as a perfect example of the conceptual intersection between puberty (sexual development) and adolescence (psychosocial development). Remodeling of the frontal lobes during the adolescent years leads to a period of short-sightedness and difficulties with impulse control, which allows the strong emotions typical of the adolescent years to usurp control over behavior and get teenagers out of the house and into the world to socialize and learn the rules of the current culture.

All of the aforementioned changes serve valuable purposes and allow adolescence to work as a stage of change. However, the modern world provides a litany of ultimately unhealthy options for rebellious and short-sighted teenagers. In addition, the changes in brain function during adolescence, particularly the shifting of control away from emotional areas to forward cognitive control centers, do not always go as planned. Collectively, the changes of adolescence provide both opportunity and risk, and development sometimes goes awry. Let us explore some of the pitfalls that developing adolescents face.

ADOLESCENT BRAIN DEVELOPMENT AND PSYCHOLOGICAL DISORDERS

During adolescence, the frontal lobes are handed executive control over behavior, and interactions with the outside world allow the adolescent to learn how to use the frontal lobes to regulate emotional expressions and make forward-thinking decisions that trade short-term reinforcement for long-term gains. Unfortunately, this transition of power does not always go according to plan. Problems with this process seem to contribute to the development of a host of psychological disorders, from depression to schizophrenia.[18]

The age range of 15 to 19 is considered a "hazard period" with regard to the development of conditions such as bipolar depression.[12] Adolescent-onset bipolar disorder is associated with a poorer prognosis and more comorbidity. As is the case with most psychiatric conditions, a combination of biology (the first hit) and experience (the second hit) seems to trigger bipolar disorder in developing young people. It is likely that basic wiring maps for the brain handed down through genetics predispose some individuals to such disorders. Maladaptive learning during the maturation of cortical circuits can serve as the catalyst that ultimately leads to the condition.

As an example of the role that learning plays in the development of disorders during adolescence, research has indicated that cognitive styles are associated with the onset of psychopathologies such as depression. Things such as ruminating about problems, making generalized statements about one's self-worth, etc, are common tendencies in those who develop these conditions. Depressive thinking involves the activity of brain circuits. As the brain learns to deal with life and solve problems, the tendencies it acquires affect how the individual interacts with the world, which in turn affects brain function and reinforces those tendencies. Circuits exercised during adolescence have the potential to become part of the default circuits used by the brain for daily functioning during adult life. As such, the acquisition of maladaptive cognitive styles is associated with, and ultimately contributes to, psychopathologies such as depression.

It remains unclear whether problems with brain circuitry come first and give rise to maladaptive cognitive styles and behaviors or if maladaptive cognitive styles and behaviors emerge first as a result of learning and then further contribute to unhealthy molding of the brain. What is clear is that brain pathology is part of these conditions one way or the other. For instance, bipolar depression during adolescence is associated with reduced frontal lobe volumes. Once bipolar adolescents reach adulthood, they perform more poorly than controls on tests of attention and vigilance and show less activation in the prefrontal cortex during the performance of such tasks. They also have trouble with working memory and with shifting attention. Similarly, bipolar adolescents show reduced activation in the prefrontal lobes during performance of the Stroop test, which requires subjects to shift attention away from reading target words and respond on the basis of the color of the words instead.[12]

MEDICATION ISSUES AND THE ADOLESCENT BRAIN

Research suggesting that various medications affect adolescents differently than adults comes as no surprise to most pediatricians. Drugs used for conditions such as depression work by causing often-subtle changes in neurotransmitter levels, including levels of serotonin (5-hydroxytryptamine), dopamine, and norepinephrine. The adolescent brain is a brain in flux and exhibits widespread changes in the levels of all 3 transmitters and their effects on neurons. Behaviorally, adolescents often have rapidly shifting baselines, which can make it difficult to assess whether medications such as those for depression are actually doing their job. For these reasons, antidepressants tend not to work well for teenagers, although they certainly do for some young patients. In their meta-analysis of clinical trials, the US Food and Drug Administration concluded that only 3 of the 15 trials they examined suggested that antidepressants are better than placebo treatment in adolescents.[19]

In cases where they are effective, there is no evidence that use of antidepressants causes long-term complications with brain and psychological development. However, because of brain-related plasticity, one could speculate that teenagers might be more prone to exhibiting the discontinuation syndromes now associated with many antidepressants.

Much has been written in the past few years about the risk of suicide in adolescents who take antidepressants. This issue is worth discussing here, because the implication is that antidepressants affect the adolescent brain in such a way that suicidal thoughts and behaviors could emerge. Do antidepressants increase the risk that a teenager will commit suicide? It does not seem so, but for a variety of reasons, kids on antidepressants are more likely to think about it.

In 2004, a 27-member panel of public representatives, psychiatrists, pediatricians, statisticians, and experts in several other fields concluded that there was no evidence of an increased risk of actual suicides among teenagers treated with antidepressants.[20] However, they did observe compelling evidence of an overall increase in suicidality, a category that includes both suicidal thoughts and suicidal behaviors, among treated teenagers (4% of treated teenagers relative to

2% of untreated teenagers). This finding led the Food and Drug Administration to issue a warning about the potential link between antidepressants and the risk of suicide in teenagers. In the years since, some researchers have challenged the block-box warning and asserted that antidepressants are safer and more effective for adolescents than earlier studies suggested.[21]

Why antidepressants might cause an increase in suicidality in adolescents is unclear. However, it is important to remember that, until adolescent brain development is complete, areas involved in emotional reactivity often hold sway over behavior. It has long been speculated that, early in the course of treatment with antidepressants, there is an activation of cognitive functions before emotional well-being is improved. As such, it would become easier for one to think about the strong emotional impulses attempting to influence behavior. If, at a deep emotional level, one feels that life is not worth living, the augmented cognitive capabilities could be spent thinking about those troubling feelings, particularly early in treatment. The hope is that emotional well-being eventually improves and frees the frontal lobes to think positive thoughts. Until that time, increased suicidality seems to be a real possibility for a small percentage of adolescents treated with antidepressants.

ADOLESCENT BRAIN DEVELOPMENT AND DRUG USE

The adolescent brain is a true learning machine. A vast array of changes occur in the brain during these years. These changes seem to be driven by genes and hormones and modified along the way by experience. As during both childhood and adulthood, the reward system plays a central role in learning during adolescence. When the reward system is activated, the behaviors that lead to its activation are reinforced and are more likely to occur again in the future. Indeed, that seems to be the main purpose of the reward system: to reinforce behaviors that the brain assumes are good for the individual's survival and/or the survival of the species. Eating food, drinking fluids, and engaging in sexual activity are examples. The intensive learning-related changes that occur in the brain during adolescence combined with strong motivation to activate the reward system during this time can easily lead to the development of bad habits that can become stubbornly imbedded in brain circuitry.

Substance use is more likely to begin during adolescence than at any other time, and the odds that such behaviors will lead to problems down the road are higher when they begin during adolescence relative to adulthood. Drugs from nicotine to heroin all act, in part, by activating the reward system and essentially tricking the brain, and the brain's owner, into thinking something important and adaptive just happened. As such, each time an adolescent, or an adult, activates the reward system with drugs, the odds go up that the individual will repeat this behavior in the future. Each time the urge to repeat the rewarded behavior is expressed behaviorally and not prevented by the frontal lobes, the odds go down that the individual will be able to muster the necessary frontal lobe strength to stop the behavior the next time the urge emerges. It is this learning related process that likely culminates in the loss of control that is characteristic of serious drug problems.

Adults with fully functioning frontal lobes are typically capable of keeping themselves from going back to drugs that activate the reward pathway in exchange for pursuing long-term goals. Strong emotional impulses that lead to reinforced behavior combined with still-fragile cognitive control centers makes it easier for adolescents to head down pathways involving substance abuse and other risky activities and to keep coming back for more. Because the brain learns so quickly during adolescence, the odds seem higher that substance abuse will become a lifelong problem if it begins, and is repeated, during the adolescent years. The behaviors can become firmly rooted in brain circuitry and are difficult to override once the window of enhanced malleability closes.

In addition to being at greater risk for developing drug habits through learning, it also seems that several drugs affect the brain differently during the adolescent years than during adulthood, and many of these differences do not bode well for teenagers. For instance, in rats, the reinforcing effects of nicotine are much stronger during early adolescence than during late adolescence or adulthood,[22] a finding that could help explain why most adult smokers actually become dependent on nicotine during adolescence.

Of the drugs known to affect adolescents and adults differently, alcohol is the most well studied. Research with humans has suggested that alcohol abuse during the adolescent years is capable of knocking normal development off track and can lead to lingering cognitive impairments. Brown et al[23] compared 15- to 16-year-old adolescents in an inpatient substance abuse treatment program to controls from the community on a battery of neuropsychological tests. Frequent drinkers ($\geq$100 total drinking sessions), particularly those who had experienced alcohol withdrawal, performed more poorly than controls on several tests, including tests of learning and memory.

In a longitudinal study of subjects, aged 13 to 19, recruited from treatment programs, Tapert and Brown[24] observed that a return to drinking after the program led to further declines in cognitive abilities, particularly in tests of attention, over the next 4 years. Once again, withdrawal from alcohol was a powerful predictor of such impairments. Similarly, Tapert et al[25] assessed neuropsychological functioning and substance use involvement at 7 time points during an 8-year period in subjects beginning, on average, at the age of 16 and ending at 24. Many of the subjects were assessed initially while in treatment and then tracked after their stay in the facility ended. Others were recruited from the community and then followed during the 8-year period. Cumulative levels of substance use, including alcohol use, were correlated with impairments in verbal learning and memory during the final assessment. The findings suggested that heavy use of alcohol and other drugs during the teenage years predicts lower scores on tests of memory and attention when one is in their early to mid-20s and highlights the disruptive effects that substance abuse can have on healthy neuropsychological development during adolescence.

Additional research by Tapert et al explored the brain mechanisms underlying such developmental impairments. In 1 study,[26] alcohol-dependent young women and healthy controls between the ages of 18 and 25 performed tests of working memory and vigilance (attention) while brain oxygen levels were measured by using functional MRI. The sample sizes were not quite big enough to detect significant impairments in working memory, although a clear trend toward such impairments was observed. However, alcohol-dependent subjects exhibited significantly less brain activity while performing the working-memory task. Weaker activity was observed in several parts of the frontal lobes and in the parietal lobes.

A subsequent study with alcohol-dependent young women showed that alcohol-related cues, such as words associated with drinking, elicited craving and led to greater increases in brain activity in a variety of regions relative to controls,[27] thus establishing a link between craving for alcohol and brain function in key areas and yielding further evidence that the brains of alcohol-dependent young women function differently than those of their peers. Given that the adolescent brain is built to learn and that brain plasticity diminishes once the adolescent years end, it seems likely that these strong reactions to alcohol-related cues could stick around for quite some time and increase the risk of relapse down the road.

Additional studies with rats supported the differential effects of alcohol on brain function during adolescence relative to the adult years. For instance, the hippocampus, which is central to the formation of memories for facts and events, is far more sensitive to alcohol in adolescent rats than in adult rats. Less alcohol is required to suppress memory circuits in the adolescent, relative to adult, hippocampus.[28] Exposing rats to high levels of alcohol across a period of several days causes cell death in the hippocampus, frontal lobes, and other brain regions and does so at lower levels in adolescents relative to adults, although the mechanisms underlying such damage remain unclear. In addition, alcohol suppresses the birth of new neurons in the hippocampus and does so with greater ease in adolescent brains.[29] In humans, the hippocampus is smaller in alcohol-abusing adolescents.[30] Whether this is a result of the suppression of cell birth, the death of existing cells, both, or an alternative cause is unclear.

The particularly negative effects of alcohol on hippocampal function in adolescent brains could help explain why memory blackouts, amnesia for events that take place while one is drinking, are so common during the adolescent years. Research by White and Swartzwelder[31] suggested that ~50% of college students have experienced at least 1 blackout. A survey of >5000 recent high school graduates during the summer before they started college revealed that more than half consumed alcohol in the 2 weeks before the survey, and of those who drank, 12% of males and females experienced at least 1 memory blackout during that 2-week period.[32]

Other structures seem to suffer from the negative effects of alcohol on adolescent brain development, as well. For instance, alcohol abuse during adolescence is associated with reduced sizes of both the amygdala and the corpus callosum. It also seems that alcohol interferes with the maturation of white-matter tracts in the frontal lobes, perhaps by suppressing the activity of genes associated with the creation of the myelin sheath.[30] Research with rats has suggested that glial cell functioning affected by alcohol during adolescence only partially recovers with prolonged abstinence.[33]

The ease with which the adolescent brain learns seems to apply to learning about alcohol at a neurochemical level, not just at a social and behavioral level. It has long been known that the earlier an adolescent is exposed to alcohol, the greater his or her odds of becoming dependent on the drug down the road. It seems that the rapid learning made possible by heightened brain plasticity during the adolescent years can work against healthy development when it applies to drinking alcohol and, perhaps, using other substances.[34] For instance, the initial development of tolerance to alcohol, a process that involves learning at a neurochemical level, is faster during adolescence than adulthood, and such tolerance remains evident for a much longer period of time in adolescent subjects compared with adults.[35]

The good news is that the enhanced brain plasticity of adolescence seems to lend itself to recovery and not just to the development of the initial problem. Research indicates that adolescent substance abuse treatment works, particularly when adolescents are motivated to improve.[36]

KEEPING ADOLESCENT BRAIN DEVELOPMENT ON TRACK

The changes that occur in the adolescent brain seem to unfold as part of the larger, gene-encoded, hormone-aided developmental plan. However, the outcomes of these changes are strongly influenced by interactions between the individual and the outside world. Strong emotional impulses help propel kids out of their basements and into the world. How the individual regulates these strong emotional impulses is influenced by learning. Some learn to exercise effective restraint over their urges, whereas others learn to do what they feel like doing when they feel like doing it.

At any stage of development, individuals are motivated to meet particular psychological needs. The needs of adolescents are similar in many ways to those of children and adults, with accentuated needs to push away from family members, explore the world, take risks, maintain privacy, and spend increasing amounts of time with their peers. Similar to children and adults, adolescents need to feel safe and secure, feel loved and accepted by those around them, and have a sense of purpose and meaning in life. These needs exist against the backdrop of rampant hormonal changes and physical development, as well as the neurologic metamorphosis explored above. When adolescents have outlets for their deep emotional urges to explore, take chances, and socialize, the odds increase that they will make it through the teenage years unscathed. Adolescents, and their parents, should be encouraged to explore healthy outlets for these urges, lest they translate into unhealthy behaviors aimed at satisfying them, such as substance abuse, risky sexual practices, aggression, bullying, and so on. Quite simply, when teenagers are busy doing activities that make them feel validated and independent, they are less likely to engage in unhealthy, misguided behaviors. Extracurricular activities such as sports, music, drama, and volunteer work are all good ideas for keeping adolescents busy and helping to guide their development in healthy directions. When healthy behaviors are modeled by the adults in a home, adolescents are more likely to develop healthy habits without the need for special interventions. Parents should be encouraged to explore options for engaging their adolescents in extracurricular activities and to ensure that the behaviors they model are healthy.

It is paramount that adolescents learn to recognize and regulate their emotional impulses. By the end of the teenage years, the frontal lobes will be firmly in the driver's seat and should be capable of providing the right balance of gas and brakes. Until that time, any activities that help teenagers learn to take responsibility for, and hopefully pride in, their actions will be useful in keeping frontal lobe development on a healthy course. Similarly, activities that teach teenagers to delay gratification, such as saving money for a desired purchase, can serve as useful exercises for the frontal lobes and useful training for adult life in general. Educating parents about the changes taking place in their adolescents' bodies and brains can help diffuse the tension that normally exists in such households and, hopefully, increase their patience with the often-unfamiliar teenagers living in their homes.

CONCLUSIONS

As we enter the second decade of life, begin to test drive adult behaviors, and inch our way toward autonomy, our bodies, including our brains, enter a very unique and tumultuous period of flux that culminates in physical maturation and the development of neurologic circuits capable of governing responsible adult behaviors. The changes that take place in the brain during adolescence shift behavioral control away from emotional regions (amygdala, nucleus accumbens, cingulate) to cognitive control centers (the frontal lobes). These changes culminate in improved abilities to regulate emotional impulses and make rational, forward-thinking decisions.

In the years that lead up to adolescence, an overabundance of synapses are created in the frontal lobes and between neurons in the frontal lobes and the brains structures with which they communicate. Early in the second decade of life, the brain simultaneously begins to shift control over behavior toward the frontal lobes and places synapses formed by frontal lobe neurons and neurons in other brain regions on the chopping block. This kind of malleability allows each successive wave of adolescents to adapt to a unique and increasingly complex world.

Once we leave adolescence and enter adulthood, the malleability of the brain decreases, and it becomes increasingly difficult to make changes. Although it is certainly possible to teach an old dog new tricks, it is much easier to learn new tricks when we are young. The good news, although sometimes bad news, is that the way the teenaged brain is molded depends in large part on the environments in which teenagers grow. By constructing healthy environments, the potential inherent in the changing adolescent brain can be harnessed, and the odds that a given adolescent will make it into young adulthood cognitively and emotionally prepared for the rigors of adult life can be maximized.

REFERENCES

1. Giedd J. Structural magnetic resonance imaging of the adolescent brain. *Ann N Y Acad Sci.* 2004;1021:77–85
2. Ernst M, Mueller SC. The adolescent brain: insights from functional neuroimaging research. *Dev Neurobiol.* 2008;68(6):729–743
3. Chugani H. Biological basis of emotions: brain systems and brain development. *Pediatrics.* 1998;102(5 suppl E):1225–1229
4. Schweinsburg AD, Nagel BJ, Tapert SF. fMRI reveals alteration of spatial working memory networks across adolescence. *J Int Neuropsychol Soc.* 2005;11(5):631–644
5. Rubia K, Overmeyer S, Taylor E, et al. Functional frontalisation with age: mapping neurodevelopmental trajectories with fMRI. *Neurosci Biobehav Rev.* 2000;24(1):13–19
6. Marsh R, Zhu H, Schultz RT, et al. A developmental fMRI study of self-regulatory control. *Hum Brain Mapp.* 2006;27(11):848–863
7. Rubia K, Smith AB, Taylor E, Brammer M. Linear age-correlated functional development of right inferior fronto-striato-cerebellar networks during response inhibition and anterior during error-related processes. *Hum Brain Mapp.* 2007;28(11):1163–1177
8. Shaw P, Greenstein D, Lerch J, et al. Intellectual ability and cortical development in children and adolescents. *Nature.* 2006;440(7084):676–679
9. Lenroot RK, Schmitt JE, Ordaz SJ, et al. Differences in genetic and environmental influences on the human cerebral cortex associated with development during childhood and adolescence. *Hum Brain Mapp.* 2009;30(1):163–174
10. Casey BJ, Jones RM, Hare TA. The adolescent brain. *Ann N Y Acad Sci.* 2008;1124:111–126
11. Eaton DK, Kann L, Kinchen S, et al. Youth risk behavior surveillance: United States, 2005. *J Sch Health.* 2006;76(7):353–372
12. Alloy LB, Abramson LY, Walshaw PD, Keyser J, Gerstein RK. A cognitive vulnerability-stress perspective on bipolar spectrum disorders in a normative adolescent brain, cognitive, and emotional development context. *Dev Psychopathol.* 2006;18(4):1055–1103
13. Coplan JD, Moreau D, Chaput F, et al. Salivary cortisol concentrations before and after carbon-dioxide inhalations in children. *Biol Psychiatry.* 2002;51(4):326–333
14. Walker EF, Sabuwalla Z, Huot R. Pubertal neuromaturation, stress sensitivity, and psychopathology. *Dev Psychopathol.* 2004;16(4):807–824
15. Nagy Z, Westerberg H, Klingberg T. Maturation of white matter is associated with the development of cognitive functions during childhood. *J Cogn Neurosci.* 2004;16(7):1227–1233

16. Fryer SL, Frank LR, Spadoni AD, et al. Microstructural integrity of the corpus callosum linked with neuropsychological performance in adolescents. *Brain Cogn*. 2008;67(2):225-233
17. Nelson EE, Leibenluft E, McClure EB, Pine DS. The social re-orientation of adolescence: a neuroscience perspective on the process and its relation to psychopathology. *Psychol Med*. 2005;35(2):163-174
18. Spessot AL, Plessen KJ, Peterson BS. Neuroimaging of developmental psychopathologies: the importance of self-regulatory and neuroplastic processes in adolescence. *Ann N Y Acad Sci*. 2004;1021:86-104
19. Newman TB. A black-box warning for antidepressants in children? *N Engl J Med*. 2004;351(16):1595-1598
20. Lock J, Walker LR, Rickert VI, Katzman DK; Society for Adolescent Medicine. Suicidality in adolescents being treated with antidepressant medications and the black box label. *J Adolesc Health*. 2005;36(1):92-93
21. Bridge JA, Iyengar S, Salary CB, et al. Clinical response and risk for reported suicidal ideation and suicide attempts in pediatric antidepressant treatment: a meta-analysis of randomized controlled trials. *JAMA*. 2007;297(15):1683-1696
22. Belluzzi JD, Lee AG, Oliff HS, Leslie FM. Age-dependent effects of nicotine on locomotor activity and conditioned place preference in rats. *Psychopharmacology*. 2004;174(3):389-396
23. Brown AS, Tapert SF, Granholm E, Delis DC. Neurocognitive functioning of adolescents: effects of protracted alcohol use. *Alcohol Clin Exp Res*. 2000;24(2):164-171
24. Tapert SF, Brown SA. Neuropsychological correlates of adolescent substance abuse: four-year outcomes. *J Int Neuropsychol Soc*. 1999;5(6):481-493
25. Tapert SF, Granholm E, Leedy NG, Brown SA. Substance use and withdrawal: neuropsychological functioning over 8 years in youth. *J Int Neuropsychol Soc*. 2002;8(7):873-883
26. Tapert SF, Brown GG, Kindermann SS, Cheung EH, Frank LR, Brown SA. fMRI measurement of brain dysfunction in alcohol-dependent young women. *Alcohol Clin Exp Res*. 2001;25(2):236-245
27. Tapert SF, Brown GG, Baratta MV, Brown SA. fMRI BOLD response to alcohol stimuli in alcohol dependent young women. *Addict Behav*. 2004;29(1):33-50
28. White AM, Swartzwelder HS. Hippocampal function during adolescence: a unique target of ethanol effects. *Ann N York Acad Sci*. 2004;1021:206-220
29. Monti PM, Miranda R, Nixon K, et al. Adolescence: booze, brains, and behavior. *Alcohol Clin Exp Res*. 2005;29(2):207-220
30. Clark DB, Thatcher DL, Tapert SF. Alcohol, psychological dysregulation, and adolescent brain development. *Alcohol Clin Exp Res*. 2008;32(3):375-385
31. White AM. What happened? Alcohol, memory blackouts, and the brain. *Alcohol Res Health*. 2003;27(2):186-196
32. White AM, Swartzwelder HS. College bound students drink heavily during the summer before their freshman year. *Am J Health Educ*. 2009; In press
33. Evrard SG, Duhalde-Vega M, Tagliaferro P, Mirochnic S, Caltana LR, Brusco A. A low chronic ethanol exposure induces morphological changes in the adolescent rat brain that are not fully recovered even after a long abstinence: an immunohistochemical study. *Exp Neurol*. 2006;200(2):438-459
34. Carpenter-Hyland EP, Chandler LJ. Adaptive plasticity of NMDA receptors and dendritic spines: implications for enhanced vulnerability of the adolescent brain to alcohol addiction. *Pharmacol Biochem Behav*. 2007;86(2):200-208
35. White AM, Bae JG, Truesdale MC, Ahmad S, Wilson WA, Swartzwelder HS. Chronic-intermittent ethanol exposure during adolescence prevents normal developmental changes in sensitivity to ethanol-induced motor impairments. *Alcohol Clin Exp Res*. 2002;26(7):960-968
36. White AM, Jordan JD, Schroeder KM, Acheson S, Hanusa B, Swartzwelder HS. Predictors of relapse and treatment completion among marijuana-dependent adolescents in an intensive outpatient substance abuse program. *Subst Abus*. 2004;25(1):53-59

An Approach to Obesity Management in Primary Care: Yes, We Can Make a Difference

Kathy Love-Osborne, MD*

Department of Pediatrics, Section of Adolescent Medicine, Denver Health and Hospitals, University of Colorado Denver Health Sciences Center, 501 28th Street, Denver, CO 80220, USA

Childhood and adolescent obesity is associated with multiple medical problems including type 2 diabetes mellitus (T2DM), future cardiovascular disease, dyslipidemia, hypertension, obstructive sleep apnea (OSA), and nonalcoholic fatty liver disease (NAFLD). It has also been associated with poor school performance and attendance.[1] The definition of obesity is BMI at >95th percentile for age and gender. Overweight is defined as a BMI between the 85th and 95th percentiles. The incidence of T2DM in children and adolescents has increased dramatically over the last 2 decades in the United States.[2] Now recognized in the pediatric population worldwide,[3] T2DM is likely to be a major global public health problem in the coming decades. Vascular complications resulting from diabetes, such as retinopathy, nephropathy, and heart disease, are clearly related to the duration of diabetes and the severity of hyperglycemia. Recent studies have indicated that the time to occurrence of complications is as fast or faster in adolescents compared with adults with T2DM.[4] Thus, it can be anticipated that adolescents who develop T2DM will develop symptomatic vascular complications in early adulthood. Furthermore, it can be expected that the increasing number of children and youth diagnosed with T2DM will dramatically add to the economic burden of this disease over the upcoming decades. The long-term complications and costs associated with T2DM make preventing or delaying the onset in obese adolescents imperative.

The prevalence of impaired glucose tolerance (IGT) (2-hour glucose level >140 mg/dL) in adolescents is relatively low. A large study of 1740 middle school students, 49% of whom had a BMI at >85th percentile, showed only 2% to have IGT.[5] On the other hand, the progression rate from IGT to diabetes in adolescents is high, reported in 1 study to be 24% over 2 years.[6] Thus, it is critical to screen obese adolescents regularly for the development of IGT or overt diabetes. In adults, prevention of weight gain is associated with decreased likelihood of

---
*Corresponding author.
E-mail address: kathryn.love-osborne@dhha.org (K. Love-Osborne).

Copyright © 2009 American Academy of Pediatrics. All rights reserved. ISSN 1934-4287

developing T2DM. The rate of progression from IGT to T2DM in adults depends on change in weight over time, with reversal of IGT to normal glucose tolerance (NGT) predicted by the ability to avoid weight gain with aging. In a study of first-degree relatives of patients with T2DM, subjects who developed T2DM 5 to 8 years later gained 5 to 10 kg, whereas subjects with continued NGT maintained or lost weight. Thus, a modest goal of arresting weight gain in adolescence may substantially lower the risk of progression to T2DM in adulthood.[7]

The presence of fatty liver as determined by ultrasound and abnormal liver-associated enzyme levels was measured in a study of 50 obese adolescents with elevated fasting insulin levels. The prevalence of fatty liver was 74% and of elevated alanine aminotransferase (ALT) levels was 14%. Fatty liver was more common in male and Hispanic subjects, and elevated ALT levels were more common in Hispanic subjects. Subjects with fatty liver seemed more insulin resistant (higher fasting insulin and triglyceride levels, lower high-density lipoprotein cholesterol levels) and had higher ALT levels.[8]

Treatment of adolescent obesity is difficult, with many well-intentioned interventions showing at best the modest result of weight maintenance. Most effective treatment programs have been conducted in academic centers through an interdisciplinary approach.[9] The US Preventive Services Task Force's statement on screening and intervention for overweight in children and adolescents revealed insufficient evidence for the effectiveness of family-based or individual approaches that can be conducted in primary care settings with overweight children.[10]

A 2007 report from the Childhood Obesity Action Network Expert Committee on the Assessment, Prevention, and Treatment of Childhood Overweight and Obesity showed equivocal results.[11] Although consistent evidence exists regarding prevention of obesity, there is little evidence regarding efficacy of interventions aimed at treating adolescents who are already obese. Only involving the family in lifestyle changes and decreasing screen time have been consistently shown to improve obesity. Interventions that have shown mixed efficacy include increasing the intake of fruits and vegetables, minimizing sugar-sweetened beverage intake, increasing physical activity to 1 hour/day or more, increasing family meals, and eating breakfast.

Many providers may feel a sense of frustration when reading reports such as the one by the expert committee; however, a closer look at the literature provides some hope for strategies that may be effective in at least slowing weight gain.

SCHOOL-BASED INTERVENTIONS

Most school-based obesity interventions are preventive in nature and implemented in all students, not just those with obesity.[12,13] One study of 1140 middle school students showed improvement in blood pressure (BP) and less increase in skinfold measurements (but not BMI) with an exercise intervention compared with the control and education-only groups.[14] A study of 50 obese middle school children (mean age: 12 years old) evaluated a lifestyle-focused, fitness-oriented gym class and showed a decrease in body fat and increase in cardiovascular fitness along with improvement in fasting insulin levels.[15] School-based health centers (SBHCs) provide a potential setting for obesity interventions with greater ease of access to students than in the traditional office-based setting.[16] Some projects have been implemented in SBHCs but have not been scientifically evaluated. One SBHC implemented a "junk-free zone" that prohibited chips, soda, and candy in the clinic and offered a weekly cooking lesson for families for 6 weeks.[16,17]

GOAL SETTING

Although goal-setting techniques have not been studied extensively in adolescents, they are effective tools for promoting behavior change in adults.[17] The literature suggests that goals should be proximal (short-term), specific, and difficult yet attainable to result in higher success rates. Guided goal setting has been proposed as most appropriate for adolescents, with the practitioner designing multiple goal choices and the participant choosing 1 goal.[18]

INTENSIVE BOARDING SCHOOL INTERVENTIONS

These types of interventions are expensive and not available to most patients. However, studies in this area have provided insight into predictors of successful maintenance of weight loss, and some of these strategies may lend themselves to being incorporated into a primary care setting. One long-term study evaluated children 1½ years after a 10-month intervention. The intervention included a low-calorie diet, structured physical activity, and psychological support. The subjects successfully lost weight at 10 months; at 1½ years they regained weight but were still significantly leaner that at the beginning of the intervention. The study assessed eating and exercise behavior after the intervention was complete. Those with healthy eating and exercise behavior at follow-up were 138% overweight, whereas those with unhealthy eating and exercise were 183% overweight (more than baseline). The study found that either healthy eating with unhealthy exercise or unhealthy eating with healthy exercise patterns were associated with similar rates of overweight (150% vs 156%).[19] Another study showed behavior changes in the follow-up period including increase in fat and sucrose intake, smaller percentage of calories consumed at breakfast, more snacking, decreased activity, and increased television viewing.[20]

INTERNET/COMPUTER INTERVENTIONS

Because most adolescents are computer savvy, the Internet is a potentially powerful tool for delivering interventions for obesity. One study used an Internet intervention in middle school students with computer-generated, tailored feedback based on stage of change (ie, whether students were precontemplative, contemplative, or actually prepared for change) for physical activity and dietary fat intake. Intervention students that completed at least half of 8 sessions delivered over 1 month (some with activity feedback and others with dietary feedback) increased moderate/vigorous exercise by 22 minutes/week. No long-term follow-up was performed to assess maintenance of this behavior change.[21] A study conducted in primary care settings used computerized assessments in the waiting room for 875 adolescents coming for a well-care visit in which subjects selected 1 nutritional and 1 physical activity goal. During their visit, providers endorsed the goals. Additional interventions included follow-up by telephone and mail. The authors reported improvement in some areas: reduced sedentary behavior, more active days per week (boys), and less consumption of saturated fat (girls). Unfortunately, no change in BMI was reported for the 46% of subjects who were overweight or obese at baseline.[22]

GLYCEMIC INDEX

In many countries, low-glycemic-index diets are very popular. Low-glycemic-index carbohydrates (eg, oatmeal) do not raise blood glucose as much as high-glycemic-index foods (such as white bread). There are limited data for obese adolescents to support the use of this approach, although results have been promising. A small study of 16 obese adolescents randomly assigned the subjects to an ad-lib low-glycemic-index diet versus a calorie-restricted low-fat diet. The low-glycemic-index group had a BMI change of -1.3 kg/m^2 compared with an increase of 0.7 kg/m^2 in the low-fat-diet group. Most interestingly, although subjects in the low-fat-diet group maintained their weight during the 6-month intervention, they gained weight over the 6-month follow-up period. In contrast, the low-glycemic-index group lost weight over the intervention and maintained that weight over the 6-month follow-up period. This implies that teenagers were able to continue the diet without intensive support and that they maintained weight loss, a rarity in obesity studies.[23]

WHAT ABOUT MEDICATIONS?

Several medications have been studied specifically for weight loss in adolescents.

Orlistat

Orlistat works by blocking the uptake of approximately one third of ingested fat and is marketed over-the-counter in the United States as "Alli." A multicenter 54-week study randomly assigned 539 obese adolescents to orlistat 120 mg or placebo 3 times per day. Subjects also were prescribed a mildly hypocaloric diet, exercise, and behavioral therapy. Both groups lost weight in the first 12 weeks, and by the end of 1 year BMI had decreased by 0.55 kg/m^2 with orlistat and increased by 0.31 with placebo. Among those taking the active drug, 26.5% had at least a 5% decrease in BMI, and 13% had at least a 10% decrease in BMI. The behavioral intervention was relatively intense, with visits every 2 weeks for 4 months and then monthly for the remainder of the study. Adverse gastrointestinal effects were common but led to discontinuation of the study for only 2% of the subjects. A weight loss of >5% after 12 weeks of orlistat was associated with a mean decrease in BMI of 3.7 kg/m^2 at 1 year.[24] A smaller study of orlistat followed 42 patients (mean age: 12 years old) for 5 to 15 months (average: 1 year). The orlistat group lost a mean of 6.3 kg compared with 4.2 kg gain in controls. Subjects were prescribed 20% reduction in calories and 30 minutes of exercise per day. Seven of 22 orlistat subjects dropped out in the first month because of adverse effects. The most common adverse effects (oily stools, fecal incontinence) are generally not serious and may be minimized by not taking the medication if a fatty meal is consumed, which may also lead to lower efficacy. Subjects were seen monthly by a dietician.[25]

On the basis of these studies, orlistat seems to have some efficacy, especially if patients respond in the first 3 months. Adverse gastrointestinal effects may be prohibitive; more subjects dropped out because of adverse effects in the study with less-intensive support. Orlistat is taken 3 times per day with meals, which makes it difficult for the average teenager to remain adherent. Cost of the medication, typically more than $50 for a 1-month supply, may be prohibitive to many adolescents.

Sibutramine

Sibutramine works by inhibiting reuptake of serotonin and norepinephrine and is contraindicated in patients with eating disorders. A large multicenter trial of 498 adolescents used behavior therapy plus sibutramine 10 mg or placebo (3:1)[26] for 1 year. The sibutramine dose was increased to 15 mg at 6 months if initial BMI was not reduced by 10%. At the outset of the study, mean BMI was 36 kg/m^2, and mean age was 13.7 years. BMI decreased by a mean of 3.1 kg/m^2 in the sibutramine group compared with 0.3 kg/m^2 in the placebo group. At 1 year, BMI reduction of 5% was attained by 70% of sibutramine-treated subjects, and 46% attained a 10% reduction. Tachycardia occurred in 13% of the treated subjects (versus 6% in placebo subjects). Hypertension was slightly more common in subjects taking sibutramine than in those taking placebo (11% vs 8%).

Another study randomly assigned 60 obese adolescents (BMI: 30–45 kg/m^2) to placebo or sibutramine 10 mg for 6 months. Subjects had a 4-week placebo run-in period and were counseled to decrease their intake by 500 cal/day (2092 J/day) and to exercise 30 minutes/day. The sibutramine group lost a mean of 10.3 kg (versus 2.4 kg in the placebo group). BMI decreased by a mean of 3.6 kg/m^2 in the sibutramine group and 0.9 in the placebo group. Among the sibutramine-treated subjects, 73% reduced BMI by 5%, 47% by 10%, and 23% by 15%. This study did not show clinically significant increases in pulse or BP.[27]

On the basis of these studies, sibutramine seems to be effective, but concerns include increase in BP and/or pulse.

Metformin

Metformin, a biguanide antihyperglycemic agent, has been used extensively in the treatment of T2DM in adults. Whether metformin may be effective in treatment of obesity in adolescents has been less clearly demonstrated. In general, studies to date that explored the use of metformin in obese adolescents without T2DM have been small (<100 subjects). Many of these studies have not included lifestyle modification and used short treatment duration (in the range of 8 weeks to 6 months). In a study of 15 adolescents with polycystic ovarian syndrome (PCOS) and IGT, the use of metformin without significant lifestyle intervention for 3 months resulted in improvement in glucose tolerance (with 8 reverting to NGT) and a mean decrease in BMI of 1.4 kg/m^2.[28] A study of 45 children and adolescents with obesity used metformin without lifestyle intervention for 6 to 16 months. Metformin was found to be more effective in producing weight loss in white girls and in those subjects with more severe insulin resistance at baseline without insulin hypersecretion.[29] Another study examined the use of metformin in conjunction with personal goal setting in a 6-month study of 85 insulin-resistant obese (mean BMI: 40 kg/m^2) adolescents (mean age: 15.7 years).[30] Of the metformin-treated subjects, 23% had a BMI decrease of ≥5%. Subjects who were adherent with metformin decreased BMI to the greatest extent (mean loss: 0.32 kg/m^2), although even subjects with lower adherence to metformin gained less weight than adherent subjects on placebo. Girls were twice as likely as boys to decrease their BMI by ≥5%. Among female subjects with good metformin adherence, only 10% gained weight, whereas 50% of male subjects with good metformin adherence gained weight. Subject report of decrease in portion size was associated with weight loss.

CONCLUSIONS FROM THE LITERATURE

1. Both exercise and a healthy diet are important for maintenance of weight loss.
2. Low-glycemic-index diets have shown promise in adolescents.
3. Behaviors such as increasing the percentage of calories eaten at breakfast, less snacking, eating less sugar and less fat, increasing activity, and decreasing television/computer/video game time are associated with maintenance of weight loss.
4. Medications have shown promise but are still experimental.

Table 1
Age and gender-based BMI cut-offs (kg/m^2)

Age, y	Male >85%	Female >85%	Male >95%	Female >95%
13	21.8	22.6	25.2	26.2
14	22.6	23.4	26.0	27.2
15	23.4	24.0	26.8	28.0
16	24.2	24.6	27.6	28.8
17	24.9	25.0	28.2	29.6

Data from CDC growth curves.

WHAT SHOULD WE DO IN THE CLINICAL SETTING?

Our main goals of obesity tracking and management in primary care are to:

- identify the problem of overweight or obesity;
- assess patient motivation for change;
- identify comorbidities of obesity;
- use every visit as an opportunity to make a brief intervention;
- tailor intervention frequency to the motivation level of the patient; and
- promote weight loss or, at least, stabilization of weight gain.

Identify Obesity or Overweight as a Problem

This should be done at every visit, whether for immunizations, acute illness, or routine health care. A common issue in office-based treatment of obesity is low rates of follow-up over time. Thus, addressing the problem at every visit provides more opportunities for motivating patients to change their lifestyle.

Record BMI

If height is routinely measured in your practice setting, BMI is ideal for tracking obesity. Especially in adolescent boys, height may change significantly over time, so following weight alone may underestimate a patient's progress. In adolescent girls who are postmenarcheal, height is less likely to change dramatically over several months. In some settings, BMI curves may not be readily available. Tables 1 and 2 may be used to estimate whether a patient falls into the overweight or obese category.

A BMI of >25 kg/m^2 is always considered to be >85th percentile, because it merges with the adult definition of overweight. In patients with a BMI between the 85th and 95th percentiles, it may be helpful to measure a waist circumference (Table 2); if it is normal (most commonly seen in athletes), the student is probably not overweight (and should not be labeled as such) but is just muscular. Consider checking the waist circumference in a patient with a BMI at >85th

Table 2
Ninetieth percentile for waist circumference according to age and demographic (in cm)[33]

Age, y	Black Boys	Black Girls	Hispanic Boys	Hispanic Girls	White Boys	White Girls
8	69	72	74	73	71	70
9	73	76	78	76	74	73
10	76	80	81	79	78	76
11	79	83	85	82	81	78
12	82	87	88	85	85	81
13	85	91	92	89	88	84
14	89	94	95	92	91	87
15	92	98	98	95	95	90
16	95	102	102	98	98	93
17	98	105	105	101	102	96
18	101	109	109	104	105	98

percentile who seems to be very muscular or to have little abdominal obesity on physical examination. Although the data in pediatric patients are not conclusive, elevated waist circumference in overweight (but not obese) women has been associated with increased risk of cardiac disease.[31] Waist-circumference measurement is less commonly useful in patients with a BMI at >95th percentile, because most will be have a BMI at >90th percentile. A BMI of >30 kg/m^2 is always considered obese, because this merges with the adult definition of obesity.[32]

How to Approach Adolescents Regarding Obesity

Many providers avoid bringing up a patient's obesity for fear of alienating patients or families. Most providers still prefer to avoid the term "obese" when speaking with patients. Motivational interviewing techniques can be helpful when working with obese teens.[33] Possible approaches include:

- "Tell me how you feel about your weight."
- "Are you doing anything to work on losing weight?"
- "Are you interested in help with losing weight?"

Keep in mind the patient's readiness for change. If patients are not ready to make changes, it is generally not helpful to spend significant time talking about lifestyle changes. However, it is appropriate to let patients know that you are concerned about the medical complications of obesity: "Being overweight for your height means you may be at higher risk for medical problems such as diabetes, heart disease, or liver problems; I would like to check your blood to make sure everything is okay."

Remember to offer support and keep the door open for future visits: "I understand that you aren't ready to work on your weight right now, but if you want help in the future, feel free to set up an appointment."

Check the Records

One of the most important pieces of information to have when approaching a patient with obesity is the patient's most recent weight. The approach to a patient is very different if he or she has lost 2 lb since the last visit or gained 10 lb.

Personal Goal Setting

Make an effort to try to start with 2 simple goals even if the visit is for shots or an acute illness. This can be done in as little as a few minutes; for patients who are very motivated or have many questions, they can come back for a separate visit, but always try to briefly address obesity at every visit. Goals should be very concrete: 1 related to exercise and 1 to nutrition.

Exercise

Walking does not result in weight loss for most adolescents. Most need moderate-to-vigorous exercise and need to work up a sweat. If they are very sedentary, walking can be a first step. For girls, dancing (which can be done at home and does not require going to a club) may be an option. Initially, aim for 150 minutes/week. Ask the patient whether he or she thinks it would be easier to exercise for 30 minutes 5 times per week or 45 minutes to 1 hour 3 times per week. Remember that if patients are doing no exercise at all, setting a goal of even 15 to 20 minutes of walking twice per week is an improvement. Weight lifting also helps build muscle (which increases metabolism) and should be encouraged if teens are interested. The long-term goal advised by the American Academy of Pediatrics is 60 minutes of moderate-to-vigorous exercise daily.

Nutrition

Rather than asking teenagers what they want to work on, help guide them toward evidence-based goals that may lead to weight loss (Table 3). An easy first target is limiting sugary drinks including soda, juices, fruit-flavored beverages, sports drinks, sweetened teas, and coffees. Complete elimination may seem too lofty of a goal; reduction to 1 serving per day may be more attainable.

Write the goals down in your assessment and plan. Help patients understand a reasonable weight loss goal: ½ lb/week, or 2 lb in 1 month. Make sure patients understand that this will lead to 24 lb of weight loss in 1 year. Adolescents often have unrealistic expectations and want to lose 20 lb in a few weeks. Schedule a follow-up visit in 1 month (with fasting laboratory tests if indicated).

Future Visits With a More Specific Obesity Focus

- Consider using patient and family questionnaires that screen for comorbidities such as OSA as well as other disorders related to obesity.

Table 3
Types of nutrition goals

Type of Goal	Sample Goals
Smaller portions	I will eat 3 tortillas instead of 5 at dinner
Fewer second helpings	I will only have seconds once a week
Fewer sugared beverages	I will only drink soda once per day
Less fast food	I will only go out for fast food twice per week
	I will get a small burger rather than a quarter-pounder
	I will choose fries or soda but not both
Fewer "junk-food" snacks	I will only have chips or candy twice per week
No skipped meals	I will eat breakfast 5 d/wk

- Measure weight and let the patient know how he or she is doing. Reinforce that most teenagers gain weight on an ongoing basis, and provide positive feedback for those who maintain or lose even just a small amount of weight.
- Follow-up on previous goals, and set new goals for the next month. Check in on how the goals are going and modify them if they seem too unrealistic.

Tier 1 Laboratory Screening

The American Academy of Pediatrics Task Force on Obesity has recommended screening obese children and adolescents beginning at age 10 for comorbidities of obesity including diabetes, dyslipidemia, and NAFLD.

Who? Patients with a BMI at >85th percentile starting at the age of 10 (or pubertal). How Often? Every 2 years is the standard recommendation. Consider annual screening of:

- patients with previous abnormal laboratory test results; and/or
- patients who have gained a significant amount of weight (≥10 lb) in the year since their laboratory tests were performed.

What? Tests to order depend on the practice setting, volume of obese patients in the practice, and the likelihood that the patient can (or will) return for fasting laboratory tests. It is reasonable to start with basic screening (Table 4). For patients who have not returned as recommended on previous visits, random laboratory testing may be necessary.

Tier 2 Laboratory Screening

With most abnormalities identified on initial screening, it is reasonable to work with patients on lifestyle modification before repeat laboratory testing in 2 to 3

Table 4
Tier 1 strategies for laboratory screening of obese adolescents

Option 1	Option 2	Option 3
Cost-effective (basic)	More thorough	Last resort (basic)
Fasting lipid panel	Fasting lipid panel	Random cholesterol
Fasting glucose	Fasting glucose	Random glucose
ALT	Fasting insulin	ALT
	Liver function panel	
	Thyrotropin	

months. This gives patients an opportunity to improve their test results and, thus, reinforce positive behavior change. Exceptions include evidence of overt diabetes or significant elevation of ALT levels in excess of 3 times the upper limit of normal, which requires identification of possible etiologies for liver dysfunction other than NAFLD. Patients with abnormal glucose values or evidence for metabolic syndrome should have more formal testing for abnormal glucose regulation (Table 5).[34] If the oral glucose tolerance test (OGTT) results are normal, glycosylated hemoglobin (HbA1c) can be used in the future in conjunction with a fasting or random glucose test to track patients. If the HbA1c level remains stable, a repeat OGTT may not be necessary.

Metabolic syndrome in adolescents is defined as ≥3 of the following:[35]

1. Elevated BP for age/gender/height[36]
2. BMI at >95th percentile or waist circumference at >90th percentile
3. Fasting triglyceride level of >110 mg/dL
4. High-density lipoprotein cholesterol level of <40 mg/dL
5. Impaired fasting glucose, IGT, or diabetes (diabetes mellitus is defined by a random or 2-hour glucose level of >200 mg/dL or a fasting glucose level of >126 mg/dL [abnormal glucose results need to be confirmed]; IGT is defined as a 2-hour glucose level of 140–199 mg/dL; and impaired fasting glucose is defined as a fasting glucose level of 100–125 mg/dL).

Table 5
TIER 2 laboratory screening for abnormal glucose regulation

Indications	Tests
Fasting glucose >100 mg/dL	OGTT (fasting glucose, 75 g of glucose, followed by 2-h glucose)
Random glucose >140 mg/dL	
Metabolic syndrome	Fasting lipid panel (if not performed previously)
	Liver function panel (if not performed previously); consider HbA1c (for tracking purposes)

Nonalcoholic Fatty Liver Disease

NAFLD is more common in obese male adolescents, especially Latinos. It can (rarely) progress to cirrhosis and liver failure. The most common abnormal laboratory value is the ALT, which is typically 1½ to 3 times the upper limit of normal. Patients with a screening ALT level of 1½ to 3 times the upper limit of normal should be instructed on lifestyle modification to encourage weight loss, with a complete liver function panel test repeated 3 months later. Additional evaluation should be considered for persistence of an ALT level of more than twice the upper limit of normal 3 months after instruction on lifestyle change or for patients with an ALT level of >4 times the upper limit of normal at any time. Additional testing includes those for hepatitis B (surface antigen and antibody), hepatitis C antibody, ceruloplasmin (elevated in Wilson disease), α-1-antitrypsin level, antinuclear antibody (ANA) and anti–smooth muscle antibody, autoimmune hepatitis), iron and total iron-binding capacity (elevated in hemochromatosis), and liver ultrasound (structural abnormalities or cholelithiasis). If no other etiology of abnormal liver transaminases is established, one may presume NAFLD. Follow liver function tests every 3 months, and if there is no improvement after 1 year, consider a referral to gastroenterology for possible liver biopsy and/or metformin therapy. Make sure these patients have been vaccinated against hepatitis A and B, because NAFLD will worsen with acute hepatitis.

Abnormal Lipid Levels

Patients with a random cholesterol level between 170 and 240 mg/dL (<18 years old) or between 200 and 240 mg/dL (≥18 years old) should be instructed on lowering cholesterol in their diet. Identify 1 or 2 specific problem areas in the diet and set goals such as "change from whole milk to 2%" or "trim fats from meat." Then, have the patient return for a fasting lipid panel 2 months after lifestyle-change counseling. For diagnosed mild hypercholesterolemia (low-density lipoprotein [LDL] = 100–130 mg/dL), provide dietary counseling regarding a lower-cholesterol diet and recommend returning in 1 year for a repeat fasting lipid panel. For moderate (LDL = 130–160 mg/dL) or severe (LDL >160 mg/dL) hypercholesterolemia, it is reasonable to be more aggressive with more detailed diet history and counseling, and have patients return in 3 months for a repeat fasting lipid panel. For persistent LDL levels of >190 mg/dL (or >160 mg/dL with ≥2 risk factors including male gender, obesity, metabolic syndrome, smoking, hypertension, medical conditions such as diabetes, systemic lupus erythematosis, HIV infection, organ transplantation, or survivors of childhood cancer or a family history of early cardiovascular disease), consider medications.[37] Statins inhibit cholesterol synthesis and are the most commonly used medication in adolescents. The choice of statin is a matter of preference and, of course, insurance formulary. Medication should be started at the lowest dose and given once daily, usually at bedtime. Laboratory studies should be performed at baseline and at 1 month (Table 6). Patients should report symptoms of possible

Table 6
Medication guidelines

	Laboratory Tests	Dose	Side Effects/Warnings
Metformin	Creatinine; liver function (baseline and annual)	500 mg extended release; increase by 500 mg weekly to 2 g daily	Diarrhea, nausea, and bloating (common) and lactic acidosis (rare); hold medications for surgery, contrast studies, vomiting, or planned alcohol use
Orlistat	None; recommend vitamin supplement with fat-soluble vitamins and β-carotene (take 2 h before or after a meal)	120 mg 3 times per day with meals	Oily stools; fecal incontinence
Sibutramine	None	10 mg daily; increase dose to 15 mg daily if weight loss is <4 lb at 1 mo	Dry mouth; insomnia; tachycardia; elevated BP; PVCs
Statins	Baseline CK, ALT, and AST; repeat CK if signs of myopathy occur; hold if CK is >10 × ULN; after 1 mo, check lipids, CK, ALT, and AST	Start with lowest dose once daily at bedtime	Need effective contraception; myopathy: muscle cramps, weakness, or asthenia; drug interactions include erythromycin and antifungal agents

PVC indicates premature ventricular contractions; CK, creatine kinase; AST, aspartate aminotransferase; ULN, upper limit of normal.

myopathy (muscle cramps, weakness, asthenia) immediately. If myopathy is present, the medication should be stopped and the creatine kinase level assessed. Medication may be restarted when symptoms and laboratory abnormalities resolve. Adolescent girls should be educated regarding the need for contraception. Drug interactions include cyclosporine, fibric acid derivatives, niacin, erythromycin, azole antifungal agents, nefazodone, and many HIV protease inhibitors. The minimal treatment goal is to decrease the LDL level to <130 mg/dL. If target LDL levels are achieved, repeat laboratory tests in 2 months and then every 3–6 months. If not at target, double the dose and recheck laboratory tests in 1 month. Continue increasing the dose as needed to the maximum recommended dose until the target LDL level is reached or there is evidence of toxicity.

Hypertension

Systolic and/or diastolic BP at >95th percentile for gender, age, and height[36] on ≥3 separate occasions is a standard criterion for diagnosing hypertension. Make sure to use the correct cuff size, which may be difficult with severely obese patients. Thigh cuffs are often too long and may result in inaccurate measurements. Prehypertension is defined as BP at the 90%–95th percentile for gender, age, and height. Stage 1 hypertension is defined as BP from the 95th percentile to 5 mm Hg above the 95th percentile. Stage 2 hypertension is generally ≥12 mm Hg above the 95th percentile and should trigger urgent evaluation within 1 week. Patients with hypertension should be instructed on dietary modifications including the reduction of sodium, limited consumption of high-salt processed foods, and increased consumption of fresh vegetables and fruits and low-fat dairy foods. Additional evaluation for patients with stage 2 hypertension or other comorbidities may include an echocardiogram to screen for left ventricular hypertrophy and obtaining a plasma renin level. Routine screening by obtaining a urine microalbumin level is not recommended.[37] Indications for medication include symptomatic hypertension, secondary hypertension, left ventricular hypertrophy, diabetes, and persistent hypertension after lifestyle change. The choice of medication depends on specific patient characteristics. Diuretics and β-adrenergic blockers have a long history of safety and efficacy. Angiotensin-converting enzyme inhibitors or angiotensin-receptor blockers are preferred for adolescents with diabetes and microalbuminuria or proteinuria. The β-adrenergic blockers or calcium-channel blockers are more often used for patients with migraine headaches. Medication should be started with the lowest recommended dose and increased until the desired BP goal is achieved. Once the highest recommended dose is reached, or if adverse effects occur, a second drug from a different class should be added.

Polycystic Ovarian Syndrome

Criteria for making the diagnosis include ≥2 of the following:

- oligomenorrhea or anovulation: fewer than 6 to 8 menstrual periods per year (usually in the setting of a teenager who established regular cycles after menarche but then became oligomenorrheic);

- clinical or laboratory evidence of hyperandrogenism including acne, hirsutism, or elevated free testosterone level; and/or
- polycystic ovaries on ultrasound (not necessary for diagnosis if the other 2 criteria are present).

If any of the following are present, consider other diagnoses:

- premature adrenarche (consider adrenal hyperandrogenism);
- significantly elevated testosterone levels (rule out tumor); and
- oligomenorrhea starting at menarche and not improving after 2 to 3 years (consider adrenal hyperandrogenism).

Additional laboratory testing that may be helpful includes the evaluation of luteinizing hormone and follicle-stimulating hormone (FSH) levels. Elevation of FSH suggests ovarian failure, whereas an elevated luteinizing hormone/FSH ratio of >2.5 suggests PCOS.

Obstructive Sleep Apnea

Five or more of the following symptoms suggest the diagnosis of OSA:

- snoring;
- sleepiness during the day;
- restless sleep;
- difficulty breathing;
- frequent waking from sleep;
- gasping for air or cessation of breathing during sleep;
- mouth breathing;
- morning headaches; and
- nocturnal enuresis (new onset).

If at all possible, try to obtain additional history information from a family member (either by telephone or screening questionnaire), because these symptoms are difficult for patients to report. Patients with OSA are at risk for systemic hypertension, pulmonary hypertension, and cor pulmonale. In the office, initial management includes an electrocardiogram to rule out right ventricular hypertrophy. The gold standard for diagnosis of OSA is a sleep study; however, if this test is not easily available, consultation with an ear, nose, and throat (ENT) specialist is an appropriate option. ENT physicians often recommend a trial of nasal steroids before considering surgical intervention with a tonsillectomy/adenoidectomy; thus, it may be reasonable to initiate a nasal steroid 1 to 2 months before ENT evaluation.

Other Considerations

Obese children are also at risk for orthopedic problems (hip/knee pain, foot pain), gallstones, pseudotumor cerebri, and mental health problems such as depression, eating disorders, violence/bullying, and anxiety.

TREATMENT: WHEN TO CONSIDER MEDICATION OR CONSULTATION WITH SPECIALIST

Medication or referral to a specialist should be considered with persistence after 3 months of lifestyle modification of:

- impaired fasting glucose, or IGT;
- PCOS;
- ALT levels of more than twice the upper limit of normal;
- severe hypercholesterolemia (LDL level of >190 mg/dL or >160 mg/dL with other risk factors)[38]; or
- stage 2 hypertension.

CONCLUSIONS

Treatment of adolescent obesity remains challenging, whether it is in the primary care or research setting. The bottom line is that as primary care providers we often see these patients for years, and in that capacity we may have many opportunities to help motivate them to change, one visit at a time. Teaching our patients realistic goals for weight loss and lifestyle change, promoting arrest of weight gain, and screening for comorbidities are all critical to the long-term health of obese adolescents.

REFERENCES

1. Shore SM, Sachs ML, Lidicker JR, Brett SN, Wright AR, Libonati JR. Decreased scholastic achievement in overweight middle school students. *Obesity (Silver Spring)*. 2008;16(7):1535–1538
2. Fagot-Campagna A, Pettitt DJ, Engelgau MM, et al. Type 2 diabetes among North American children and adolescents: an epidemiologic review and a public health perspective. *J Pediatr*. 2000;136(5):664–672
3. Pinhas-Hamiel O, Zeitler P. The global spread of type 2 diabetes mellitus in children and adolescents. *J Pediatr*. 2005;146(5):693–700
4. Pinhas-Hamiel O, Zeitler P. Acute and chronic complications of type 2 diabetes mellitus in children and adolescents. *Lancet*. 2007;369(9575):1823–1831
5. Baranowski T, Cooper DM, Harrell J, et al. Presence of diabetes risk factors in a large U.S. eighth-grade cohort. *Diabetes Care*. 2006;29(2):212–217
6. Weiss R, Taksali SE, Tamborlane WV, Burgert TS, Savoye M, Caprio S. Predictors of changes in glucose tolerance status in obese youth. *Diabetes Care*. 2005;28(4):902–909
7. Osei K, Rhinesmith S, Gaillard T, Schuster D. Impaired insulin sensitivity, insulin secretion, and glucose effectiveness predict future development of impaired glucose tolerance and type 2 diabetes in pre-diabetic African Americans. *Diabetes Care*. 2004;27(6):1439–1446

8. Nadeau KJ, Ehlers LB, Zeitler PS, Love-Osborne K. Treatment of non-alcoholic fatty liver disease with metformin versus lifestyle intervention in insulin-resistant adolescents. *Pediatr Diabetes*. 2008; In press
9. Caprio S. Treating child obesity and associated medical conditions. *Future Child*. 2006;16(1): 209-224
10. US Preventive Services Task Force. Screening and interventions for overweight in children and adolescents: recommendation statement. *Pediatrics*. 2005;116(1):205-209
11. Barlow SE; Expert Committee. Expert committee recommendations regarding the prevention, assessment, and treatment of child and adolescent overweight and obesity: summary report. *Pediatrics*. 2007;120(suppl 4):S164-S192
12. Jain A. What works for obesity? A summary of the research behind obesity interventions. Available at: http://unitedhealthfoundation.org/obesity.pdf. Accessed February 13, 2009
13. Stice E, Shaw H, Marti CN. A meta-analytic review of obesity prevention programs for children and adolescents: the skinny on interventions that work. *Psychol Bull*. 2006;132(5):667-691
14. McMurray RG, Harrell JS, Bangdiwala SI, Bradley CB, Deng S, Levine A. A school-based intervention can reduce body fat and blood pressure in young adolescents. *J Adolesc Health*. 2002;31(2):125-132
15. Carrel AL, Clark RR, Peterson SE, Nemeth BA, Sullivan J, Allen DB. Improvement of fitness, body composition, and insulin sensitivity in overweight children in a school-based exercise program: a randomized, controlled study. *Arch Pediatr Adolesc Med*. 2005;159(10):963-968
16. Scudder L, Papa P, Brey LC. School-based health centers: a model for improving the health of the nation's children. *J Nurse Pract*. 2007;3(10):713-720
17. Shilts MK, Horowitz M, Townsend MS. Goal setting as a strategy for dietary and physical activity behavior change: a review of the literature. *Am J Health Promot*. 2004;19(2):81-93
18. Shilts MK, Horowitz M, Townsend MS, Shilts MK, Horowitz M, Townsend MS. An innovative approach to goal setting for adolescents: guided goal setting. *J Nutr Educ Behav*. 2004;36(3):155
19. Deforche B, De Bourdeaudhuij I, Tanghe A, Debode P, Hills AP, Bouckaert J. Role of physical activity and eating behaviour in weight control after treatment in severely obese children and adolescents. *Acta Paediatr*. 2005;94(4):464-470
20. Rolland-Cachera MF, Thibault H, Souberbielle JC, et al. Massive obesity in adolescents: dietary interventions and behaviours associated with weight regain at 2 y follow-up. *Int J Obes Relat Metab Disord*. 2004;28(4):514-519
21. Frenn M, Malin S. Diet and exercise in low-income culturally diverse middle school students. *Public Health Nurs*. 2003;20(5):361-368
22. Patrick K, Calfas KJ, Norman GJ, et al. Randomized controlled trial of a primary care and home-based intervention for physical activity and nutrition behaviors: PACE+ for Adolescents. *Arch Pediatr Adolesc Med*. 2006;160(2):128-136
23. Ebbeling CB, Leidig MM, Sinclair KB, Hangen JP, Ludwig DS. A reduced-glycemic load diet in the treatment of adolescent obesity. *Arch Pediatr Adolesc Med*. 2003;157(8):773-779
24. Chanoine JP, Hampl S, Jensen C, Boldrin M, Hauptman J. Effect of orlistat on weight and body composition in obese adolescents: a randomized controlled trial [published correction appears in *JAMA*. 2005;294(12):1491]. *JAMA*. 2005;293(23):2873-2883
25. Ozkan B, Bereket A, Turan S, Keskin S. Addition of orlistat to conventional treatment in adolescents with severe obesity. *Eur J Pediatr*. 2004;163(12):738-741
26. Berkowitz RI, Fujioka K, Daniels SR, et al. Effects of sibutramine treatment in obese adolescents: a randomized trial. *Ann Intern Med*. 2006;145(2):81-90
27. Godoy-Matos A, Carraro L, Vieira A, et al. Treatment of obese adolescents with sibutramine: a randomized, double-blind, controlled study. *J Clin Endocrinol Metab*. 2005;90(3):1460-1465
28. Arslanian SA, Lewy V, Danadian K, Saad R. Metformin therapy in obese adolescents with polycystic ovary syndrome and impaired glucose tolerance: amelioration of exaggerated adrenal response to adrenocorticotropin with reduction of insulinemia/insulin resistance. *J Clin Endocrinol Metab*. 2002;87(4):1555-1559

29. Lustig RH, Mietus-Snyder ML, Bacchetti P, Lazar AA, Velasquez-Meyer PA, Christensen ML. Insulin dynamics predict body mass index and z-score response to insulin suppression or sensitization pharmacotherapy in obese children. *J Pediatr*. 2006;148(1):23-29
30. Love-Osborne K, Sheeder J, Zeitler P. Addition of metformin to a lifestyle modification program in adolescents with insulin resistance. *J Pediatr*. 2008;152(6):817-822
31. Freiberg MS, Pencina MJ, D'Agostino RB, Lanier K, Wilson PW, Vasan RS. BMI vs waist circumference for identifying vascular risk. *Obesity (Silver Spring)*. 2008;16(2):463-469
32. Fernandez JR, Redden DT, Pietrobelli A, Allison DB. Waist circumference percentiles in nationally representative samples of African-American, European-American, and Mexican-American children and adolescents. *J Pediatr*. 2004;145(4):439-444
33. Gold MA, Kokotailo PK. Motivational interviewing strategies to facilitate adolescent behavior change. Available at: www.hcet.org/resource/postconf/08/MI4FPpros/GOLD/AHUOct07GoldKokotailo.pdf. Accessed February 13, 2009
34. Love-Osborne KA, Nadeau KJ, Sheeder J, Fenton LZ, Zeitler P. Presence of the metabolic syndrome in obese adolescents predicts impaired glucose tolerance and nonalcoholic fatty liver disease. *J Adolesc Health*. 2008;42(6):543-548
35. Cook S, Weitzman M, Auinger P, Nguyen M, Dietz WH. Prevalence of a metabolic syndrome phenotype in adolescents: findings from the third National Health and Nutrition Examination Survey, 1988-1994. *Arch Pediatr Adolesc Med*. 2003;157(8):821-827
36. National Heart, Lung, and Blood Institute. Blood pressure levels by age and height percentile. Available at: www.nhlbi.nih.gov/health/prof/heart/hbp/hbp_ped.pdf. Accessed February 13, 2009
37. Falkner B, Daniels SR. Summary of the fourth report on the diagnosis, evaluation, and treatment of high blood pressure in children and adolescents. *Hypertension*. 2004;44(4):387-388
38. McCrindle BW, Urbina EM, Dennison BA, et al. Drug therapy of high-risk lipid abnormalities in children and adolescents: a scientific statement from the American Heart Association Atherosclerosis, Hypertension, and Obesity in Youth Committee, Council of Cardiovascular Disease in the Young, with the Council on Cardiovascular Nursing. *Circulation*. 2007;115(14):1948-1967

The Metabolic Syndrome in Children and Adolescents: A Clinician's Guide

Christel A. Biltoft, MD, FAAP*[a,b], Andrew Muir, MD[c]

[a]*Pediatric Center of Stone Mountain, LLC, 5405-D Memorial Drive, Stone Mountain, GA 30083, USA*

[b]*Kids Health First Pediatric Alliance, 2814 New Spring Road, Suite 104, Atlanta, GA 30339, USA*

[c]*Division of Endocrinology, Department of Pediatrics, Emory University School of Medicine, 2015 Uppergate Drive NE, Atlanta, GA 30322, USA*

You are taking care of a black family that has just joined your practice. They are bringing their 2 children, a 14-year-old girl and a 9-year-old boy, to see you. Past medical history for both children is negative. Family history is significant for the 48-year-old father who is obese and was recently diagnosed with type 2 diabetes and hypertension. Their mother is 38 years old and is pregnant at 28 weeks' gestation and has gestational diabetes.

The 14-year-old girl weighs 160 lb, is 63 in tall, and has a BMI of 28 (>95th percentile). Her blood pressure is 130/78 mm Hg. Physical examination shows an obese abdomen. Puberty has progressed to Tanner stage 4 breast and Tanner stage 3 pubic hair. She has thick, velvety, hyperpigmented skin on the back of her neck and in her axillae. She has no acne or hirsuitism. Menarche was at age 11. She has a regular menstrual cycle.

The little brother is 9 years old, weighs 94 lb, is 56 in tall, and has a BMI of 21 (95th percentile). His blood pressure is 110/67 mm Hg. He, too, has an obese abdomen. He is at Tanner stage 1 for pubic hair and testicular development.

From history and physical alone, you are concerned about this family's risk for insulin resistance and the metabolic syndrome. How are you going to manage, treat, and advise this family?

---

*Corresponding author.
E-mail address: christelbiltoft@yahoo.com (C. A. Biltoft).

The metabolic syndrome and its association with type 2 diabetes and cardiovascular disease is becoming an increasingly common concern for pediatricians in clinical practice. As a concept, the metabolic syndrome is not new. In 1988, Reaven[1] described a "syndrome X" that linked insulin resistance and central obesity to the development of hypertension, dyslipidemia, hyperuricemia, and cardiovascular disease. Since the 1980s, the metabolic syndrome in adult medicine has been thought of as a constellation of modifiable risk factors that are predictive for the development of type 2 diabetes and cardiovascular disease. Obesity has become a problem of increasing concern in pediatric medicine. The National Health and Nutrition Examination Survey (NHANES) began collecting data on childhood obesity in the 1970s. At that time, the prevalence of obesity (defined as a BMI at >95th percentile) was ~5% among children and adolescents aged 2 to 19 years.[2] The most recent NHANES data from 2003–2006 show that the prevalence of obesity is up to 16.3% for those in the same age group.[2,3] Furthermore, children and adolescents with the metabolic syndrome are at increased risk for developing juvenile-onset type 2 diabetes and adult-onset cardiovascular disease.[4,5]

As pediatricians begin to focus on the epidemic of childhood and adolescent obesity and the possibility of juvenile metabolic syndrome, a new perspective is already emerging in adult medicine. Many experts have begun to question the utility of designating the metabolic syndrome as a true "syndrome." Specifically, it is unclear whether the combination of the risk factors used to define the metabolic syndrome is more helpful in assessing a patient's risk for diabetes or cardiovascular disease than the individual components.[6,7] For example, someone with hyperlipidemia and hypertension may not meet the criteria for the metabolic syndrome but is, nonetheless, at risk for cardiovascular disease. Also, a fasting blood glucose level by itself may predict type 2 diabetes more accurately than a diagnosis of metabolic syndrome.[7] Reaven[8] himself argued against labeling a patient with a syndrome when treatment options merely address each of the individual derangements. Others have argued that the advent of preventive treatments for subjects at high risk validates consideration of the metabolic syndrome as a clinically important diagnosis.[9]

The objective of this article is to review the components of the metabolic syndrome and the theory behind the combined negative effects of insulin resistance and obesity and to discuss the clinical utility of this concept in pediatrics. The latest diagnostic criteria for obesity, dyslipidemia, and hypertension in children and adolescents, as well as management and prevention strategies, will be reviewed also.

DEFINITIONS AND EPIDEMIOLOGY

Unfortunately, there are many definitions for the metabolic syndrome. Some of the most cited definitions come from the World Health Organization, the Inter-

Table 1
Comparing 2 adaptations of the diagnostic criteria for the metabolic syndrome for pediatrics with the ATPIII criteria

Risk Factor	Defining Level per the NCEP ATPIII[11]	Defining Level per Cook et al[15]	Defining Level per Weiss et al[16]
Central obesity	Men: >102 cm; women: >88 cm	Waist circumference > 90th percentile for age and gender from sample population	BMI ≥ 97th percentile for age and gender
Triglycerides	≥150 mg/dL	≥110 mg/dL	≥95th percentile for age and gender
HDL cholesterol	Men: <40 mg/dL; women: <50 mg/dL	≤40 mg/dL	≤5th percentile for age and gender
Blood pressure	≥130/≥85 mm Hg	≥90 percentile for age, gender, and height	≥95th percentile for age, gender, and height
Fasting glucose	≥110 mg/dL	≥110 mg/dL	Impaired glucose tolerance

national Diabetes Federation, and the National Cholesterol Education Program (NCEP). Pediatric researchers have modified many of these definitions to be used for children and adolescents, but there is no consensus on a pediatric definition either. A study that reviewed the definition of the metabolic syndrome in children found that authors used 40 different definitions in 27 publications.[10] Differences included definitions of obesity (BMI versus waist circumference), the inclusion of uricemia, the method of determining insulin resistance, and the number of criteria required for diagnosis. In this article we discuss the definition by the NCEP Expert Panel on Detection, Evaluation, and Treatment of High Blood Cholesterol in Adults (Adult Treatment Panel III [ATPIII])[11] because it is relatively easy to modify for implementation in a pediatric clinical practice. The metabolic syndrome is defined by the ATPIII as having 3 or more of 5 risk factors: central obesity, high blood pressure, dyslipidemia characterized by high serum triglyceride levels and low serum high-density lipoprotein (HDL) cholesterol levels, and evidence of insulin resistance as manifested by elevated fasting glucose levels (Table 1).

Even with an acceptable definition, the metabolic syndrome remains a challenge in childhood and adolescence because there are no well-established age- and gender-specific values for many of the diagnostic criteria. For example, it is difficult to define central obesity in childhood, because adiposity distribution differs on the basis of age, ethnicity, gender, and pubertal development. In the past decade, however, advances have been made in the availability of some pediatric-specific parameters. Age- and gender-specific normal values for BMI and hypertension are readily available.[12,13] More recently, pediatric lipid-screening recommendations with age-specific lipid profile values were published.[14]

The diagnostic heterogeneity described above has confounded estimates of the prevalence of metabolic syndrome in children. One of the most widely cited prevalence estimates comes from the NHANES III survey (1988–1994), which used a modified ATPIII definition of the metabolic syndrome with reference values for children and adolescents. The overall prevalence rate among adolescents was 4.2%, with slightly higher rates in male adolescents (6.1%).[15] It was found that nearly 30% of adolescents who met criteria for overweight also met criteria for the metabolic syndrome.[15] These data are thought to underestimate the current prevalence of the pediatric metabolic syndrome because of the rising prevalence of overweight among children. A more recent study of a multiethnic, multiracial cohort of 439 overweight children and adolescents identified metabolic syndrome in 50% of those who were "severely obese" (defined as a BMI at >97th percentile). Furthermore, the presence of metabolic syndrome was correlated with BMI.[16]

PATHOGENESIS

The theory behind metabolic syndrome is that obesity promotes the development of insulin resistance in some individuals. Insulin resistance is thought to be the major causal factor for the metabolic derangements of dyslipidemia, hypertension, and impaired glucose tolerance.[17,18] A genetic predisposition to developing insulin resistance is clearly important. As mentioned earlier, 30% of the overweight adolescents in the NHANES III survey had evidence of insulin resistance, leaving 70% "protected" despite their adiposity. Insulin resistance refers to the ineffective function of insulin hormone at normal serum levels. The main function of insulin is energy homeostasis through its effects on muscle, liver, and fat. Insulin resistance is clinically observed as hyperglycemia because of impaired glucose transport from blood to cells and impaired suppression of hepatic glucose output. In addition, insufficient insulin action causes aberrant synthesis of very-low-density lipoprotein and triglycerides and, consequently, dyslipidemia.[17] In adult studies, it has long been established that insulin resistance is an independent risk factor for type 2 diabetes, essential hypertension, and cardiovascular disease.[19,20] We are now finding evidence that this may also be true in children. The Cardiovascular Risk in Young Finns Study showed that a high fasting serum insulin concentration was the best predictor of metabolic syndrome and subsequent cardiovascular disease in adulthood.[18] Findings from the Bogalusa Heart Study, a longitudinal study on the natural history of cardiovascular disease beginning in childhood, found that the best predictors for the metabolic syndrome were obesity and elevated basal insulin levels.[4]

Although the epidemiology of insulin resistance as a risk factor for developing type 2 diabetes and cardiovascular disease is clear, the pathogenesis of insulin resistance from adiposity is complicated and poorly understood. There seem to be many pathways in energy homeostasis that are disrupted with increased adiposity. Our understanding of the metabolic roles and interactions of the adipocyte and insulin is increasing. Adipocytes were once thought merely to be storage sites for glycerin and free fatty acids as triglycerides. It is now known that adipocytes are complicated endocrine cells that secrete hormones, cytokines, vasoactive substances, and other metabolically active proteins.[19] The exact role that the adipocyte plays in insulin resistance is still under investigation, but many simultaneous processes are likely occurring. Some of the current research is examining substances secreted directly from adipocytes, such as the cytokine tumor necrosis factor α, the adipocytokine adiponectin, and free fatty acids. Tumor necrosis factor α impairs insulin signaling and reduces *GLUT4* gene expression, the major insulin-responsive glucose transporter of muscle and fat cells.[19] Adiponectin, an adipocytokine that is exclusively expressed by adipocytes, is thought to be a protective factor against the development of atherosclerosis and type 2 diabetes via incompletely understood antiproliferative and antiinflammatory effects.[21] Adiponectin levels are suppressed with increased adiposity, and low levels may strongly predict the presence of metabolic derangements.[21] An elevated plasma free fatty acid concentration is linked to many of the derangements of insulin resistance, including increased hepatic triglyceride output, impaired suppression of hepatic glucose output, impaired glucose uptake in skeletal muscle, and inhibited insulin secretion from pancreatic β cells. It is now becoming clear that fatness is not benign.[19–22]

CLINICAL ASSESSMENT

The absence of well-defined criteria for diagnosing the metabolic syndrome in childhood makes the clinical assessment in a pediatric setting difficult. However, it is becoming easier as parameters for each component are becoming standardized for childhood. The 5 components of the metabolic syndrome defined by the ATPIII and suggestions on how to measure them in a pediatric practice are as follows.

1. Central obesity: defined as excessive abdominal distribution of fat, central obesity is correlated with visceral adiposity and associated with worse cardiovascular risk.[15] The ATPIII definition used adult waist circumference as one of the criteria for the metabolic syndrome, but waist circumference is problematic in the pediatric setting because normative values for American children are not readily available. In the NHANES III study, waist circumference was measured at the midpoint between the bottom of the rib cage and above the top of the iliac crest at minimal respiration. Because there are no standardized reference values for waist circumference in childhood, the NHANES III defined abnormal as >90th percentile for age and gender of the sample population.[15] Other major studies of the metabolic syndrome in childhood, however, used BMI in their definition, citing the fact that waist circumference is too difficult to interpret in children because it is heavily affected by pubertal development and ethnicity[16] (Table 1).

Although its correlation to abdominal adiposity in childhood is not as reliable as in adults, BMI is an accepted way of measuring obesity and overweight in both children and adults. BMI is measured by weight in kilograms divided by the square of height in meters squared. Obesity has been defined as a BMI at >95th percentile for age and gender on the basis of the standard 2000 Centers for Disease Control and Prevention growth curves, and the BMI of overweight children falls between the 85th and the 95th percentiles.[23]

2. Hypertension: normal blood pressure ranges according to percentiles for age, gender, and height can be found in tables published in 2004 by the National High Blood Pressure Education Program Working Group on High Blood Pressure in Children and Adolescents.[13] Hypertension is defined as an average systolic and/or diastolic blood pressure reading measured on 3 or more occasions at >95th percentile for height, age, and gender. Children are considered prehypertensive if their blood pressure is between the 90th and 95th percentiles. Adolescents with a blood pressure of ≥120/80 mm Hg but <95th percentile should be considered prehypertensive.[13] Factitious hypertension is common among obese children when an undersized arm cuff is used.

3 and 4. Dyslipidemia: dyslipidemia is characterized by elevated triglyceride and low HDL levels. The characteristic dyslipidemia of the metabolic syndrome of hypertriglyceridemia and low HDL levels is a result of insulin resistance. High insulin levels promote triglyceride release from the liver and suppression of HDL.[24] In the NHANES III study, the reference values for pediatric cholesterol levels were taken from the NCEP Report of the Expert Panel on Blood Cholesterol Levels in Children and Adolescents.[11,15] An elevated fasting triglyceride level was defined as >90th percentile (≥110 mg/dL), and a low HDL level was defined as <10th percentile (≤40 mg/dL). In July 2008, the American Academy of Pediatrics (AAP) published new guidelines for lipid screening in childhood and published reference values for fasting lipid levels according to percentiles that were age and gender specific. The AAP recommended fasting serum lipid screening for all children at risk, starting at 2 years of age. Risk factors include family history of cardiovascular disease and/or diabetes, unknown family history, and obesity.[14]

5. Evidence of insulin resistance: in research settings, insulin sensitivity is measured by invasive studies such as the euglycemic insulin clamp with a constant insulin-infusion rate and variable glucose-infusion rate. There are surrogates of insulin resistance that are more clinically practical. The ATPIII and the NHANES III used an elevated fasting glucose level of >110 mg/dL as evidence of insulin resistance. As mentioned earlier, insulin resistance causes the characteristic dyslipidemia of elevated triglyceride and low HDL levels. A study that evaluated metabolic markers in identifying overweight individuals who are insulin resistant suggested that measuring the fasting plasma triglyceride level, the fasting plasma triglyc-

eride/HDL ratio, and the fasting plasma insulin level were all clinically useful surrogate measurements of insulin resistance.[20] Our ability to predict future disease in individual insulin-resistant children remains poor. Furthermore, safe therapies beyond healthy lifestyle interventions for preventing progression of insulin resistance to overt disease have not been validated in children. Thus, the question remains as to whether a diagnosis of insulin resistance offers more useful information than is provided by direct measures of blood pressure, serum lipids, and glucose.

MANAGEMENT

The management of metabolic syndrome in childhood is as difficult a task as defining it. The concept seems simple: lose weight by improving diet and participating in more vigorous exercise. However, lifestyle and long-term behavior change is very hard to implement. It seems intuitive that the younger one starts, the better. The goal should be to have a target weight at ≤85th-percentile BMI for age and gender. A stepped approach with intermediate goals may be best for those children with morbid obesity or with medical complications of being overweight.

Initial evaluation should establish whether (1) weight gain is the consequence of a primary disease and (2) complications of obesity exist. Thus, a complete history and physical examination are needed. It is important to remember that diet recall or logs are notoriously unreliable for establishing caloric intake. Questions regarding physical activity should include an evaluation of type, duration, and frequency of activity. Some guideline of exercise tolerance may be useful. Specific enumeration of daily "screen time" (hours per day spent on recreational use of computers and television) is important. The physical examination should be punctuated by calculation of BMI and a careful skin examination. In addition to acanthosis nigricans and striae, one should search for abscesses (especially intertriginous, perianal, axillary, inguinal, and upper thigh). In general, the height of children with exogenous obesity is >50th percentile for age and gender. Overweight caused by endocrinologic or genetic conditions is almost always associated with short stature or slow linear growth velocity. A careful search for dysmorphia may provide a clue to a genetic cause of obesity (eg, Prader-Willi syndrome). Laboratory evaluations should be ordered when the clinical presentation increases the index of suspicion for a specific condition. Routine testing panels should be avoided, because the interpretation of such investigations can be confounded by obesity itself. For example, serum thyrotropin concentrations are modestly elevated in some 10% to 15% of overweight children as a result of (not as a cause of) obesity.[25] In addition to traditional evaluations, a psychological assessment may discover treatable conditions that either underlie a weight problem or are the result of obesity (eg, affect disorders, eating disorders).

Weight management should first focus on whether the patient and the family have acknowledged the importance of obesity and are ready to institute necessary changes. The diagnosis of a complication, regardless of whether it is related to the metabolic syndrome (eg, sleep apnea, worsening asthma, leg pain), can serve as a focus to reinforce the importance of weight control. Successful intervention in willing families often requires input from a team of providers that may include 1 or more physicians, a dietitian, an exercise trainer, and a psychologist. Long-term commitment from both the family members and the providers is vital to the success of all treatments.[26] Diet interventions should begin by adopting the most simple steps to eliminate obviously unhealthy eating habits (eg, skipping breakfast, drinking sugar-sweetened beverages, eating on an erratic schedule, and frequent restaurant meals). Recommend starting a daily light exercise routine such as walking with light handheld weights. Excluding time for schoolwork, screen time should be reduced to 1 to 2 hours/day. Organized weight-loss programs such as Weight Watchers can be very helpful. Note that adolescents younger than 16 years will need a prescription with goal weight parameters to sign up for Weight Watchers. A clinical psychologist can often identify underlying causes of overeating. Specific weight goals should be set, and progress should be monitored weekly at home and at 1- to 4-month intervals in the office. The initial goal should be for weight maintenance while lifestyle changes are put in place, then try for moderate but consistent weight loss such as 1 or 2 lb/month.[27] Adolescents with obesity-induced complications that are refractory to initial management should be considered for aggressive treatments supervised by a subspecialist.

Early pharmacotherapy for weight control is controversial. There is limited evidence to support the use of metformin to augment weight loss and improve insulin sensitivity. A trial of 500 mg of metformin twice daily in obese adolescents reported modest improvement in weight loss and insulin sensitivity.[28] The improvements in BMI and fasting blood glucose and insulin levels were small, and the results were more consistent with female patients than with male patients. Nonetheless, the use of metformin in conjunction with diet and exercise may be justified for obese adolescents with abnormal glucose tolerance or signs of hyperandrogenism (eg, hirsutism, menstrual irregularities). Currently, metformin has not been approved by the US Food and Drug Administration for weight loss. Metformin has a small risk of lactic acidosis and should not be used in patients with ketosis-prone diabetes or known renal, hepatic, or cardiopulmonary disease.[28]

The newest AAP guidelines for lipid screening in childhood gave diet and lifestyle change recommendations as well as when and how to start pharmacologic intervention for dyslipidemia.[14] The National High Blood Pressure Education Program Working Group on High Blood Pressure in Children and Adolescents guidelines recommended lifestyle changes for prehypertension and follow-up blood-pressure monitoring every 6 months. Pharmacotherapy, in addition to lifestyle changes, was recommended for those with blood pressure consistently measuring above the 99th percentile or those with evidence of end-organ damage such as left ventricular hypertrophy.[13] Symptomatic hyper-

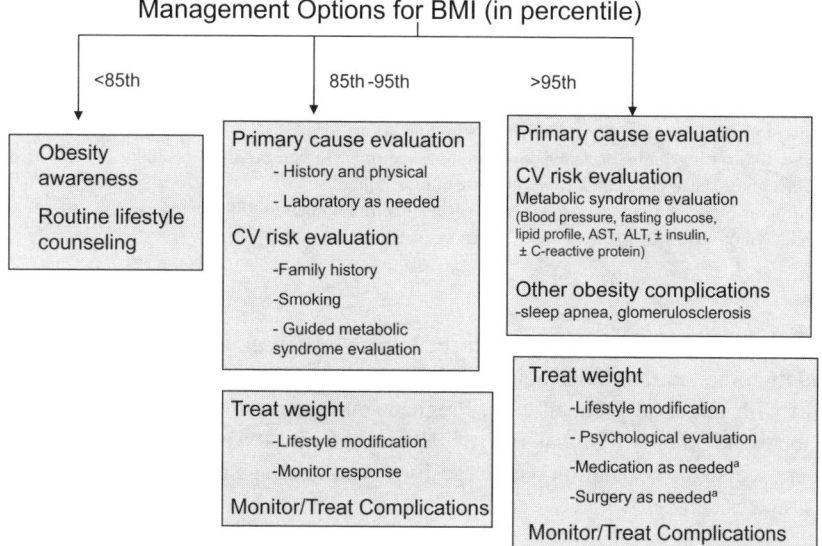

Fig 1. Management options for BMI (in percentile). [a] Consider intensive therapies if refractory to initial care or complications not responsive to traditional management. CV indicates cardiovascular; AST, aspartate aminotransferase; ALT, alanine aminotransferase.

tension needs to be managed emergently. Renal causes of hypertension should be ruled out by a complete blood count, chemistries, and urine analysis. Evaluation for aortic coarctation by 4-limb blood pressures in morbidly obese hypertensive children can be difficult at times because of inadequate cuff size or challenges with auscultation. Referral to a specialist before starting pharmacotherapy for either dyslipidemia or hypertension should be strongly considered (Fig 1).

PREVENTION

Prevention is perhaps the most attractive therapeutic tool with regard to obesity and the metabolic syndrome. Research has shown that insulin resistance begins in childhood from both genetic factors and modifiable environmental factors. A diet starting in early childhood of excess saturated fats and carbohydrates is likely an important contributor to hyperinsulinemia and obesity.[17] Pediatricians play an important role in counseling on healthy early nutrition practices. In 2003, the AAP published guidelines for obesity prevention that were reaffirmed in 2007.[29] The guidelines recommended that pediatricians (1) calculate and plot BMIs at every health check, (2) promote exclusive breastfeeding, (3) promote healthy food choices, such as avoidance of sugary drinks, (4) promote setting strict limits on television watching and other screen times, (5) encourage daily physical activity at home and in school, and (6) monitor blood pressure, lipid levels, hyperinsulinemia, impaired glucose tolerance, and symptoms of obstructive sleep apnea syndrome (Table 2). Despite recent concerns that any protective

Table 2
AAP guidelines for obesity prevention

---
1. Calculate and plot BMIs at every health check
2. Promote exclusive breastfeeding
3. Promote healthy food choices, such as avoiding sugary drinks
4. Promote setting limits on television watching and other screen times
5. Encourage daily physical activity at home and in school
6. Monitor blood pressure, lipid levels, hyperinsulinemia, impaired glucose tolerance, and symptoms of obstructive sleep apnea syndrome

---

effect of breastfeeding may be artifactual, there is mounting evidence that obesity and its complications have their roots in early life.[30] Therefore, prevention should start with maternal prenatal care. Pregnant mothers with obesity or gestational diabetes put their infants at risk of developing obesity and insulin resistance. There is also an association with large-for-gestational-age infants and subsequent insulin resistance.[31]

REIMBURSEMENT

With payers just beginning to acknowledge obesity as a disease, pediatricians must adopt billing strategies that optimize the reimbursement for work to fulfill the AAP recommendations. Counseling and promoting weight loss is complex and time consuming. In the long run, health care delivery for obesity needs to be restructured to ensure efficient delivery of indicated investigation and therapy. Until then, it is important that pediatricians be reimbursed appropriately. Specific obesity codes (278 series) are frequently denied reimbursement. Complications of obesity, such as the metabolic syndrome and acanthosis nigricans, are more likely to be recognized. The better alternative may be to bill a visit on the basis of time. Therefore, pediatricians should document the start and finish times of the office visit, as well as the time spent counseling in excess of 50% of the total visit time.

CONCLUSIONS

Understanding the impact of obesity and insulin resistance on the health of children and adolescents, as well as knowing the latest diagnostic criteria and management strategies for obesity, dyslipidemia, and hypertension, remain important. The concept underlying the metabolic syndrome remains useful in reminding physicians that cardiovascular risk factors tend to cluster within individuals and families. Therefore, screening patients at high risk for components of the metabolic syndrome is recommended. From a patient's or parent's point of view, the metabolic syndrome may provide a construct for helping them conceptualize the medical risk of obesity and the value of preventive or therapeutic weight loss.

Table 3
Summary points

- The metabolic syndrome is thought to be a clustering of modifiable risk factors for the development of cardiovascular disease and type 2 diabetes mellitus
- Obesity leads to insulin resistance and the metabolic syndrome
- Obesity in childhood and adolescence is of epidemic proportions
- Conditions causing obesity include genetic, endocrine, psychiatric, and socioeconomic factors
- Prevention should include maternal prenatal care, exclusive breastfeeding, and health maintenance with proper nutrition and exercise throughout childhood and adolescence

Pediatricians have unique influence on the prevention, early diagnosis, and early intervention of childhood obesity and its complications. Prevention is arguably the most important of these contributions. Pediatricians should actively advocate for children in the office and publicly by promoting good prenatal care, exclusive breastfeeding, early healthy nutrition, daily exercise at home and in school, limitation of screen time and sedentary activities, early complication monitoring, and more. A concerted effort from the pediatric community is needed to slow down and reverse the epidemic of childhood obesity and the impending epidemic of type 2 diabetes and cardiovascular disease (Table 3).

REFERENCES

1. Reaven GM. Role of insulin in human disease. *Diabetes.* 1988;37(12):1595–1607
2. Centers for Disease Control and Prevention, National Center for Health Statistics. Obesity prevalence. Available at: www.cdc.gov/nccdphp/dnpa/obesity/trend/index.htm. Accessed February 17, 2009
3. Ogden CL, Carroll MD, Flegel KM. High body mass index for age among US children and adolescents, 2003–2006. *JAMA.* 2008;299(20):2442–2443
4. Li S, Chen W, Srinivasan S, et al. Childhood cardiovascular risk factors and carotid vascular changes in adulthood: the Bogalusa Heart Study [published correction appears in *JAMA.* 2003; 290(22):2943]. *JAMA.* 2003;290(17):2271–2276
5. Mattsson N, Rönnemaa T, Juonala M, Viikari J, Raitakari O. Childhood predictors of the metabolic syndrome in adulthood. The Cardiovascular Risk in Young Finns Study. *Ann Med.* 2008;40 (7):542–552
6. Kahn R. Metabolic syndrome: what is the clinical usefulness? *Lancet.* 2008;371(9628):1892–1893
7. Sattar N, McConnachie A, Shaper AG, et al. Can metabolic syndrome usefully predict cardiovascular disease and diabetes? Outcome data from two prospective studies. *Lancet.* 2008; 371(9628):1927–1935
8. Reaven GM. The metabolic syndrome: is this diagnosis necessary [published correction appears in *Am J Clin Nutr.* 2006;84(5):1253]? *Am J Clin Nutr.* 2006;83(6):1237–1247
9. Grundy S. Does a diagnosis of metabolic syndrome have value in clinical practice? *Am J Clin Nutr.* 2006;83:1248–1251
10. Ford E, Li C. Defining the metabolic syndrome in children and adolescents: will the real definition please stand up? *J Pediatr.* 2008;152(2):160–164
11. Expert Panel on Detection, Evaluation, and Treatment of High Blood Cholesterol in Adults. Executive summary of the third report of the National Cholesterol Education Program (NCEP) Expert Panel on Detection, Evaluation, and Treatment of High Blood Cholesterol in Adults (Adult Treatment Panel III). *JAMA.* 2001;285(19):2486–2496
12. Centers for Disease Control and Prevention, National Center for Health Statistics. 2000 CDC growth charts: United States. Available at: www.cdc.gov/growthcharts. Accessed March 18, 2004

13. National High Blood Pressure Education Program Working Group on High Blood Pressure in Children and Adolescents. The fourth report on the diagnosis, evaluation, and treatment of high blood pressure in children and adolescents. *Pediatrics.* 2004;114(2 suppl 4th report):555–576
14. Daniels S, Greer F; American Academy of Pediatrics, Committee on Nutrition. Lipid screening and cardiovascular health in childhood. *Pediatrics.* 2008;122(1):198–208
15. Cook S, Weitzman M, Auringer P, Nguyen M, Dietz W. Prevalence of a metabolic syndrome phenotype in adolescents: findings from the Third National Health and Nutrition Examination Survey, 1988–1994. *Arch Pediatr Adolesc Med.* 2003;157(8):821–827
16. Weiss R, Dziura J, Burgert T, et al. Obesity and the metabolic syndrome in children and adolescents. *N Engl J Med.* 2004;350(23):2362–2374
17. Ten S, Maclaren N. Insulin resistance syndrome in children. *J Clin Endocrinol Metab.* 2004; 89(6):2526–2539
18. Mattsson N, Rönnemaa T, Juonala M, Viikari JS, Raitakari OT. Childhood predictors of the metabolic syndrome in adulthood. The Cardiovascular Risk in Young Finns Study. *Ann Med.* 2008;40(7):542–552
19. Kahn B, Flier J. Obesity and insulin resistance. *J Clin Invest.* 2000;106(4):473–481
20. McLaughlin T, Abbasi F, Cheal K, Chu J, Lamendola C, Reaven G. Use of metabolic markers to identify overweight individuals who are insulin resistant. *Ann Intern Med.* 2003;139(10):802–809
21. Körner A, Kratzsch J, Gausche R, Schaab M, Erbs S, Kiess W. New predictors of the metabolic syndrome in children: role of adipocytokines. *Pediatr Res.* 2007;61(6):640–645
22. Raitakari OT, Porkka KV, Rönnemaa T, et al. The role of insulin in clustering of serum lipids and blood pressure in children and adolescents. The Cardiovascular Risk in Young Finns Study. *Diabetologia.* 1995;38(9):1042–1050
23. August GP, Caprio S, Fennoy I, et al. Prevention and treatment of pediatric obesity: an Endocrine Society clinical practice guideline based on expert opinion. *J Clin Endocrinol Metab.* 2008; 93(12):4576–4599
24. Toledo F, Sniderman A, Kelley D. Influence of hepatic steatosis (fatty liver) on severity and composition of dyslipidemia in type 2 diabetes. *Diabetes Care.* 2006;29(8):1845–1850
25. Reinehr T, de Sousa G, Andler W. Hyperthyrotropinemia in obese children is reversible after weight loss and is not related to lipids. *J Clin Endocrinol Metab.* 2006;91(8):3088–3091
26. Boon CS, Clydesdale FM. A review of childhood and adolescent obesity interventions. *Crit Rev Food Sci Nutr.* 2005;45(7–8):511–525
27. Schneider MB, Brill SR. Obesity in children and adolescents. *Pediatr Rev.* 2005;26(5):155–187
28. Freemark M, Bursey D. The effects of metformin on body mass index and glucose tolerance in obese adolescents with fasting hyperinsulinemia and a family history of type 2 diabetes. *Pediatrics.* 2001;107(4). Available at: www.pediatrics.org/cgi/content/full/107/4/e55
29. Krebs NF, Jacobson MS; American Academy of Pediatrics, Committee on Nutrition. Prevention of pediatric overweight and obesity. *Pediatrics.* 2003;112(2):424–430
30. Butte NF. Impact of infant feeding practices on childhood obesity. *J Nutr.* 2009;139(2):412S–416S
31. Boney C, Verma A, Tucker R, Vohr B. Metabolic syndrome in childhood: association with birth weight, maternal obesity, and gestational diabetes mellitus. *Pediatrics.* 2005;115(3). Available at: www.pediatrics.org/cgi/content/full/115/3/e290

Primary Immunodeficiencies Presenting in Adolescence

Lisa J. Kobrynski, MD, MPH*

Departments of Pediatrics, Allergy/Immunology Section, Emory University School of Medicine, 1648 Pierce Drive, Atlanta, GA 30322, USA

Primary immunodeficiency diseases (PIDDs) are a heterogeneous group of more than 120 disorders, many of which are caused by a single gene defect.[1] The genetic mutations usually result in a loss of function of the affected gene. Deficiencies in all parts of the immune system causing PIDDs have been described. Molecular studies of PIDDs have identified new genes that play critical roles in host defense, and the study of family kindreds with PIDDs has also elucidated the function of other previously identified genes. The study of this group of disorders has expanded our knowledge of how the immune system works to clear specific pathogens, make antibodies, and evade tumors. Despite the large number of distinct immunodeficiency syndromes, all individuals with PIDDs have in common an increased susceptibility to infection.

The true prevalence of PIDDs is not known, but it is estimated that 1 in 1200 individuals in the United States has been diagnosed with a PIDD.[2] This number is in contrast to previous estimates of 1 in 10 000 to 1 in 500 000 based on data from disease registries[3–8] and suggests that many cases of PIDD remain undiagnosed. Web-based registries developed in Europe (European Society for Immunodeficiencies), the United States (Immune Deficiency Foundation), and Australia will assist clinical immunologists in obtaining more accurate estimates of PIDD prevalence. PIDDs are typically classified by the nature of the immune defect, whether it affects antibody production by B cells (humoral immunity), T-cell function (cellular immunity), both T- and B-cell function (combined immune defect), killing of bacteria by neutrophils (phagocytic defect), or complement. Figure 1 shows the breakdown of PIDDs according to the underlying defect.[9] The largest proportion of PIDDs affect antibody production. Individuals with these diseases may develop symptoms at any age. Approximately 60% of individuals with PIDD present with infections or other findings of PIDD in the first few years of life. The most severe defects, such as severe combined

---

*Corresponding author.
E-mail address: lkobryn@emory.edu (L. J. Kobrynski).

Copyright © 2009 American Academy of Pediatrics. All rights reserved. ISSN 1934-4287

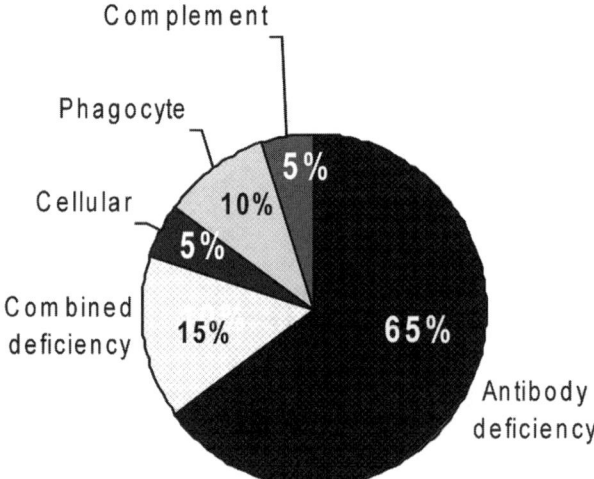

Fig 1. Breakdown of primary immunodeficiencies according to underlying defect. Shown is the relative frequency of different types PIDDs.[9]

immunodeficiency (SCID), are fatal in early childhood if not treated and will not be discussed further in this review. Diagnosis of PIDD, even with symptoms starting early in childhood, may be delayed until adolescence because of a lack of clinical suspicion. Other PIDDs have a late onset of symptoms, even into the third or fourth decade of life. Left untreated, recurring infections of the lungs and sinuses can lead to significant morbidity, and untreated patients are at risk for death resulting from overwhelming infection. Therefore, it is important for clinicians to be aware that these disorders have a variable phenotype and may present with their onset during adolescence. On the basis of the clinical presentation, practitioners should be able to initiate the evaluation of patients with suspected PIDD. In this article I discuss the clinical presentation of PIDDs in adolescent patients and provide a current update on their diagnosis and management.

CLINICAL PRESENTATION

By adolescence, the immune system is fully developed. Maternal immunoglobulin G (IgG) antibodies that cross the placenta during the third trimester disappear by 6 to 9 months of age, and production of specific antibody with the development of immunologic memory begins during the end of the first year of life. Adult levels of IgG in the serum are reached by 6 years of age.[10] The capability to produce specific antibody, to clear organisms through neutrophil phagocytosis, cytotoxic T cells, and natural killer (NK) cells, and to kill pathogens using complement is fully functional by late childhood. The slow maturation of the immune system explains, in part, why young children have an increase in respiratory infections compared with older children and adolescents. The hallmark of PIDD is an increased frequency or severity of infections or infections with unusual organisms. The types of infections and their severity will vary depending on the nature of the immune defect (Table 1).

B-CELL DEFECTS

Hypogammaglobulinemia

Primary immune defects in antibody production, or humoral immunodeficiencies, result in recurring bacterial infections of the ears, sinuses, and lungs with pyogenic bacteria commonly found in the respiratory tract and gastrointestinal infections with *Giardia lamblia*. A complete absence of specific antibody production occurs in defects such as X-linked agammaglobulinemia (XLA) or X-linked hyper-IgM (XHIGM1) syndrome. In these disorders, the onset of infections often begins after 6 months of age, although there have been reports of milder variants diagnosed in adolescents and adults. In XLA, a defect in *Bruton tyrosine kinase* (*btk*) causes the absence of mature B cells in peripheral blood and, subsequently, a lack of circulating immunoglobulins. All affected individuals are male and typically have recurring infection with pyogenic bacteria starting in the first year of life. XHIGM1 syndrome is, in fact, caused by the lack of CD40L on T cells, which leads to the inability of B cells to undergo class-switch recombination (CSR) and produce IgA, IgG, or IgE antibodies. Serum IgM levels are normal or elevated, and affected individuals have recurrent bacterial infections and frequently have infection with *Pneumocystis jiroveci* (*carinii*) early in life. Neutropenia is also seen in patients with XHIGM.[11,12] Only a few cases have been diagnosed in older children and young adults.[13]

Common Variable Immunodeficiency

By far the most significant immune defect diagnosed in adolescents and young adults is common variable immunodeficiency (CVID), which has also been called adult-onset hypogammaglobulinemia and acquired hypogammaglobulinemia. Diagnostic criteria defined by the World Health Organization includes having a serum IgG level of <2 SD below normal, accompanied by variably low levels of other serum immunoglobulins and decreased specific antibody production.[14] Most patients with CVID have normal numbers of T and B cells, but the phenotype can be variable. CVID likely represents a group of disorders with variable age of onset and severity. In 1 series of patients, the average age at diagnosis was 25 years,[15] with a lag period of 4 to 6 years between the onset of symptoms and diagnosis. At least 10% of CVID cases are familial, with either autosomal dominant (AD) or autosomal recessive (AR) inheritance.[16] One subset of patients with CVID has mutations in the inducible T-cell costimlator gene (*ICOS*). This molecule is expressed on the surface of T cells, and its interaction with the ICOS ligand on B cells is important in antibody responses. ICOS deficiency is inherited as an AR defect, and patients with this deficiency have

Table 1.
Presentation of PIDD by infection site and organism

PIDD	Site of Infection	Organisms	Age at Onset
B cell defects: XLA, CVID, IgA deficiency, SAD IgG subclass deficiency, HIGM 2 and 3 syndromes	a. Lung, sinuses, ear b. Gastrointestinal tract c. Skin d. Sepsis/meningitis	a. Pyogenic bacteria: *Staphylococcus, S pneumoniae, H influenza, Mycoplasma* b. Enterovirus, *Giardia, Camplysbacter* c. *Staphylococcus* d. Pyogenic bacteria	Early onset: (after 6 months): XLA, HIGM1 and 2 syndromes Late onset (childhood, adolescence, young adult): CVID, HIGM2 and 3 syndromes, IgA deficiency, SAD, IgG subclass deficiency
T cell defects: DiGeorge Combined Defects SCID, HIGM1, WAS, NEMO, IPEX Other IFNγR deficiency, IL12 deficiency	a. Lung, sinuses b. GI tract c. Skin d. Sepsis	a. Bacterial, fungal, viral, opportunistic, mycobacteria b. Enterovirus, protozoa c. Bacterial, fungal, papilloma virus, HSV d. Epstein Barr virus, cytomegalovirus, herpes simplex virus, fungi, bacteria	Early onset (from birth): DGS, SCID, HIGM1, WAS Variable onset: NEMO, IPEX syndrome, IFNγR deficiency, IL12 deficiency, CMC/AIRE Late onset: ADA-deficiency
Phagocyte defects CGD, LAD1, congenital neutropenia	Lung GI tract Skin Lymph nodes Abscesses	Pyogenic bacteria (All) catalase positive bacteria (CGD) *Staphylococcus, Pseudomonas, Serratia, Aspergillus, Nocardia*	Early onset (from infancy): X-linked CGD, LAD1, congenital neutropenia Late onset: AR CGD, LAD1
Complement defects	Sepsis/bacteremia Meningitis	Encapsulated bacteria: *S pneumoniae, H influenza, N meningitidis*	Early onset: C1-C8, Alt pathway defects Late onset: partial defects, C9 deficiency, Mannose binding lectin deficiency

panhypogammaglobulinemia and impaired antibody responses to polysaccharide antigens.[17] Other patients with CVID have been found to have mutations in the gene for the transmembrane activator and CAML interactor (TACI), part of the tumor necrosis factor (TNF) receptor family. This genetic defect can be inherited in an AD or AR fashion. TACI is expressed on peripheral B cells and is important in the activation of B cells and specific antibody formation. The same mutation in TACI can result in CVID or IgA deficiency.[18,19] Data from large cohorts of patients with CVID show that mutations in TACI account for 8% to 10% of cases.[20]

Affected individuals have recurring infections of the sinuses, lungs, and gastrointestinal tract with bacterial pathogens such as *Streptococcus pneumoniae*, *Haemophilus influenzae*, *Moraxella catarrhalis*, *and Mycoplasma* sp. Recurring infections of the lungs frequently lead to the development of bronchiectasis and are a cause of significant morbidity and mortality in patients with CVID. In addition, autoimmune diseases occur in ~22% of patients with CVID.[21] The most common autoimmune diseases are immune thrombocytopenia (ITP), hemolytic anemia, arthritis, autoimmune hepatitis, and vasculitis. Arthritis caused by *Mycoplasma hominis* or *Ureaplasma urealyticum* responds well to gammaglobulin therapy and antibiotics. Infection of the gastrointestinal tract may be caused by *Campylobacter*, *Yersinia*, or *Giardia*. Lymphoid hyperplasia of the small bowel is frequently seen on radiographic studies (computed tomography, upper gastrointestinal series with small bowel follow-through) or endoscopy. Nonmalignant lymphoproliferative disease and granuloma formation occur in up to one third of patients with CVID.[15] Lymphoma occurs with a greater frequency in older individuals with CVID, particularly those who are female. Opportunistic infections occur infrequently in this disorder (<5%), and their presence indicates a significant defect in T-cell function.[21]

IgA Deficiency

Individuals with selective IgA deficiency, defined as a serum IgA level of <7 mg/dL, may be asymptomatic until adolescence; indeed, the majority of individuals with selective IgA deficiency do not have significant infections. IgA deficiency has been estimated to occur in 1 in 328 individuals on the basis of data from blood donors.[22] IgA deficiency is frequently associated with atopic disease, and individuals with the deficiency may have asthma that is difficult to control with standard treatment.[23] Recurring sinus disease is particularly troublesome for these patients, and many are subjected to multiple surgical procedures in an effort to cure their sinus disease. Some patients with IgA deficiency will have chronic or recurrent gastrointestinal infections, particularly with *G lamblia*, causing persistent diarrhea and even weight loss. IgA-deficient individuals are able to produce protective IgG antibodies against protein and polysaccharide antigens, and some may produce secretory monomeric IgM, which can provide some protection against infection.[23] As with other immunodeficiencies, autoimmune diseases are seen more frequently in IgA-deficient individuals. These diseases include arthritis, ITP, inflammatory bowel disease, hypothyroidism, and celiac(-like) disease.[23–26] One additional risk faced by these IgA-deficient individuals is anaphylactoid transfusion reactions caused by IgG antibodies in the patients' blood directed against IgA in the serum of the transfused product.[27,28]

Selective Antibody Deficiency/IgG Subclass Deficiency

Individuals with more lacunar defects, such as IgG2 subclass deficiency or a selective antibody deficiency (SAD), may not develop problems with recurring infections until later in childhood. These children have recurring respiratory infections despite having normal total serum immunoglobulin levels and normal responses to protein antigens such as tetanus toxoid. Deficiency of IgG subclasses can occur without a decrease in total serum IgG level. In IgG2 deficiency or SAD, infections of the respiratory tract with encapsulated bacteria such as *S pneumoniae* and *H influenzae* type b are the most prominent. These individuals do not meet clinical or laboratory criteria for CVID but generally have defects in antibody production against encapsulated organisms such as *S pneumoniae*. Recurring or chronic sinopulmonary infections start during childhood and continue through adolescence, long after the adolescent's peers have begun to be able to successfully defend themselves against these organisms.

IgG2 and IgG4 are the antibody isotypes formed in response to infection with polysaccharide-encapsulated organisms. Responses to protein antigens are intact, and cellular immune responses against viral pathogens are normal. IgG2 deficiency can occur alone or in combination with IgG4 or IgA deficiency. IgG2 production matures later than the other subclasses and does not reach adult levels until a child is 8–10 years of age, so a diagnosis of IgG2 subclass deficiency is difficult to make with certainty before 10 years of age. Selective IgG4 deficiency is rarely of any clinical significance.[29]

SAD is a distinct disorder with normal or increased serum immunoglobulins and intact antibody production to protein antigens. Immune responses to polysaccharide antigens, usually *S pneumoniae*, are absent or profoundly impaired.[30,31] Recurring or chronic sinus infections, purulent rhinitis, and otitis media occur most frequently. Bronchitis and pneumonia may be seen also. Individuals with SAD usually respond to extended courses of antibiotics but frequently undergo multiple surgical procedures in an attempt to resolve their sinus disease. Allergic disease may occur concurrently, but these patients do not develop autoimmune disease or other complications seen with CVID. Most individuals with SAD develop responses to pneumococcal vaccines at some point, so repeat assessment of antibody responses after immunization should be performed.[32] Occasionally, individuals will develop IgG subclass deficiency or CVID.

HIGM Types 2, 3, and 4 and Uracil-DNA Glycosylase Deficiency

These AR-inherited disorders are characterized by elevated levels of IgM with low levels of IgG and IgA. The underlying problem is a deficiency in CSR and somatic hypermutation (SHM) in B cells. CSR and SHM are the processes by which interaction with antigen-specific T cells causes gene recombination in the Ig heavy chain in B cells to generate specific IgG, IgA, or IgE antibodies (CSR) and point mutation in the variable regions of the Ig chains to create high-affinity antibody (SHM). In AR HIGM syndrome, T-cell responses are intact. HIGM2 syndrome is caused by a defect in activation-inducing cytidine deaminase,[33] HIGM3 syndrome is caused by the absence of CD40 on the surface of B cells,[34] and the defect in HIGM4 syndrome is unknown. HIGM syndrome with a deficiency of uracil-DNA glycosylase resembles HIGM2 and HIGM4.[35] The clinical phenotype in all forms of HIGM syndrome is recurrent pyogenic infections of the sinopulmonary and gastrointestinal tract, often with their onset in the second or third decade of life. Lymphonodular hyperplasia is frequently seen in this disorder. T-cell immunity is intact, and opportunistic infections are unusual except in HIGM3.

COMPLEMENT DEFECTS

Defects in other arms of the immune system, particularly phagocytes (neutrophils) and complement, also predispose individuals to recurring infection, although the pattern of infection is often different from that seen in patients with humoral immunodeficiencies. Patients with congenital complement deficiency are unusually susceptible to infection with encapsulated organisms such as *S pneumoniae*, *H influenza*, and *Neisseria meningitidis*. Complement is a serum protein, part of the innate immune system, which is activated during infection and results in the complement cascade and formation of the membrane-attack complex. Destruction of bacteria occurs through lysis mediated by the membrane-attack complex. There are 3 complement pathways: the classical, the alternative, and the lectin pathways.[36,37] Inherited or genetic defects in complement typically cause the absence of 1 component of a pathway leading to a complete lack of function. Nearly all are inherited in an AR fashion, with an estimated prevalence of 0.03%.[38] Defects in the classical or alternative pathway lead to infections (bacteremia, meningitis) occurring during the first few years of life, but there are many cases in which the onset of infections occurs during adolescence.[39] Complications of complement deficiency include systemic lupus erythematosus (SLE) and glomerulonephritis, which may have their onset during adolescence. Individuals with SLE should be screened for complement deficiency, because it occurs with much greater frequency in patients with deficiency. Ninety percent of C1q-deficient and 40% of C4-deficient patients will develop SLE.[40] Mannose-binding lectin deficiency is also seen more frequently in individuals with lupus and causes an increase in infections in these patients.[41] A complete deficiency of C3 or factor H results in membranous glomerulonephritis.[42,43]

PHAGOCYTIC DEFECTS

Chronic Granulomatous Disease

The presentation of a disorder may vary depending on the location of the genetic defect (X-linked versus AR) and the penetrance of the disorder (AD with variable penetrance [eg, CVID]). One example of this is chronic granulomatous disease (CGD), which results from the absence of 1 component of reduced nicotinamide-adenine dinucleotide phosphate oxidase. All affected individuals lack the ability to generate the superoxide anion radicals needed to kill certain catalase-positive bacteria such as *Staphylococcus aureus*, *Serratia*, *Pseudomonas cepacia* (*Burkholderia*), *Nocardia*, and *Aspergillus*.[44–46] Patients with the AR form of CGD, which accounts for 22% of patients with CGD, have a milder form of the disease than those with the X-linked form. In a report of 368 patients with CGD, 24% of them were diagnosed during late childhood and adolescence, and 10% were diagnosed after the age of 20 years.[47] In several series, the most frequent presenting infection is pneumonia, mostly caused by *Aspergillus*.[47–49] Abscesses (perirectal and liver) and suppurative adenitis are the next most frequent infections, followed by osteomyelitis, bacteremia, cellulitis, and meningitis.[47]

Cyclic Neutropenia

Cyclic neutropenia is an AD condition caused by a defect in neutrophil elastase 2, which causes cyclic fluctuations in neutrophil counts.[50] Periods of severe neutropenia occur every 14 to 30 days and can last for 3 to 10 days. During these periods patients may have fever, oral ulcers, lymphadenopathy, and skin lesions. Older patients and those with a milder phenotype may have recurring oral ulcers and chronic gingivitis leading to tooth loss. Bone marrow aspiration will show an arrest of granulocyte maturation during periods of neutropenia.

Leukocyte Adhesion Deficiency Type 1

Leukocyte adhesion deficiency type 1 (LAD1) is a defect in neutrophil migration caused by a lack of expression of the β_2-integrin common chain (CD18) on the surface of neutrophils. In this AR disorder, individuals with the severe phenotype have the early onset of severe infections, especially of the skin, characterized by the absence of pus and poor wound healing. Patients with the moderate phenotype of LAD1 have partial expression of CD18 on neutrophils and tend to have a milder clinical course. They are diagnosed later in life and usually present with severe periodontal disease, poor wound healing, and viral infections.[51]

Hyper-IgE Syndrome

Hyper-IgE syndrome (HIES), or Job's syndrome, is an AD PIDD characterized by severe recurrent *Staphylococcal* infections of the lungs and skin causing pneumatoceles and abscesses. These infections are accompanied by eczematous skin, coarse features, delayed shedding of the primary teeth, hyperextensibility, scoliosis, long bone fractures, eosinophilia, and an elevated IgE level. A clinical scoring system has been developed to aid in the diagnosis of this disorder.[52] Infections usually begin early in childhood. However, many of the clinical features are not seen until later; thus, the diagnosis of this disorder may be delayed into adolescence. AD HIES was previously classified as a phagocyte disorder, but the underlying immune defect was not known until recently. The discovery of a mutation in the intracellular signaling molecule STAT3[53] in patients with AD HIES will help further our understanding of this immunodeficiency and facilitate earlier diagnosis.

CELLULAR IMMUNE DEFECTS

DiGeorge/22q11.2 Deletion Syndrome

Patients with cellular immune defects (T-cell defects) generally present in infancy with severe viral, fungal, or opportunistic infections. Complete DiGeorge syndrome (DGS), which refers to patients with an absent thymus and a complete lack of functional T cells, fits this picture. Although diagnosis is frequently delayed in individuals with a mild phenotype, few infants with a complete absence of thymic tissue survive infancy without immune reconstitution. DGS, or 22q11.2 deletion syndrome (also known as velocardiofacial syndrome), affects between 1 in 3900 and 1 in 5600 live births.[54,55] The congenital abnormalities seen are the result of a field defect affecting midline structures. The phenotype can include conotruncal heart defects, hypoparathyroidism, thymic hypoplasia or aplasia, cleft palate, hypernasal speech, gastroesophageal reflux, hypothyroidism, vertebral anomalies, speech delay, learning disorders, and renal anomalies.[56,57] A microdeletion of 3.5 megabases in chromosome 22q11.2 is seen in up to 90% of patients with DGS.[58] Although an absent thymus is found in <1% of individuals with DGS, two thirds of patients have some degree of thymic defect.[59–61] Between 8% and 28% of the deletions are inherited from a parent,[56,57,62] and affected parents typically have a milder phenotype than their child and seldom have a significant immune defect.[58,63] Diagnosis of DGS/22q11 deletion syndrome is frequently delayed for children without a cardiac defect. Adolescents and older children may be diagnosed on the basis of characteristic facial features, speech abnormalities, hypernasal speech, and, occasionally, late-onset hypocalcemia. Individuals with thymic defects may have a reduced number of peripheral T cells, which remains consistent through childhood and adolescence.[64] The restricted T-cell repertoire and impaired T-cell regulatory function causes affected patients to have an increased risk of developing IgA deficiency and autoimmune diseases, particularly juvenile rheumatoid arthritis and ITP.[59,61,65,66]

Immune Dysregulation, Polyendocrinopathy, Enteropathy, X-linked

Some cellular defects affect the regulation of cellular immune responses but do not cause T-cell lymphopenia. The immune dysregulation, polyendocrinopathy, enteropathy, X-linked (IPEX) syndrome is caused by mutations in the gene for *FOXP3*, which result in a deficiency of regulatory T cells. The most common clinical features of IPEX are early onset of endocrinopathy, usually type 1 diabetes mellitus, eczematous dermatitis, chronic diarrhea caused by enteropathy, and recurrent infections with bacteria.[67] The clinical phenotype can vary depending on the location of the mutation, and milder variants may be diagnosed later in childhood and adolescence.

Other Cellular Defects

Adolescents who develop recurrent thrush, disseminated herpetic infections, or infections with cytomegalovirus or pneumocystis or other opportunistic organisms should have a thorough evaluation of their cellular immunity. The most common cause of an isolated deficiency in T-cell number or function in adolescents and adults is secondary to another infection, such as HIV, or because of immunosuppressive drug therapy for a malignancy or to prevent organ rejection after transplant. However, lymphopenia in adolescents and adults may be caused by an inherited deficiency of adenosine deaminase (ADA)[68] or idiopathic CD4 lymphopenia.[69] These disorders cause recurrent infections with bacteria and opportunistic organisms in adolescents and adults. Early-onset complete ADA deficiency accounts for 10% to 15% of cases of SCID, but in approximately one fifth of patients the defect leads to a severe but incomplete deficiency in ADA resulting in late-onset immunodeficiency, usually in the second or third decades of life.[70] Individuals develop recurrent respiratory infections leading to pulmonary insufficiency as well as other disorders of immunoregulation.

Interferon γ Receptor/Interleukin 12/Interleukin 12 Receptor Deficiency

Mutations in the interferon γ receptor (IFNγR) chains, interleukin (IL)12p40, and IL-12 receptor (IL-12R) β1 chain result in an increased susceptibility to nontuberculosis mycobacteria, herpes viruses (all), and *Salmonella* (IL-12 defects only). IFNγR deficiency can be inherited in an AD or AR fashion. The AD form has a milder phenotype, with the onset of atypical mycobacterial infections of the bones and lungs occurring later in childhood and adolescence. Infections with *Salmonella* and herpes viruses (cytomegalovirus, herpes simplex virus, varicella zoster virus) occur more frequently and are more severe in these patients. In the AD form of IFNγR deficiency, the extracellular domain of the IFNγR is present on the cell surface, but upregulation of IFNγ-induced genes does not occur because of the loss of intracellular signaling sites.[71] IL-12p40 and IL-12R deficiencies are inherited in an AR fashion. IL-12 signaling causes IFNγ secretion by T cells, so the clinical phenotype is very similar to that of IFNγR deficiency.[72,73]

Autoimmune Polyendocrinopathy Candidiasis Ectodermal Dystrophy Syndrome/Chronic Mucocutaneous Candidiasis

One clinical variant of chronic mucocutaneous candidiasis (CMC) is the autoimmune polyendocrinopathy candidiasis ectodermal dystrophy syndrome (APECED). APECED is caused by an AR-inherited defect in the autoimmune regulator (*AIRE*) gene.[74,75] Affected individuals have a variable onset of endocrinopathies, primarily hypoparathyroidism and/or adrenal insufficiency, but insulin-dependent diabetes mellitus, hypothyroidism, and hypogonadism may also occur. They frequently develop other autoimmune diseases such as ITP, hemolytic anemia, alopecia, vitiligo pernicious anemia, and chronic active hepatitis. The disease is characterized by recurring and persistent mucocutaneous infections with *Candida albicans*. Patients with late onset of the manifestations of the syndrome have a milder variant.[74] *AIRE* is expressed in some thymic epithelial cells and plays a critical role in immunotolerance and the negative selection of autoreactive T cells.[76] The immune defect is characterized by poor T-cell responses to candida. Serum immunoglobulins and specific antibody responses are usually normal early in the course of the disease.[77]

COMBINED DEFECTS

Nuclear Factor κB Essential Modulator Defects (NEMO)

In recent years, several new disorders with defective transcription factors have been described. The onset of infections and the pattern of infections are generally similar to those of other antibody deficiencies. However, frequently, these disorders are associated with other manifestations, and the severity of infection may depend on the location of the gene mutation.

Patients with a genetic mutation in *IKKG*, which causes inappropriate activation of nuclear factor κB (NF-κB)–mediated transcription, have immunodeficiency associated with ectodermal dysplasia (NF-κB essential modulator [NEMO]). There is an increased susceptibility to bacterial infections in infancy and childhood and mycobacterial infections in childhood and adolescence. In the classic phenotype of this X-linked disorder, the ectodermal dysplasia with hypohidrosis is accompanied by conical-shaped teeth.[78] Recently, individuals with NEMO defects lacking the ectodermal dysplasia have been described.[79] Individuals with NEMO defects have hypogammaglobulinemia, with low IgG and low or normal IgA levels, deficient specific antibody production to tetanus and other antigens, and impaired lymphocyte proliferation in response to antigen stimulation. Defects in NK cell activation and cytotoxicity are characteristic of NEMO defects.[78]

X-Linked Lymphoproliferative Disease

Fulminant infectious mononucleosis from uncontrolled B-cell lymphocytosis is the hallmark of X-linked lymphoproliferative disease (XLP), also known as

Purtilo or Duncan's disease.[80] The clinical picture is one of sudden onset of fever, hepatosplenomegaly, lymphocytosis, lymphadenopathy, and hematologic abnormalities. The median age of presentation is 3 to 4 years,[81] but up to 40% do not develop fulminant mononucleosis, so diagnosis may occur at any age. Most individuals have normal immune responses before Epstein-Barr virus infection, but up to 30% can have abnormal serum immunoglobulins or inverted CD4/CD8 ratios with median age of onset of 7 to 9 years. In some cases, patients with XLP have been diagnosed as having CVID or HIGM syndrome.[82] The fulminant form of XLP is frequently fatal. However, milder forms may be managed successfully with gammaglobulin replacement therapy. The risk of their developing lymphoma or nonmalignant lymphoproliferative disease is 200-fold greater than that of the general population.[83] A mutation in the *SH2D1A* gene on the X chromosome, which encodes for a signaling lymphocyte-activation molecule (SLAM)-binding protein (SAP), is responsible for the majority of cases.[84-86] Males with the XLP phenotype without mutations in *SH2D1A* have been described. Binding of SLAM molecules by SAP during infection with Epstein-Barr virus regulates lymphocyte proliferation, cytokine secretion, cytotoxicity, and antibody production.[81]

Other PIDDs typically classified as combined immunodeficiencies, such as SCID, Wiskott-Aldrich syndrome (WAS), ataxia telangiectasia, and XHIGM, uniformly present with illnesses in infancy and are not discussed further in this article.

DIAGNOSIS

Clinical

Primary immune defects should be suspected in older children and adolescents having an increased number of common infections (≥2 pneumonias within 5 years, ≥2 serious sinus infections within 1 year, >2 invasive bacterial infections), severe infections (organ abscesses, invasive infections), or infections with unusual or opportunistic organisms (*Burkholderia* pneumonia, *pneumocystis* pneumonia)[87] (Table 2). Clinical screening occurs when the clinician pursues additional evaluation on the basis of a clinical history of infection. Additional history features suggestive of a primary immune defect include recurring fevers, chronic diarrhea, weight loss, persistent lymphadenopathy, hepatosplenomegaly, persistent thrush, and a family history of primary immunodeficiency. The physical examination may yield signs of chronic infection (eg, lymphadenopathy or hepatosplenomegaly) or acute infection (eg, such as rales, otitis media, or lymphadenitis).[88] Associated signs of immunodeficiency syndromes include eczematous dermatitis, anhydrosis, thrombocytopenia, arthritis, lymphonodular hyperplasia of the intestines, granulomas in the lung, intestines, or skin, and pallor caused by anemia.[89] Figure 2 shows the 10 warning signs of primary immunodeficiency as proposed by the Jeffrey

Table 2
Clinical signs identified as having a high positive predictive value for PIDD[80]

Clinical signs of primary immunodeficiency in adolescents and adults
>2 pneumonias (chest radiograph proven)
>3 sinus infections requiring antibiotics
>1 hospitalization for treatment of an infection
Any opportunistic infection
Recurrent neisserial meningitis
A persistently abnormal white blood cell count (neutrophils or lymphocytes)
A family history of immunodeficiency
A congenital heart defect with an absent thymus

Modell Foundation, which provides reasonable guidelines for prompting the evaluation of an individual for a PIDD.

Laboratory

Laboratory evaluation of suspected primary immune defects is necessary to identify the underlying immune defect. Figure 3 shows a diagnostic algorithm for the evaluation of a patient with a suspected immunodeficiency according to the types of infections.[90] Patients with recurrent bacterial infections may have defects in humoral immunity (antibody production), neutrophils, or complement. Recurring viral infections or opportunistic infections may indicate a problem with T cells or cellular immunity.

Evaluation for humoral immunodeficiencies starts with a complete blood count (CBC) and differential, looking for leukopenia and lymphopenia, as well as anemia, which is associated with chronic disease, autoimmune disease, or blood loss from the gastrointestinal tract. Next, measurement of serum immunoglobulins (IgG, IgA, IgM, and IgE) will identify individuals with hypogammaglobulinemia. An elevated IgE level is usually a sign of atopic disease, but levels >5000 IU/mL with no symptoms of allergic disease may be seen in HIES. Normal serum immunoglobulin levels do not rule out a humoral immunodeficiency, so B-cell function should be assessed through the measurement of protective IgG antibodies after vaccination. Titers to protein antigens (tetanus, diphtheria, measles) and polysaccharide antigens (*H influenza*, *S pneumoniae*, and *meningococcus*) can be measured. It should be noted that the current immunization schedule in North America uses conjugate vaccines against these bacterial polysaccharides. The antibody production is, in effect, an immunologic response to a protein antigen and not a measure of responsiveness to polysaccharides or carbohydrate antigens. Children older than 2 years of age can be vaccinated by using polysaccharide vaccines for pneumococcus (23 valent) or meningococcus (4 serotypes). Low levels of antibody titers can be seen with vaccine failure, but titers naturally decrease over time. Protective levels of

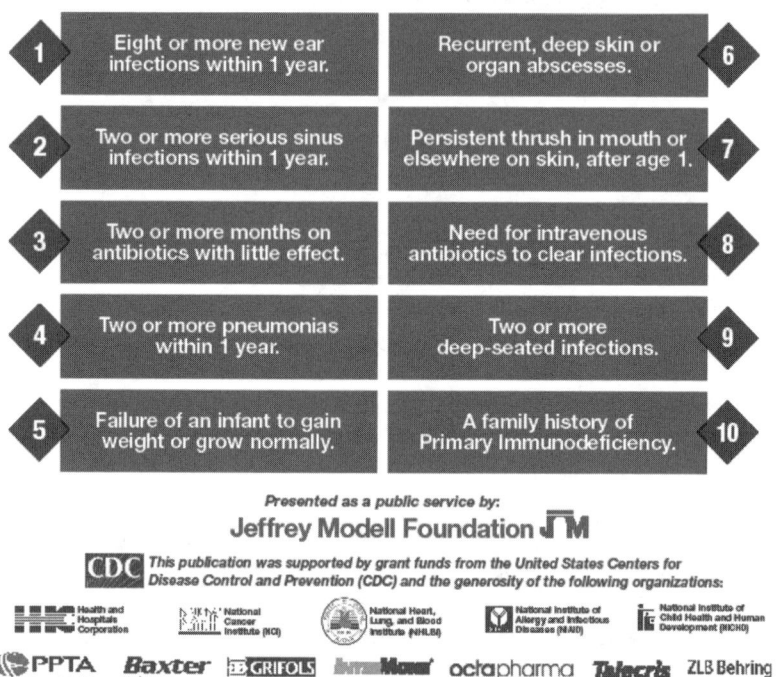

Fig 2. Ten warning signs of primary immunodeficiency. (Reprinted with permission from the Jeffrey Modell Foundation. 10 warning signs of primary immunodeficiency. Available at: www.info4pi.org/patienttopatient/pdf/10_warnings_poster_eng.pdf.)

antibody to many protein antigens are established by most reference laboratories. Postimmunization antibody titers of 1.3 μg/mL or 200 ng/mL are considered protective against *S pneumoniae*.[91] Normal children should have protective titers to all 7 serotypes in the Prevnar vaccine or 50% of the serotypes in the 23-valent polysaccharide vaccine.[92] Older adolescents and adults should mount a response to 70% of the serotypes in the polysaccharide vaccine.[32] If nonprotective antibody titers are found, patients should be revaccinated and titers repeated 3 to 4 weeks after vaccination. Other specialized tests for identifying specific B-cell

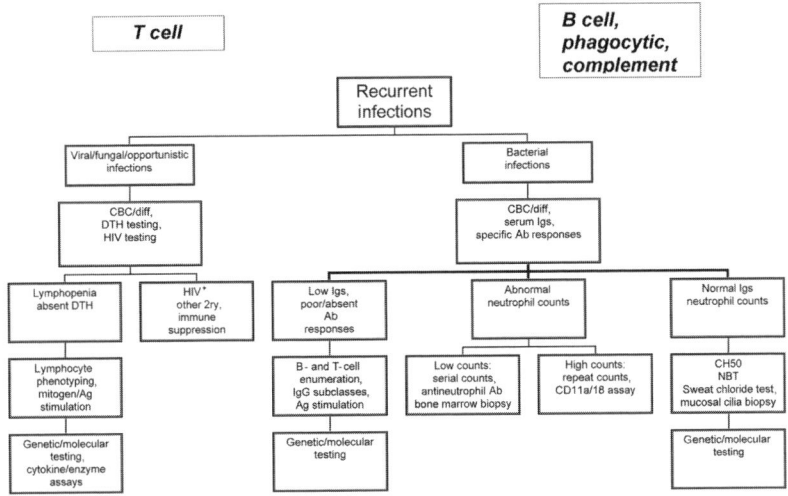

Fig 3. Algorithm for testing for suspected PIDDs. diff indicates differential; Igs, immunoglobulins; Ab, antibody; Ag, antigen; NBT, nitroblue tetrazolium.

defects include flow cytometry to measure the number of peripheral B cells and the number of memory B cells, enzyme-linked immunospot assays to evaluate secretion of immunoglobulin by peripheral B cells, and genetic testing to identify mutations in known genes associated with specific PIDDs (eg, *btk* on the X chromosome, TACI for CVID, *NFkB* for NEMO). In the absence of any humoral immune defect, other disorders such as cystic fibrosis or immotile cilia syndrome should be considered.

In cellular defects caused by T-cell disorders, lymphopenia is a frequent finding. Therefore, the presence of persistent lymphopenia on a CBC should prompt additional evaluation of T-cell number by flow cytometry and function. Normal absolute lymphocyte counts in older children and adolescents are comparable with normal values for adults. The majority of peripheral lymphocytes are T cells, and the proportion of T-helper (CD4) and T-suppressor (CD8) cells and the absolute number are easily measured by flow cytometry. Individuals with ADA deficiency will have low numbers of all lymphocytes, whereas defects that affect predominantly thymic function will cause low numbers of T cells, predominantly CD4 T cells. T-cell function can be assessed in vivo through the use of delayed-type hypersensitivity (DTH) responses to recall antigens such as tetanus toxoid or *C albicans*. In DTH testing, a small amount of antigen (0.1 mL) is placed intradermally and read at 48 hours in the same manner as purified protein derivative (PPD) testing. A normal response produces skin induration and erythema at the site. DTH testing may be attenuated by a lack of exposure (no previous vaccination) or treatment with immunosuppressive medications (eg, systemic steroids). In vitro assays measure proliferation of T lymphocytes after stimulation with a mitogen (a plant lectin such as pokeweed mitogen, phytohemagglutinin, or concavalin A) or an antigen (such as tetanus toxoid or *C albicans*). Measurement of specific antibody titers after vaccination is another measure to assess T-cell–B-cell interactions, because B cells require help from T cells for specific immunoglobulin production and isotype class switching to IgG or IgA antibodies. Additional testing may be performed to measure enzymes (ADA), other cell-surface proteins (Foxp3, SAP), intracellular cytokines (IL-2, IL-12, IFNγ), and cytokine receptors (IL-2R, IFNγR). Fluorescent in situ hybridization is used to identify a microdeletion in chromosome 22q11.2, which is associated with DGS. Gene sequencing may identify mutations in genes associated with specific cellular immunodeficiencies (ADA deficiency, XLP, NEMO defect, IPEX syndrome). Laboratory evaluation of NK cell defects includes flow-cytometry measurement of NK cell numbers and functional assays of NK cell killing of radiolabeled target cells.

Assessment of patients with a suspected neutrophil defect begins with a CBC with manual differential. Additional testing depends on the absolute neutrophil counts (ANCs). Patients with a low ANC require additional evaluation for cyclic neutropenia with biweekly measurements of ANCs. Diagnosis of autoimmune neutropenia requires measurement of antineutrophil antibodies. A persistently elevated ANC (usually >20 000 cells per μl) is characteristic of LAD1. Diagnosis of LAD1 is confirmed by demonstrating absent or decreased expression of CD11a and CD18 on the surface of neutrophils by flow cytometry. A normal ANC does not rule out a functional defect of neutrophils. Additional assessment should include measurement of the oxidative or respiratory burst through dye-reduction tests, either nitroblue tetrazolium or dihydrorhodamine. Both tests measure the ability of neutrophils to reduce a dye or fluorescent molecule after stimulation of the cells. Patients with X-linked CGD will demonstrate no response, whereas patients with AR CGD will have a markedly reduced response. Dihydrorhodamine is a more quantitative test than nitro blue tetrazolium and can be used to distinguish X-linked from AR CGD and to identify maternal carriers of the X-linked form.[93]

A CH_{50} (total hemolytic complement) is the only test needed to screen for complement defects in the classical and alternative pathways. This test measures the amount of serum needed to hemolyze 50% of target red blood cells and provides a quantitative measure of complement function. In congenital complement deficiency, the CH_{50} is 0, except in C9 deficiency, with which there may still be partial activity.[94] If the CH_{50} is 0, then the specific defect can be identified through measurement of individual complement levels, starting with C1q, C1r, C1s, and C2. The alternative complement pathway can be assessed by using an alternative hemolytic assay (AH_{50}). A normal CH_{50} but absent AH_{50} should prompt evaluation of terminal complement components, factor H, and factor I levels. As with other PIDDs, mutational analysis of the gene encoding the specific complement component can confirm the diagnosis.

Most of the first-line tests can be performed by a commercial clinical laboratory, either through the local hospital or commercial private laboratories. Because normal levels of immunoglobulins and lymphocytes vary with age, it is critical to obtain age-appropriate normal ranges. In addition, some tests require special handling to ensure the integrity of the test. The CH_{50} assay should be performed on plasma that has been frozen shortly after collection and not allowed to thaw until the assay is performed; otherwise, falsely low values will occur from consumption of the complement proteins. Tests of lymphocyte or neutrophil function require live cells that are kept at room temperature and received by the testing laboratory within 24 hours of collection. One challenge in assessing individuals with a suspected PIDD is that recurrent bacterial infections can occur with normal serum immunoglobulins and specific antibody production. If a strong clinical suspicion of a primary immunodeficiency remains, then evaluation by a clinical immunologist is warranted for more specialized testing.[92]

THERAPY

The mainstay of therapy for PIDD is to prevent infection to avoid end-organ damage and death. Current treatment modalities use replacement of immunoglobulins, antibiotics, and other agents to prevent infection; ultimately, however, reconstitution of the immune system either through hematopoietic stem cell transplantation (HSCT) or gene therapy is curative for many PIDDs. Table 3 summarizes the current therapies for various PIDD.

Humoral Immune Defects

Replacement of immunoglobulins through intravenous or subcutaneous administration is the mainstay of therapy for XLA, CVID, HIGM types 1 through 4, IgG2 subclass deficiency NEMO, and for some patients with SAD.[95] Gammaglobulin products contain >95% IgG collected from human plasma, which is further treated to kill viruses and other pathogens. There are numerous products available that differ in the viral inactivation steps and osmolality. Table 4 shows a comparison of the different γ-globulin products approved for use in the United States. Dosing for replacement of serum immunoglobulins is 400 mg/kg given every 3 to 4 weeks intravenously or 137 mg/kg given weekly by the subcutaneous route. Generally, serum trough IgG levels (for intravenous immunoglobulin) should be maintained at >500 mg/dL.[96] Higher doses may be beneficial for patients with chronic lung disease.[97] Gammaglobulin replacement is also used in several combined immunodeficiencies (WAS, ataxia telangiectasia, SCID) but is contraindicated for selective IgA deficiency. It may be used in patients with SAD and IgG subclass deficiency whose conditions have failed to respond to other therapies.[95]

Acute infections should be treated promptly with antibiotics. However, patients with repeated or chronic infections of the sinuses and lungs may benefit from

Table 3
Therapies for primary immunodeficiencies

Therapy	Antibody Deficiency	Cellular Deficiency	Combined Deficiency	Phagocyte Defect	Complement Deficiency
Antibiotics	Treatment/prophylaxis	Treatment/prophylaxis	Treatment/prophylaxis	Treatment/prophylaxis	Treatment/prophylaxis
Gammaglobulin	All except Sel IgA deficiency	Selected defects	All	NA	NA
IFNγ	No	IFNγR and IL-12 defects	No	CGD	No
Vaccination	Selected antibody deficiencies IgA deficiency	No live vaccines	No live vaccines	No live vaccines	Polysaccharide vaccines
Enzyme replacement	NA	NA	PEG-conjugated ADA	NA	NA
HSCT/BMT	HIGM1 syndrome, CVID (severe)	Thymus transplant (DGS), ADA deficiency	SCID, NEMO, WAS, XLP syndrome, IPEX	CGD, LAD1	No

NA indicates not applicable.

Table 4
Comparison of gammaglobulin products

Product	Form and Concentration, %	IgA Content	Viral Inactivation	Sugar Content	Osmolality/Osmolarity	Na Content
Carimune NF	Lyophilized 3%, 6%, 9%, or 12%	<720 μg/mL	pH 4, pepsin nanofiltration	Sucrose	384–690 mosM/kg	<20 mg/g
Flebogam	Liquid 5%	<50 μg/mL	S/D, pasteurization nanofiltration	Sorbitol	240–350 mosM/L	<3.2 mEq/L
Gammagard	Liquid 10%	<37 μg/mL	S/D, low pH, heat nanofiltration	None	240–300 mosM/kg	None
Gammagard S/D	Lyophilized 5% or 10%	<2.2 μg/mL	S/D	Glucose	636/1250 mosM/L	0.85%
Gamunex	Liquid 10%	46 μg/mL	Low pH, caprylate filtration	None	258 mosM/kg	Trace
Octagam	Liquid 5%	<100 μg/mL	S/D, low pH	Maltose	380 mosM/kg	<30 mmol/L
Polygam S/D	Lyophilized	<2.2 μg/mL	S/D	Glucose	636/1250 mosM/L	0.85%
Privigen	Liquid 10%	<25 μg/mL	Low pH depth filtration	None	320 mosM/kg	<5 mmol/L
Vivaglobin	Liquid 16%	1700 μg/mL	Pasteurization, low pH	None	440 mosM/kg	3 mg/mL

S/D indicates solvent/detergent.

chronic therapy with systemic or inhaled antibiotics. In patients with milder humoral immune defects (SAD, IgA, IgG subclass deficiency), prophylactic antibiotic therapy should be the initial therapy. Therapy of acute and chronic sinus disease should include saline lavage of the nose and mucolytics. Patients with bronchiectasis should have aggressive pulmonary treatments including postural drainage, inhaled antibiotics, and mucolytics. Pulmonary function should be monitored regularly, and symptomatic patients should have imaging to look for the development and monitor the progression of bronchiectasis. If disease is not controlled by aggressive medical therapy, consideration should be given to surgical interventions. For patients with CVID with impaired T-cell function, treatment with polyethylene glycol (PEG)-conjugated IL-2 has been shown to improve T-cell function.[98]

Those patients who have some ability to produce specific antibodies (CVID, SAD, IgG subclass and IgA deficiency) can benefit from vaccination to boost protective antibodies to respiratory pathogens such as *H influenza* and *S pneumoniae*, including yearly vaccination with the inactivated influenza vaccine. The pneumococcal conjugate vaccine should be given to older patients with poor responses to the 23-valent polysaccharide vaccine. Generally, vaccination with live vaccines is not recommended for patients with CVID, XLA, HIGM syndrome, NEMO defects, or combined immunodeficiencies.[92] Specific antibody titers should be monitored to help guide the practitioner in scheduling booster immunizations.

Cellular or Combined Immunodeficiencies

Because severe defects in cellular immunity generally lead to problems producing specific antibodies, replacement therapy with gammaglobulin (intravenous or subcutaneous) is used to help prevent infections. Antibiotic prophylaxis with trimethoprim/sulfamethoxazole or pentamidine against *Pneumocystis*, acyclovir against HSV, or gancyclovir against cytomegalovirus may be needed if T-cell numbers are low or proliferative responses are impaired. Treatment with systemic antifungal agents may be necessary to decrease infections with *Candida* and prevent fungemia. Live viral vaccines should not be used in any patient with a suspected cellular or combined immune defect. All blood products should be leukodepleted, cytomegalovirus-negative, and irradiated. Despite immunoglobulin replacement and prophylactic antibiotics, these patients will continue to have recurrent infections with a variety of bacterial and viral illnesses. Nearly all patients with primary cellular immune defects and most with combined immunodeficiencies will require immune reconstitution to correct their immunodeficiency. Immune reconstitution can be performed by using thymus transplantation for DGS or HSCT for SCID and other cellular/combined immunodeficiencies (HIGM syndrome, WAS, XLP). ADA deficiency may be treated by using PEG-conjugated ADA.[99,100]

Phagocyte Defects

Treatment of phagocyte defects is directed at treating the underlying defect. For cyclic neutropenia, granulocyte colony-stimulating factor can lead to normal or near-normal numbers of neutrophils, although many individuals improve spontaneously with age. HSCT or bone marrow transplantation (BMT) is the only corrective therapy for LAD1. However, individuals with a mild clinical variant may be managed with early and aggressive treatment of infections with antibiotics and intensive dental treatment to preserve dentition. For CGD, therapies are directed at improving host clearance of catalase-positive bacteria through the use of IFNγ injected subcutaneously 3 times per week, prophylactic trimethoprim/sulfamethoxazole, and itraconazole to prevent disease with *Aspergillus* sp.[101] A large, multicenter, placebo-controlled trial demonstrated a 70% reduction in severe infections for patients who were receiving IFNγ.[102,103] Treatment of infections should be aggressive, with prolonged intravenous antibiotic therapy. Identification of the causative organism is crucial for treating infections and may require open biopsy of the infected tissue to obtain a proper specimen. Debridement of abscesses is essential, and intralesional instillation of granulocytes has been used in the treatment of hepatic abscess.[104] In addition, leukocyte transfusions may be used for severe infections that do not respond to antibiotic therapy. In the past 10 years, an increasing number of patients with CGD have undergone HSCT or BMT with moderate success.[105,106] Transplantation usually requires the use of myeloablative regimens, and the risk of graft-versus-host disease remains high for haploidentical (half-matched) or matched unrelated-donor transplants.[107]

Complement Deficiency

Currently, replacement of individual components of the complement cascade is not possible. Long-term therapy is directed toward reducing the risk of infection either by repeat vaccination to obtain high levels of specific antibodies or by using prophylactic antibiotics. Individuals with complement deficiency should receive pneumococcal and meningococcal vaccines and have their titers checked at regular intervals. Older children and adolescents should be vaccinated with the 23-valent pneumococcal vaccine to provide protection to other serotypes not contained in the 7-valent conjugate vaccine. Because antibody titers seem to wane more rapidly in these patients, they should be reimmunized whenever titers fall below the protective range. Antibiotic prophylaxis may be more effective than immunization in preventing bacteremia. However, the emergence of resistant organisms, particularly pneumococcus, requires careful surveillance by the clinician.

IMMUNE RECONSTITUTION

Ultimately, the only curative therapies for PIDDs are HSCT/BMT or gene therapy. HSCT/BMT has been used to treat many PIDDs but is not generally a consideration for milder diseases such as IgA deficiency, SAD, IgG subclass deficiency, or XLA. In cellular/combined immune defects and phagocyte defects, HSCT/BMT is often the therapy of choice because of the limited success of treatment using antibiotics, cytokines, and gammaglobulins. HSCT/BMT therapy in all these disorders, except SCID, requires a myeloablative regimen, and the clinical course is frequently complicated by failure of engraftment, graft-versus-host disease, and infection. HSCT/BMT has been moderately successful in treating CGD, LAD1, ADA deficiency, HIGM1 syndrome, NEMO defects, IPEX syndrome, WAS, and XLP. Survival rates vary from 42% to 71%, depending on the donor and the underlying disorder.[108] Age at transplant and the type of donor are the most important variables affecting long-term engraftment and survival. Survival rates are best when the donor is an HLA-identical sibling. Fewer than 15% of patients have an HLA-identical sibling. In several centers, use of a matched unrelated donor has yielded better outcomes than using an HLA-mismatched relative.[107–110] The use of HSCT is limited in older populations because of active inflammatory states and chronic infections causing end-organ damage.

Because most PIDDs are caused by a single gene defect affecting hematopoietic cells, these disorders should be amenable to gene therapy. The target gene can be inserted into the host gene in peripheral or bone marrow stem cells by using a viral vector. The transfected stem cells are infused back into the patient where these corrected cells function to restore normal immune responses. Gene therapy has been successful in correcting the immune defects in patients with ADA deficiency[111] and X-linked SCID[112] and is under investigation for the treatment of CGD,[113,114] WAS,[115] and LAD.[116]

GENETIC COUNSELING

Molecular diagnosis is possible for many PIDDs. Because most of them are caused by single gene defects, genetic counseling should be offered to patients with PIDDs and their families. Even in CVID, in which only a small proportion of patients have an identifiable genetic defect, family members have an increased risk of developing CVID or selective IgA deficiency. Identification of the genetic defect allows for better genetic counseling, including the possibility of prenatal testing. In addition, siblings should be screened for the disorder. For PIDDs inherited in an AR fashion, the main concern is usually for future siblings. Affected patients should be informed that all their offspring will be carriers for the disease and that subsequent generations will have an increased risk of having affected offspring. The exact risks will depend on the frequency of the gene in the population. As with all AR-inherited disorders, the risk is increased for consanguineous partners. For X-linked disorders, all daughters of the affected individual will be carriers. For these women, the risk of having an affected child is 50% for male offspring.

CONCLUSIONS

The prevalence of PIDDs is likely much higher than previous estimates. These diseases may be even more prevalent than other inherited disorders such as cystic fibrosis. Newborn screening is now available for a multitude of inherited disorders and inborn errors, including cystic fibrosis. Presently, the only method of screening for PIDDs is through clinical evaluation. Because a large proportion of PIDDs will not present to the clinician until the patient is in late childhood or adolescence, a high level of clinical suspicion is needed to make a timely diagnosis. Early diagnosis and initiation of treatment will decrease the morbidity associated with these diseases and can result in an increase in life expectancy. Initiation of treatment early in the course of PIDDs has been shown to reduce health care costs overall and improve the quality of life for these patients. Genetic counseling is also important for addressing a critical issue for adolescents as they enter their reproductive years.

REFERENCES

1. Notarangelo L, Casanova JL, Fischer A, et al. Primary immunodeficiency diseases: an update. *J Allergy Clin Immunol.* 2004;114(3):677–687
2. Boyle JM, Buckley RH. Population prevalence of diagnosed primary immune deficiency in the United States. *J Clin Immunol.* 2007;27(5):497–502
3. Baumgart KW, Britton WJ, Kemp A, French M, Roberton D. The spectrum of primary immunodeficiency disorders in Australia. *J Allergy Clin Immunol.* 1997;100(3):415–423
4. Fasth A. Primary immunodeficiency disorders in Sweden: cases among children, 1974–1979. *J Clin Immunol.* 1982;2(2):86–92
5. Matamoros Florí N, Mila Llambi J, Español Boren T, Raga Borja S, Fontan Casariego G. Primary immunodeficiency syndrome in Spain: first report of the National Registry in Children and Adults. *J Clin Immunol.* 1997;17(4):333–339
6. Ryser O, Morrell A, Hitzig WH. Primary immunodeficiencies in Switzerland: first report of the national registry in adults and children. *J Clin Immunol.* 1988;8(6):479–485
7. Smith CIE, Ochs HD, Puck JM. Genetically determined immunodeficiency diseases: a perspective. In: Ochs HD, Smith CIE, Puck JM, eds. *Primary Immunodeficiency Diseases: A Molecular and Genetic Approach.* New York, NY: Oxford University Press; 1999:3–11
8. Stray-Pedersen A, Abrahamsen TG, Froland SS. Primary immunodeficiency diseases in Norway. *J Clin Immunol.* 2000;20(6):477–485
9. Stiehm ER, Ochs HD, Winkelstein JA. Immunodeficiency disorders: general considerations. In: Stiehm ER, Ochs HD, Winkelstein JA, eds. *Immunologic Disorders in Infants and Children.* Philadelphia, PA: Elsevier Saunders; 2004:289–355
10. Schur PH, Rosen F, Norman ME. Immunoglobulin subclasses in normal children. *Pediatr Res.* 1979;13(3):181–183
11. Allen RC, Armitage RJ, Conley ME, et al. CD40 ligand gene defects responsible for X-linked hyper-IgM syndrome. *Science.* 1993;259(5097):990–993
12. Aruffo A, Farrington M, Hollenbaugh D, et al. The CD40 ligand, gp39, is defective in activated T cells from patients with X-linked agammaglobulinemia, hyperIgM syndrome, and severe combined immunodeficiency in humans. *Cell.* 1993;72:291–300
13. Winkelstein JA, Marino MC, Lederman HM, et al. X-linked agammaglobulinemia: report on a United States registry of 201 patients. *Medicine (Baltimore).* 2006;85(4):193–202
14. Primary immunodeficiency diseases: report of a WHO scientific group. *Clin Exp Immunol.* 1997;109(suppl 1):1–28

15. Cunningham-Rundles C. Clinical and immunologic analyses of 103 patients with common variable immunodeficiency. *J Clin Immunol.* 1989;9(1):22-33
16. Hammarström L, Vorechovsky I, Webster D. Selective IgA deficiency (SIgAD) and common variable immunodeficiency (CVID). *Clin Exp Immunol.* 2000;120(2):225-231
17. Grimbacher B, Hutloff A, Schlesier M, et al. Homozygous loss of ICOS is associated with adult-onset common variable immunodeficiency. *Nat Immunol.* 2003;4(3):261-268
18. Castigli E, Wilson SA, Garibyan L, et al. TACI is mutant in common variable immunodeficiency and IgA deficiency. *Nat Genet.* 2005;37(8):829-834
19. Salzer U, Chapel HM, Webster AD, et al. Mutations in TNFRSF13B encoding TACI are associated with common variable immunodeficiency in humans. *Nat Genet.* 2005;37(8):820-828
20. Bacchelli C, Buckridge S, Thrasher A, Gaspar H. Translational mini-review series on immunodeficiency: molecular defects in common variable immunodeficiency. *Clin Exp Immunol.* 2007;149(3):401-409
21. Cunningham-Rundles C, Bodian C. Common variable immunodeficiency: clinical and immunological features of 248 patients. *Clin Immunol.* 1999;92(1):34-48
22. Clark JA, Callicoat PA, Brenner NA, Bradley CA, Smith DM Jr. Selective IgA deficiency in blood donors. *Am J Clin Pathol.* 1983;80(2):210-213
23. Ammann A, Hong R. Selective IgA deficiency: presentation of 30 cases and a review of the literature. *Medicine (Baltimore).* 1971;50(3):223-236
24. Heneghan MA, Stevens FM, Cryan EM, Warner RH, McCarthy CF. Celiac sprue and immunodeficiency states: a 25-year review. *J Clin Gastroenterol.* 1997;25(2):421-425
25. Schaffer FM, Monteiro RC, Volanakis JE, Cooper MD. IgA deficiency. *Immunodefic Rev.* 1991;3(1):15-44
26. Strober W, Sneller MC. IgA deficiency. *Ann Allergy.* 1991;66(5):363-375
27. Schmidt AP, Taswell HF, Gleich GJ. Anaphylactic transfusion reactions associated with anti-IgA antibody. *N Engl J Med.* 1969;280(4):188-193
28. Vyas GN, Perkins HA, Fudenburg HH. Anaphylactoid transfusion reactions associated with anti-IgA. *Lancet.* 1968;2(7563):312-315
29. Bird D, Duffy S, Isaacs D, Webster AD. Reference ranges for IgG subclasses in preschool children. *Arch Dis Child.* 1985;60(3):204-207
30. Herrod HG. Follow-up of pediatric patients with recurrent infection and mild serologic immune abnormalities. *Ann Allergy Asthma Immunol.* 1997;79(5):460-464
31. Sorensen RU, Moore C. Antibody deficiency syndromes. *Pediatr Clin North Am.* 2000;47(6):1225-1252
32. Hidalgo H, Moore C, Leiva LE, Sorensen RU. Preimmunization and postimmunization pneumococcal antibody titers in children with recurrent infections. *Ann Allergy Asthma Immunol.* 1996;76(4):341-346
33. Revy P, Muto T, Levy Y, et al. Activation-induced cytidine deaminase (AID) deficiency causes the autosomal recessive form of the hyper-IgM syndrome (HIGM2). *Cell.* 2000;102(5):565-575
34. Ferrari S, Giliani S, Insalaco A, et al. Mutations of *CD40* gene cause an autosomal recessive form of immunodeficiency with hyper IgM. *Proc Natl Acad Sci U S A.* 2001;98(22):12614-12619
35. Imai K, Slupphang G, Lee WI, et al. Human uracil-DNA glycosylase deficiency associated with profoundly impaired immunoglobulin class-switch recombination. *Nat Immunol.* 2003;4(10):1023-1028
36. Walport MJ. Complement: first of two parts. *N Engl J Med.* 2001;344(14):1058-1066
37. Walport MJ. Complement: second of two parts. *N Engl J Med.* 2001;344(15):1140-1144
38. Morley BJ, Walport MJ. *The Complement Facts Book.* San Diego, CA: Academic Press; 2000
39. Figueroa JE, Densen P. Infectious diseases associated with complement deficiencies. *Clin Microbiol Rev.* 1991;4(3):359-395
40. Pickering M, Walport MJ. Links between complement abnormalities and systemic lupus erythematosus. *Rheumatology (Oxford).* 2000;39(2):133-141

41. Kilpatrick DC. Mannan-binding lectin: clinical significance and applications. *Biochim Biophys Acta*. 2002;1572(2–3):401–413
42. Ault BH. Factor H and the pathogenesis of renal diseases. *Pediatr Nephrol*. 2000;14(10–11): 1045–1053
43. West CD, McAdams AJ. The alternative pathway C3 convertase and glomerular deposits. *Pediatr Nephrol*. 1999;13(5):448–453
44. Curnutte JT. Chronic granulomatous disease: the solving of a clinical riddle at the molecular level. *Clin Immunol Immunopathol*. 1993;67(3 pt 2):S2–S15
45. Evans TJ, Buttery LD, Carpenter A, Springall DR, Polak JM, Cohen J. Cytokine-treated human neutrophils contain inducible nitric oxide synthase that produces nitration of ingested bacteria. *Proc Natl Acad Sci U S A*. 1996;93(18):9553–9558
46. Klebanoff SJ. Role of the superoxide anion in the myeloperoxidase-mediated antimicrobial system. *J Biol Chem*. 1974;249(12):3724–3728
47. Winkelstein JA, Marino MC, Johnston RB Jr, et al. Chronic granulomatous disease: report on a national registry of 368 patients. *Medicine (Baltimore)*. 2000;79(3):155–169
48. Gallin JI, Buescher ES, Seligmann BE, Nath J, Gaither T, Katz P. Recent advances in chronic granulomatous disease. *Ann Intern Med*. 1983;99(5):657–674
49. Mouy R, Fischer A, Vilmer E, Seger R, Griscelli C. Incidence, severity and prevention of infections in chronic granulomatous disease. *J Pediatr*. 1989;114(4 pt 1):555–560
50. Horwitz M, Benson KF, Person RE, Aprikyan AG, Dale DC. Mutations in ELA2, encoding neutrophil elastase, define a 21-day biological clock in cyclic haematopoiesis. *Nat Genet*. 1999;23(4):433–436
51. Anderson DC, Schmalstieg FC, Finegold MJ, et al. The severe and moderate phenotypes of heritable Mac-1, LFA-1 deficiency: their quantitative definition and relation to leukocyte dysfunction and clinical features. *J Infect Dis*. 1985;152(4):668–689
52. Grimbacher B, Schäffer AA, Holland SM, et al. Genetic linkage of hyper-IgE syndrome to chromosome 4. *Am J Hum Genet*. 1999;65(3):735–744
53. Holland SM, DeLeo FR, Elloumi HZ, et al. STAT3 mutations in the hyper-IgE syndrome. *N Engl J Med*. 2007;357(16):1608–1619
54. Botto LD, May K, Fernhoff PM, et al. A population-based study of the 22q11.2 deletion: phenotype, incidence, and contribution to major birth defects in the population. *Pediatrics*. 2003;112(1 pt 1):101–107
55. Goodship J, Cross I, LiLing J, Wren C. A population study of chromosome 22q11 deletions in infancy. *Arch Dis Child*. 1998;79(4):348–351
56. McDonald-McGinn DM, Kirschner R, Goldmuntz E, et al. The Philadelphia story: the 22q11.2 deletion—report on 250 patients. *Genet Couns*. 1999;10(1):11–24
57. Ryan AK, Goodship JA, Wilson DI, et al. Spectrum of clinical features associated with interstitial chromosome 22q11 deletions: a European collaborative study. *J Med Genet*. 1997; 34(10):798–804
58. Kobrynski L, Sullivan K. Velocardiofacial syndrome, DiGeorge syndrome: the chromosome 22q11.2 deletion syndromes. *Lancet*. 2007;370(9596):1443–1452
59. Jawad AF, McDonald-McGinn DM, Zackai E, Sullivan KE. Immunologic features of chromosome 22q11.2 deletion syndrome (DiGeorge syndrome/velocardiofacial syndrome). *J Pediatr*. 2001;139(5):715–723
60. Kornfeld SJ, Zeffren B, Christodoulou CS, Day NK, Cawkwell G, Good RA. DiGeorge anomaly: a comparative study of the clinical and immunologic characteristics of patients positive and negative by fluorescence in situ hybridization. *J Allergy Clin Immunol*. 2000; 105(5):983–987
61. Sullivan KE, McDonald-McGinn D, Driscoll D, Emanuel BS, Zackai EH, Jawad AF. Longitudinal analysis of lymphocyte function and numbers in the first year of life in chromosome 22q11.2 deletion syndrome (DiGeorge syndrome/velocardiofacial syndrome). *Clin Diagn Lab Immunol*. 1999;6(6):906–911
62. Digilio MC, Marino B, Giannotti A, Dallapiccola B. Familial deletions of chromosome 22q11. *Am J Med Genet*. 1997;73(1):95–96

63. Leana-Cox J, Pangkanon S, Eanet KR, Curtin MS, Wulfsberg EA. Familial DiGeorge/velocardiofacial syndrome with deletions of chromosome area 22q11.2: report of five families with a review of the literature. *Am J Med Genet.* 1996;65(4):309–316
64. Chinen J, Rosenblatt HM, Smith EO, Shearer WT, Noroski LM. Long-term assessment of T-cell populations in DiGeorge syndrome. *J Allergy Clin Immunol.* 2003;111(3):573–579
66. Kanaya Y, Ohga S, Ikeda K, et al. Maturational alterations of peripheral T cell subsets and cytokine gene expression in 22q11.2 deletion syndrome. *Clin Exp Immunol.* 2006;144(1):85–93
65. Junker AK, Driscoll DA. Humoral immunity in DiGeorge syndrome. *J Pediatr.* 1995;127(2):231–237
67. Gambineri E, Torgerson TR, Ochs HD. Immune dysregulation, polyendocrinopathy, enteropathy, and X-linked inheritance (IPEX), a syndrome of systemic autoimmunity caused by mutations of FOXP3, a critical regulator of T-cell homeostasis. *Curr Opin Rheumatol.* 2003;15(4):430–435
68. Hirschhorn R. Immunodeficiency disease due to deficiency of adenosine deaminase. In: Ochs HD, Smith CIE, Puck JM, eds. *Primary Immunodeficiency Diseases: A Molecular and Genetic Approach.* New York, NY: Oxford; 1999:121–139
69. Tanaka S, Teraguchi M, Hasui M, Taniuchi S, Ikemoto Y, Kobayashi Y. Idiopathic Cd4+ T-lymphocytopenia in a boy with Down syndrome: report of a patient and a review of the literature. *Eur J Pediatr.* 2004;163(2):122–123
70. Shovlin CL, Simmonds HA, Fairbanks LD, et al. Adult onset immunodeficiency caused by inherited adenosine deaminase deficiency. *J Immunol.* 1994;153(5):2331–2339
71. Dorman SE, Uzel G, Roesler J, et al. Viral infections in interferon gamma receptor deficiency. *J Pediatr.* 1999;135(5):640–645
72. Altare F, Durandy A, Lammas D, et al. Impairment of mycobacterial immunity in human interleukin-12 receptor deficiency. *Science.* 1998;280(5368):1432–1435
73. de Jong R, Altare F, Haagen IA, et al. Severe mycobacterial and *Salmonella* infections in interleukin-12 receptor-deficient patients. *Science.* 1998;280(5368):1435–1438
74. Aaltonen J. The Finnish-German APECED consortium: an autoimmune disease, APECED, caused by mutations in a novel gene featuring two PHD-type zinc-finger domains. *Nat Genet.* 1997;17(4):399–403
75. Nagamine K, Peterson P, Scott HS, et al. Positional cloning of the APECED gene. *Nat Genet.* 1997;17(4):393–398
76. Notarangelo LD, Mazza C, Forino C, Mazzolari E, Buzi F. AIRE and immunological tolerance: insights from the study of autoimmune polyendocrinopathy candidiasis and ectodermal dystrophy. *Curr Opin Allergy Clin Immunol.* 2004;4(6):491–496
77. Kirkpatrick C. Chronic mucocutaneous candidiasis. *Pediatr Infect Dis J.* 2001;20(2):197–206
78. Orange J, Jain A, Ballas Z, Schneider L, Geha R, Bonilla F. The presentation and natural history of immunodeficiency caused by nuclear factor $\kappa\beta$ essential modulator mutation. *J Allergy Clin Immunol.* 2004;113(4):725–733
79. Niehues T, Reichenbach J, Neubert J, et al. Nuclear factor kappaB essential modulator-deficient child with immunodeficiency yet without anhidrotic ectodermal dysplasia. *J Allergy Clin Immunol.* 2004;114(6):1456–1462
80. Sullivan JL, Byron KS, Brewster FE, Baker SM, Ochs HD. X-linked lymphoproliferative syndrome: natural history of the immunodeficiency. *J Clin Invest.* 1983;71(6):1765–1778
81. Nichols KE, Ma CS, Cannons JL, Schwartzberg PL, Tangye SG. Molecular and cellular pathogenesis of X-linked lymphoproliferative disease. *Immunol Rev.* 2005;203:180–199
82. Grierson HL, Skare J, Hawk J, Pauza M, Purtilo DT. Immunoglobulin class and subclass deficiencies prior to Epstein-Barr virus infection in males with X-linked lymphoproliferative disease. *Am J Med Genet.* 1991;40(3):294–297
83. Grierson H, Purtilo DT. Epstein-Barr virus infections in males with X-linked lymphoproliferative syndrome. *Ann Intern Med.* 1987;106(4):538–545
84. Nichols KE, Harkin DP, Levitz S, et al. Inactivating mutations in an SH2 domain-encoding gene in X-linked lymphoproliferative syndrome. *Proc Natl Acad Sci U S A.* 1998;95(23):13765–13770

85. Coffey AJ, Brooksbank RA, Brandau O, et al. Host response to EBV infection in X-linked lymphoproliferative disease results from mutations in an SH2-domain encoding gene. *Nat Genet.* 1998;20(2):129–135
86. Sayos J, Wu C, Morra M, et al. The X-linked lymphoproliferative-disease gene product SAP regulates signals induced through the co-receptor SLAM. *Nature.* 1998;395(6701):462–469
87. Kobrynski L. Evaluation of a clinical scoring system for the identification of patients with a possible primary immunodeficiency. *Chem Immunol.* 1992;53:102–120
88. Yarmohammadi H, Estrella L, Doucette J, Cunningham-Rundles C. Recognizing primary immune deficiency in clinical practice. *Clin Vaccine Immunol.* 2006;13(3):329–332
89. Knight A, Cunningham-Rundles C. Inflammatory and autoimmune complications of common variable immune deficiency. *Autoimmun Rev.* 2006;5(2):156–159
90. Lindegren ML, Kobrynski L, Rasmussen S, et al. Applying public health strategies to primary immunodeficiency diseases: a potential approach to genetic disorder. *MMWR Recomm Rep.* 2004;53(RR-1):1–29
91. Sorensen RU, Leiva LE, Javier FC 3rd, et al. Influence of age on the response to *Streptococcus pneumoniae* vaccine in patients with recurrent infections and normal immunoglobulin concentrations. *J Allergy Clin Immunol.* 1998;102(2):215–221
92. Bonilla FA, Bernstein IL, Khan DA, et al. Practice parameter for the diagnosis and management of primary immunodeficiency [published correction appears in *Ann Allergy Asthma Immunol.* 2006;96(3):504]. *Ann Allergy Asthma Immunol.* 2005;94(5 suppl 1):S1–S63
93. Jirapongsananuruk O, Malech HL, Kuhns DB, et al. Diagnostic paradigm for evaluation of male patients with chronic granulomatous disease, based on the dihydrorhodamine 123 assay. *J Allergy Clin Immunol.* 2003;111(2):374–379
94. Giclas P. Complement tests. In: Rose N, Conway de Macario E, Fold J, Lane HC, Nakamura R, eds. *Manual of Clinical Laboratory Immunology.* Washington, DC: ASM Press; 1997:181–186
95. Orange JS, Hossny EM, Walker CR. Use of intravenous immunoglobulin in human disease: a review of evidence by members of the Primary Immunodeficiency Committee of the American Academy of Allergy, Asthma and Immunology. *J Allergy Clin Immunol.* 2006;117(4 suppl):S525–S553
96. NIH Consensus Conference. Intravenous immunoglobulin: prevention and treatment of disease. *JAMA.* 1990;264(24):3189–3193
97. Roifman CM, Lederman HM, Lavis S, Stein LD, Levison H, Gelfand EW. Benefit of intravenous IgG replacement in hypogammaglobulinemic patients with chronic sinopulmonary disease. *Am J Med.* 1985;79(2):171–174
98. Cunningham-Rundles C, Bodian C, Ochs HD, Martin S, Reiter-Wong M, Zhou Z. Long-term low dose IL-2 enhances immune function in common variable immunodeficiency. *Clin Immunol.* 2001;100(2):181–190
99. Hershfield MS, Buckley RH, Greenberg ML, et al. Treatment of adenosine deaminase deficiency with polyethylene glycol-modified adenosine deaminase. *N Engl J Med.* 1987;316(10):589–596
100. Hershfield MS. PEG-ADA: an alternative to haploidentical bone marrow transplantation and an adjunct to gene therapy for adenosine deaminase deficiency. *Hum Mutat.* 1995;5(2):107–112
101. Gallin JI, Alling DW, Malech HL. Itraconazole to prevent fungal infections in chronic granulomatous disease. *N Engl J Med.* 2003;348(24):2416–2422
102. Ezekowitz RA, Dinauer MC, Jaffe HS, Orkin SH, Newburger PE. Partial correction of the phagocyte defect in patients with X-linked chronic granulomatous disease by subcutaneous interferon gamma. *N Engl J Med.* 1988;319(3):146–151
103. International Chronic Granulomatous Disease Cooperative Study Group. A controlled trial of interferon gamma to prevent infection in chronic granulomatous disease. *N Engl J Med.* 1991;324(8):509–516
104. Lekstrom-Himes JA, Holland SM, DeCarlo ES, et al. Treatment with intralesional granulocyte instillations and interferon gamma for a patient with chronic granulomatous disease and multiple hepatic abscesses. *Clin Infect Dis.* 1994;19(4):770–773

105. Del Giudice I, Iori AP, Mengarelli A. Allogeneic stem cell transplant from HLA-identical sibling for chronic granulomatous disease and review of the literature. *Ann Hematol.* 2003; 82(3):189–192
106. Horwitz ME, Barrett AJ, Brown MR, et al. Treatment of chronic granulomatous disease with nonmyeloablative conditioning and T-cell-depleted hematopoietic allograft. *N Engl J Med.* 2001;344(12):881–888
107. Seger RA, Gungor T, Belohradsky BH, et al. Treatment of chronic granulomatous disease with myeloablative conditioning and an unmodified hemopoietic allograft: a survey of the European experience, 1985–2000. *Blood.* 2002;100(13):4344–4350
108. Antoine C, Friedrich W, Cant A, et al. Long term survival and hematopoietic stem-cell transplantation for immunodeficiencies: a survey of the European experience 1968–99. *Lancet.* 2003;361(9357):553–560
109. Filipovich AH, Stone JV, Tomany SC, et al. Impact of donor type on outcome of bone marrow transplantation for Wiskott-Aldrich syndrome: collaborative study of the International Bone Marrow Transplant Registry and the National Marrow Donor Program. *Blood.* 2001;97(6): 1598–1603
110. Fischer A, Landais P, Friedrich W, et al. Bone marrow transplantation (BMT) in Europe for primary immunodeficiencies other than severe combined immunodeficiency: a report from the European Group for BMT and the European Group for Immunodeficiency. *Blood.* 1994;83(4): 1149–1154
111. Aiuti A, Vai S, Mortellaro A. Immune reconstitution in ADA-SCID after PBL gene therapy and discontinuation of enzyme replacement. *Nat Med.* 2002;8(5):423–425
112. Cavazzana-Calvo M, Hacein-Bey S, de Saint Basile G, et al. Gene therapy of human severe combined immunodeficiency (SCID-X) disease. *Science.* 2000;288(5466):669–672
113. Malech HL, Horwitz ME, Linton GF, et al. Extended production of oxidase normal neutrophils in X-linked chronic granulomatous disease (CGD) following gene therapy with gp91 phox transduced CD34$^+$ cells [abstract]. *Blood.* 1998;92(11):690a
114. Ott MG, Seter R, Stein S, Siler U, Hoelzer D, Grez M. Advances in the treatment of chronic granulomatous disease by gene therapy. *Curr Gene Ther.* 2007;7(3):155–161
115. Charrier S, Dupré L, Scaramuzza S, et al. Lentiviral vectors targeting WASp expression to hematopoietic cells, efficiently transduce and correct cells from WAS patients. *Gene Ther.* 2007;14(5):415–428
116. Malech HL, Hickstein DD. Genetics, biology and clinical management of myeloid cell primary immune deficiencies: chronic granulomatous disease and leukocyte adhesion deficiency. *Curr Opin Hematol.* 2007;14(1):29–36

Drop-out Crisis Impacting America: Can We Turn It Around?

Joan K. Teach, PhD*

Community Resource Center, 4105 Briarcliff Road, NE, Atlanta, GA 30345, USA

If the mission of public schools is to produce students who are intellectually competent and who are prepared for postsecondary education and/or to enter the increasingly competitive workforce,[1] why was it estimated that 1.23 million high school seniors would fail to graduate in 2008?[2] This total indicates that 30% of our adolescents are predicted to attain a lower income than those with high school diplomas and are probably destined to a lack of success in later life. Our nation's schools are raising their standards, and more and more of our teenagers are being left behind. Lawmakers and education officials are gradually adding rigor to the task of earning a high school diploma. School systems are requiring exit examinations to assess academic and workplace-readiness standards. This results in an even higher percentage of high school students who leave before attaining a diploma. This is not to say that the additional rigor is not necessary, but companion programming should be put into place to ensure that all students have the opportunity to be successful according to their level of ability.

Although states vary considerably as to their specific policies, 3 categories of indicators are common throughout: (1) coursework credentials needed for graduation; (2) a definition of college and work readiness; and (3) whether to include an exit examination to prove competency. In an effort to analyze the situation and address the nation's drop-out crisis, the National Governors Association's Honor States Grant Program initiated the American Diploma Project. Their goal was to examine the states' efforts to forge stronger connections between precollegiate and postsecondary education. Councils were formed to investigate the success of students following them from pre-kindergarten through a 4 year college degree (a P-16 Council) or on through 8 years of post-secondary study and advanced degrees (a P-20 Council). They determined that by strengthening ties between school and postsecondary education and vocational training, more students could be successful in completing their journey and avoid many of the conflicts and situations that lead to quitting school.[2]

---

*Corresponding author.
E-mail address: joankteach@bellsouth.net (J. K. Teach).

Copyright © 2009 American Academy of Pediatrics. All rights reserved. ISSN 1934-4287

The P-16 councils are charged with exploring what is being done to close the gap between education and attainment and determining the discrepancy in requirements and expectations. They are to review early learning processes, graduation requirements, and teacher quality and analyze data systems that span from prekindergarten through college. Councils vary greatly in size, focus, and the frequency of their meetings. Participants are volunteers and include members from all levels of education, state government, and business and leaders of community organizations. They are committed to a 4-year project to study educational issues. The most recent data collected by the councils were reported in *Education Week* by a grant from the Bill and Melinda Gates Foundation.[3] Forty states now have operating councils, and more than 30 have acquired support from the business community (eg, chambers of commerce, workforce-development groups, and private foundations). Representatives of labor unions join civic leaders, parents, and local educators in a mission to help raise the public's awareness and understanding of the important issues in American education.

Research indicates that the national high school graduation rate is 70.6%, with 67.8% of boys and 75.2% of girls graduating. According to ethnicity, graduate rates are 50.6% for American-Indians/Alaska Natives, 81.3% for Asians/Pacific Islanders, 57.8% for Hispanics, 55.3% for non-Hispanic blacks, and 77.6% for non-Hispanic whites.[4] Graduation rates vary by state, with the lowest reported in Nevada (45.4%) and the highest in New Jersey (83.3%). US public high schools lose ~6830 students daily, and cumulative promotion index calculations show California topping the list with a loss of 900 students per day. With statistics like these, we are in dire need of improvement if we are truly to address our nation's youth and prepare them to be successful in today's workplace.

The Educate America Act of 1993 placed a goal of having a 90% high school graduation rate by the year 2000.[5] In 2008 our figures showed that we are still way behind. With rates as they stand now, we have a long way to go. In 2001, President George W. Bush reauthorized the Educate America Act with the No Child Left Behind Act of 2001 (Pub L 107-110).[6] This focus on education drafted a goal of every individual graduating by 2010. Congress appropriated an additional $10 billion to increase reading and academic-accountability programs. The No Child Left Behind Act also made schools accountable for the students in their states and required a yearly report on their success. To get a firm grasp on the whole situation, it is necessary to find a uniform accounting method to have equitable measures with standard accountability goals. Graduation policies are inconsistent and vary greatly between states.[2]

When a student is progressing through the system, it is often the case that, if encouraged to remain in school, a struggling learner will, with tutoring and agony, finish the course requirements only to find that he or she cannot pass the exit examination and receives only a certificate of attendance that is not accepted as a right of passage to any further educational endeavor. Only the most tenacious student sticks it out and tries again by sitting for the General Educational Development (GED) credential to get a full pass out of high school. Students need to be made aware that only the American Council on Education (ACE) can provide the General Educational Development Testing Service (the GED tests), it cannot be taken online, and those presented on the Internet may be neither truthful nor honest. It is our responsibility to make our young adults and teenagers aware of the reality of this situation. ACE's Web site will enable you to contact testing centers in your area.[7]

A compounding issue is that these same struggling students are often recommended for a track in an educational system that is designed to provide vocational skills, wherein there is no expectation for the student to earn a diploma. At times, the student and family do not fully understand the implication of the result of receiving a certificate of attendance, and they are trapped into accepting a dead-end street. It is no wonder that these students feel they have no potential to be successful, so they bail out and leave school. Even with the programs designed to provide immediate readiness to work when finishing high school, the system seldom coordinates their curriculum with the local community employers. The student, although a high school graduate, is neither work-site ready nor easily employable. Being unprepared is an even greater problem when seeking entry to college.[8] Educational systems struggle over defining what readiness for college really entails, and the councils are exploring what other skills beyond academics have to be addressed for students to become well-adjusted, economically stable, balanced, and successful adults.

We have a glimpse of a horizon that shows the impact of raising consciousness of these concerns. The state of Maine has instituted a statewide standard diploma for those whose special circumstances are out of the norm. According to this new state law, one can earn a Maine diploma to recognize academic achievement despite disruption in education because of medical issues or homelessness.[9] It is time to deal with the issue. The system we have been using as our educational format is not working efficiently, so we have to determine other ways to reach and teach our youngsters. What was good enough is no longer viable. We need to determine who is dropping out of the system and why.[10]

ANALYZING THE CRISIS

Why should we be so concerned that our youngsters are not completing high school? Students who leave school without earning their diploma are more likely to become adults who are caught in a cycle of poverty, underemployment, and social despair. As a nation we are losing tax revenue, at risk of having to have the welfare system provide for these individuals, and are destined to have a reduced economy because of their underproduction.[11] This then limits our communities' role as being in a competitive position in the technologically sophisticated global market. Our social dilemma disproportionately lies on the shoulders of the poor, ethnic minorities, and those for whom English is not their native language. Race and cultural background become relevant factors as we investigate the need to change.

The National Study Group for the Affirmative Development of Academic Ability[12] has called for strategies for closing the achievement gap. They cite an urgent concern that the black, Hispanic, and Native-American populations are severely underrepresented in the high-achieving student population. It is time to respond to the challenge to address our educational approach to the multicultural, multilingual, and disadvantaged student. It is recommended that affirmative development of academic ability be nurtured by providing high-quality teaching and appropriate and focused instruction in the classroom. A trusting relationship should be made from school to community, and community programs should be developed to address local needs. Students from these populations can become outstanding students when their specific learning styles are addressed. We need to enrich the curriculum and provide experiences and opportunities already available to their more affluent peers. Poor-quality instruction with low expectations for poorer children continues the cycle of despair and lack of prosperity.

Do the currently available intervention programs designed to help high-achieving minorities provide these students a curriculum that enables them to realize their potential? It has been shown that even if a minority student manages to make it through a high school career as an outstanding student, he or she remains at very high risk for not realizing his or her academic promise beyond graduation. Such students set their goals low, because they do not see a way out. Although 76% of students placed in gifted-and-talented programs are white, other groups are severely underrepresented, with only 7% black, 8% Hispanic, 6% Asian, and 0.09% Native-American in these programs. The language barrier for some students compounds the difference and reduces any chance that these students will be recognized for their intellectual gifts and abilities.[12]

Our Hispanic population is the fastest growing subgroup in America. Within 20 years, one fourth of our students will be Hispanic. This larger presence in the workforce will lead to a severely depressed economy if we do not address the needs of this population. Less than 60% of our Hispanic students currently graduate from high school; only 53% of Hispanic high school graduates enroll in college, and those who do so are more likely to enter a 2-year community college.[12] Those who are more successful come from a more socially and economically advantaged subgroup, live with both biological parents, have educated parents, and often attend private schools. These factors contribute to success, but the language barrier and cultural differences should be addressed to provide for and support those who do not have these additional advantages.

Gándara, in her report on the Latino education crisis,[13,14] challenged school systems to consider beginning strong cognitive enrichment programs early in children's lives. This culture includes a society that lives together, and with focused support we can break the cycle of substandard living and poverty. It is time to exploit the advantage of this rich language resource into a cultural and linguistic capital that assists the workplace and international community.

Factors that affect the success of others in the gifted-and-talented population include peer influence and family support. A positive approach from individuals positively affects a student remaining in school and sustaining academic excellence and supports self-esteem. Negative peer influences derail the student, as do parents who do not see educational achievement and success as a priority. Because of strong family influence and interaction, some of our gifted minority students are compelled to become family caretakers or wage earners. These situations lead them toward dropping out of school.[15] Distracting factors may also include boy/girl relationships, loneliness, outside responsibilities, financial need, lure of ready cash from jobs, and the loss of self-confidence.

EDUCATING THE DISABLED

Another issue that should be addressed is the failure of our educational system to adequately prepare our disabled students for academic or workplace success. Mainstream educational reformers are not focusing on the failure of public schools to improve learning and educational outcomes for unidentified poor learners. When the school creates a review of quality and effectiveness, it is usually only focused on general education practices. The educational skills required in the contemporary workplace are not identified.[16] These outcomes should be valued by our society and reflect expectations culturally explicit for the student to achieve. Social and academic issues should be addressed. Early and relevant vocational experiences need to be placed into the curriculum.

Too often, special-needs students do not see the relevance of the textbook information to their everyday life and cannot relate the instruction to their work goals. Schools should develop partnerships with the employers in their community, ascertaining from them what skill set they require for hiring and what behavior constructs are expected. Therefore, our curriculum should address basic academics such as reading, writing to communicate, and math and its related operations. However, additional skills, including listening, speaking, organizing ideas, and critical thinking, enable the student to make decisions, solve problems, implement, visualize, reason, and become a self-initiated learner. Students need to understand personal qualities such as effort and perseverance; interpersonal skills and a value of self-worth will enable them as adults to work well with others.[16] Educators who determine the list of skills that indicate workplace readiness should consider all of these issues.

Some of our students with learning disabilities and behavioral disorders have the ability and possess a drive to go to college.[17] We need to help them select a situation in which the experience will be positive, give them assistance with the transition, and guide them through the admission process. Special support systems may be needed to support their adaptive learning style.

The lifelong needs of learners with disabilities mandate the need to attend to the development of active and ongoing support systems. Educational outcomes, therefore, include literacy, self-dependence, social/behavioral stability, contributory citizenship, and personal feelings of satisfaction as well as physical and mental health. This satisfaction with the educational process stabilizes the individual and provides the basis of prevention of dropping out of school. Statistically, 22% of students with disabilities drop out of school compared with 12% of their nondisabled peers.[16,18]

It is true that schools cannot address all of this by themselves. Any intervention that addresses quality of student learning needs a comprehensive framework. Educational systems need to rely on a community of support from local businesses. The emphasis should be on academic retooling, redesign, and unique delivery of curriculum. The size of the instructional group needs to be reduced. Goals, content, instruction, and evaluation need to be aligned with the skills and needs of the individual learner. Classroom management practices should be examined. More critical research is needed to examine the factors and variables that influence a student's learning. Outcomes should be valuable and focused on realistic vocational skills, academic strengths, and understanding the ethic of the workplace. To date, few studies have reported this collaborative effect and its success toward student retention and workplace intervention.[19]

Students reporting in a focus group reported that they had failed to learn self-advocacy skills and that their families were very influential in all decisions, and they felt like they were on the outside looking in. The students knew that the parental involvement was positive but wanted to have more input into decision-making. However, the students were not interested in being decision-makers before their junior or senior year, but by that time they felt that they should be called upon to make more decisions about their present situation and have more input about their future.[15,17,20,21]

Many were dismayed when they found that their hard-earned diploma was, in reality, a certificate of attendance. Those who did graduate reflected that many of their disabled peers left because of frustration, had been unable to gain the academic help they needed, felt they were failures, and gave up. At the same time, this group of friends ran with the wrong crowd and often made choices with adverse outcomes (such as incarceration). Students in the study group reported they had little idea as to how to go about finding a job and feared they would not be successful. They related stories of receiving a lot of help, developing learned helplessness during their years in school and, therefore, expected family or friends to find a job for them. We need to find a way to increase the responsibility and decision-making of the late high school student and to include self-advocacy, planning, and social skills into the curriculum.[22] Appropriate ongoing support needs to be organized for these youngsters and be put into place before, not after, graduation.

Each time an additional factor is added to the mix, the risk of noncompletion of high school rises exponentially. Add language-processing difficulty, test anxiety, depression, graphomotor difficulty, visual spatial disorganization, and poor student-teacher interaction and the rate of early school failure increases dramatically.[16,18] Lapointe et al[23] studied teacher-student interaction and determined that the student's perception of a teacher's behavior plays a significant role in a student's self-efficacy, intrinsic value to the subject, and anxiety when dealing with mathematical subject matter. A lack of self-confidence reduces the will to work and lessens motivation while increasing the feeling that he or she cannot succeed.[24]

Teachers experience different motivational problems in the classroom that are identified by the 3 important components of academic learning: skill, will, and self-regulation. Students may not contribute in class because of lack of self-confidence and may limit their classroom participation because they find classroom norms and interaction different from their social or cultural experiences. Self-efficacy includes how one believes that he or she has the capacity to learn or perform behaviors at designated levels influencing academic motivation, learning, and achievement. Achievement depends on the interaction between one's behavior and personal factors. It affects task choice, effort, and persistence. No amount of self-efficacy will produce a competent performance when prerequisite skills and knowledge are lacking. Students do not engage in activities that they believe will lead to negative outcomes; therefore, motivation and self-efficacy are a self-fulfilling prophecy.[25]

Proactive intervention includes developing the student's positive self-esteem and self-awareness. Feelings of self-worth should accompany the feeling of competence and belief in oneself. Effective motivation comes through success.[26] In this way, the student interacts effectively with his or her environment and feels in control. Teacher feedback that encourages and emphasizes what the student can do well continues to build self-confidence. The earlier and the more positive the interaction develops, the more lasting the effect.[27] The earlier a disability is detected, the greater the chance that remediation can reduce school failure. Teacher interaction on the middle and high school levels is seen to be less positive and more critical. Family dynamics play an encouraging role when role models are positive, interactions and communication are solid, and economic stability exists. Stable intact families support stable student success.

Testing and test anxiety have been reported to be significant factors in academic failure, leading to dropping out of school.[28,29] Test anxiety is characterized by an individual's disposition to react with extensive worry, intrusive thoughts, mental disorganization, tension, and physiologic arousal when exposed to evaluative situations. The stress is typically evoked when individuals believe that their intellectual, motivational, and social capabilities and capacities are taxed or exceeded by demands stemming from themselves or significant others. Disabled students describe the anxiety as coming from a lack of ability. Gifted and talented students view the anxiety from an exterior point of view, believing that teachers and systems are out to challenge their intellect. When they fail, gifted students are prone to feel that the system is out to get them or that their intellect has, in fact, diminished.[30] It is important to ask what should be done to ensure that all students participate in a way that best reflects what they know and are able to do. Test anxiety leads to test failure, which often leads to grade retention.

The question then becomes, does grade retention increase learning potential and success? Zentall[18] reported that more than half of the children with attention-deficit/hyperactivity disorder (ADHD) who were taught in regular classrooms experienced at least 1 grade failure by adolescence. In response to increasing pressures to improve school performance, the call for an "end of social promotion" with emphasis on grade retention is more prevalent than ever.[31] In reverse, systematic reviews that have examined research over the past century concluded that the evidence does not support the use of grade retention as an intervention for academic achievement or socioemotional adjustment.[32] Retention at any grade level is associated with later high school dropout, as well as other deleterious long-term effects. When comparing retained students with similarly underachieving but promoted peers, research has indicated that retained students have lower levels of academic adjustment in 11th grade and are more likely to drop out of high school by the age of 19.[10] Retention was found to be one of the most powerful predictors of high school dropout, because retained students are 2 to 11 times more likely to drop out of high school than promoted students,[32] are less likely to receive a high school diploma by the age of 20, receive poorer educational competence ratings, and are less likely to be enrolled in postsecondary education of any kind. These youth also receive lower educational and employment status ratings and are paid less per hour at the age of 20.[10,31] Retained students experience lower self-esteem and lower rates of school attendance relative to promoted peers.[33] These students find considerable difficulty finding and maintaining employment at a level of self-sufficiency and experience higher rates of mental health problems, chemical abuse, and criminal activities than do high school graduates.

It is time to stop retaining and start interventions that are meaningful. Suggestions include dynamic remedial reading programs, diagnostic summer schools, and more direct teacher-to-student instruction. Tutoring, well-designed homework activities, and after-school programs have also been demonstrated to be beneficial. A coordinated system of comprehensive support services should be aimed at addressing the academic, socioemotional, behavioral, and psychological needs of the child. These programs should be designed to help promote healthy adjustment and achievement among children who are at risk for grade retention.[34]

SOCIOEMOTIONAL CONTRIBUTIONS

In adolescence, antisocial behavior and delinquency are clearly associated with underachievement. Influences become a unidirectional path as 1 domain influences another compounded by an overlap of externalizing problems.[35] Low socioeconomic status, family adversity, subaverage intelligence, language deficits, and neurodevelopment delay are all underlying factors. A child may display difficult temperament in infancy, oppositional behavior in preschool, and detrimental acting out in adolescence with externalizing behavior that leads to trouble with society and the law. The underlying problem may not be in the aggressive behavior itself but in frustration from language delays in preschool, early linguistic deficits, reading difficulties, possibly dyslexia, reading failure, academic problems, and/or cognitive reading difficulties, leading to behavior problems. There is an identifiable link between juvenile delinquency and cognitive achievement problems. Underachievement leads to externalizing behavior, frustration, lowered self- image, demoralization, lack of school attachment, and subsequent antisocial activity.

Aggression can also be correlated with paternal psychopathology, substance abuse, maternal antisocial behavior, and somatization. There is a complex interrelationship between child social understanding and early familial variables when looking at the development of both underachievement and behavioral difficulties.[36]

To be successful, youth with depression, anxiety, disruptive behavior, and other psychiatric disorders require skillful tuning of their strengths and capacities to available academic and vocational opportunities. We are experiencing a mental health issue as those who fail to complete secondary school earn less income, experience less home and work stability, and are more likely to require public assistance than secondary school completers. As the proportion of available unskilled jobs decreased from 60% to 15% since 1950, what is out there for those who are ill prepared for employment? What do we as a society do with the 42 000 adolescents with psychiatric disorders who cross the threshold into adulthood without completing secondary school?[36]

In their longitudinal study, Garnier et al[37] indicated that dropping out of school is a multiple determination process with early influences beginning in childhood, which involves family as well as child and adolescent factors. Dropping out has been seen as a process that occurs over time and is the result of a combination of individual, family, and school experiences rather than a single-risk event.

Other issues that beset our communities include those developing from the high prevalence of adolescent risk-taking behaviors. As adolescents experience normal rapid biological, emotional, cognitive, and social changes, they are led to a period of tremendous exploration and experimentation. Seeing themselves as invulnerable to accidents and disease, they engage in a wide range of risk-taking behaviors. With their lack of experience, they anticipate the benefit without understanding the immediate, long-term, or life-threatening consequences of their actions. Motor vehicle accidents, homicides, and suicides among adolescents are responsible for major medical, psychological, and social morbidity in teenagers. Teenagers' use of illicit substances has somewhat declined, but its use still continues to be high.

Sexual promiscuity is prevalent, which leads to a pervasive and destructive level of sexually transmitted diseases (STDs) that has been recorded at more than 20 million annually. AIDS surveillance data are incomplete as to the extent that symptomatic HIV infection actually originated in adolescence. Inner-city adolescents have higher rates of STDs than their suburban peers and often lack appropriate medical care. Screening, education, and care should be increased on all levels of our communities to avoid the pervasive destruction of our young people.[21,38]

Reflective of the increasingly high level of sexual activity, pregnancy rates remain high. Up to 84% of inner-city adolescent pregnancies are reported as being without prenatal care. An epidemiologic study of high school students in grades 9 through 12 indicated that 54% were engaging in intercourse, 39% within the last 3 months and 45% with more than 4 partners. Girls reported never or rarely using condoms, and many were not aware that latex condoms were effective in reducing the risk of STDs and HIV. Black women reported that they were more likely to use oral contraceptives, whereas middle class teenagers attending family planning clinics selected oral contraceptives or hormonal implants. Neither group relied on or were consistent in using condoms for contraception.[38]

DiClemente et al,[21] along with other researchers, have reported that parental monitoring was a significant influence on adolescents' health-risk behavior. Parental monitoring was described as parents who know with whom the adolescent associated and where they spent their time when not at home or school. The less a teenager perceived parental monitoring, the greater the participation in antisocial activities and the more sexual risk and substance use. Because black adolescent girls experience a disproportionately high risk for pregnancy, STDs, and HIV infection, inner-city parental monitoring needs to be encouraged. In this population, 70% reported mother monitoring, but only 1.3% felt that there was any father monitoring. Therefore, it is necessary to increase the awareness of parents of the impact of familial influences that become vital as a point of intervention to reduce risk behavior. Therefore, the goal is to enhance parent-child communication, foster close relationships, and promote better understanding. As single-parent households increase in number, the monitoring role is more and more important. Communities need to provide extended prosocial programs to enhance the social monitoring through youth-serving organizations, churches, community agencies, and extended school-based programs. Prosocial activities enhance adolescents' self-esteem while providing positive role modeling and additional supervision to avoid adverse juvenile consequences. We need the village to raise the child.

Counselors, physicians, and other social support systems can encourage these important family attributes. These systems require time and greater involvement, but the outcomes are highly beneficial. Glascoe[27] recommended that practitioners use a waiting-room questionnaire to be filled out by families once or twice a year. The families found the questionnaires helpful and not time intensive but, rather, the foundation for vital information of a preventative nature and vital for the care of their families. The Guidelines for Adolescent Preventive Services (GAPS)[39] recommended periodic parental counseling by the primary care clinician and provided readily available questionnaires for direct use. It is time to facilitate the adoption and broad delivery of these preventative services as well as for society to provide adequate systems for financial reimbursement to the provider.

INTERVENTIONS: DO THEY WORK?

Greenberg et al[40] challenged interventions to include a broader educational agenda that should also involve enhancing students' socioemotional competence, character, health, and civic engagement. The program should be person centered and give educational and interpersonal problem-solving training, as well as provide strategies for school environmental change. It should be structured with work experiences that teach a broad complexity of skills that transfer to the workplace.[41] Longitudinal studies should immediately be put into place to document the value of the outcome of any program.

Vallerand et al[42] determined that self-determination and persistence in real-life settings went a long way toward motivating high school students to avoid dropping out. Extrinsic motivation encourages someone to engage in an activity as a means to an end and initiates excitement and motivation to try. Drop-out students had lower levels of intrinsic motivation, identification, and introjections but higher levels of motivation toward school activities than persistent students. However, drop-out students perceived themselves as being less competent and autonomous in school activities and perceived their teachers, parents, and administration as less supportive. Motivation and self-determination, or the lack thereof, lead to important real-life outcomes such as staying in or dropping out of school and inhibit risk-taking behaviors to avoid negative consequences such as incarceration.

Preston[43] reported on the high cost of incarceration but also on the beneficial intervention found at the Missouri Youth Services Institute. In 2005, Mark

Steward undertook a complete makeover of this prison-like facility. The program divided the service units into smaller groupings and placed an emphasis on therapy and schooling. The rehabilitation intervention was not cheap, but it no longer showed its previously high recidivism rate. Prison guards began to play the role of youth development specialists and worked to turn the lives of these youth around. Because of the overall success of the program and its promise, replications have been started in Louisiana, New Mexico, Santa Clara County, California, and Washington, DC. There are many people who say they want to change the system and do something for these youngsters, but in reality, when the intervention starts to get tough and financially intensive, they bow out. The question then becomes, are we willing to put the time, energy, and resources into a major overhaul of an adolescent penal system that seems to be broken?

Stern et al[44] reported on the success of the earlier California Peninsula Academy program. Academies were established as schools within schools. The initiative was designed to help more students finish high school successfully. These academies focused on a particular occupational sector with representatives of local employers relevant to the occupational field. Students could apply for admission if they showed a record of poor attendance, had low grades, and had insufficient course credits. As a whole, students performed better than their matched peers, and their drop-out rate was reduced. Speculation was that smaller classes, more teacher attention, a focused curriculum, and relevant programming kept students engaged longer, made them more successful, and, therefore, provided an incentive for them to stay in school.

Communities in Schools (CIS)[44,45] is the nation's fifth largest youth-serving organization and the leading drop-out–prevention organization delivering resources to nearly 1 million students in 3250 schools across the country. To further their network-wide commitment to evidence-based practice, CIS collaborated with the National Dropout Prevention Center/Network at Clemson University to conduct a comprehensive study of the drop-out crisis. The CIS review found that rigorous data on the effectiveness of drop-out–prevention programs are particularly lacking. Effective programs were seen to use a combination of personal assets and skill building, academic support, family outreach, and environmental/organizational change. Programming design should come from evidence-based strategies proven to affect the risk factors they are trying to address. Research and valid evaluation programs need to be designed and implemented strategically to document research-based outcome.[34,35] The actual list can be attained through the NDPC/N-CIS Web site.[34]

The Chicago-based long-term study established that early childhood intervention for low-income children was associated with better educational and social outcomes at up to 20 years of age. These findings are among the strongest evidence that established programs administered through public schools can promote children's long-term success.[46,47]

The National Center on Secondary Education and Transition created a manual for policy-makers, administrators, and educators. Their goal (in the chapter "What Works in Dropout Prevention?") was to create a document designed to assist the transition from educational policy and research into practice.[48] They cited the success of the Career Academy 3-year program using academic-career–themed classes. Participants apply to the academy in their freshman year to enter into this school-within-a-school conceptualization.

The strengths of these academy programs lie in the typically small classes and enriched curriculum, in which students may hear guest speakers from local businesses or participate in field trips to nearby workplaces and colleges. In their junior year, students are matched with mentors from local employers who serve as career-related "big brothers and sisters." Students who are performing well enough to be on track for graduation are placed in summer or part-time school-year jobs. Students must submit résumés, complete applications, and participate in interviews as would any other job candidate. Participating companies are responsible for realistic hiring and firing decisions. Coming from typical inner-city settings, many program participants are black and Latino, are often from low-income families, and are likely to have poor attendance and grades. Students are recruited for participation but must apply and voluntarily attend.[49]

Teachers typically request to participate in the program and must be willing to work with other teachers and a group of students interested in the given career field. The teachers in each academy should have the same planning period and meet regularly to work on program activities and curriculum, coordinate with employer partners, meet with parents, and discuss student progress. It is a time-intensive position, but it is well rewarding.

The overall effectiveness indicates that career academies reduce the rate of school dropout and increase attendance, credits earned, grade-point averages, and graduation rates. One study also showed increased college attendance and completion rates in comparison with similar students from the same district when matched before academy entry.[50]

One longitudinal study that examined outcomes for 11 academy programs in California found that academy participants performed better overall than non-academy students. Of the 43 state-supported academies in California for the 1995–1996 school year, 42 demonstrated lower rates of school dropout and higher rates of attendance among the participants compared with nonparticipants. A longitudinal study of 10 academies found statistically significant gains in employment outcomes 4 years after high school.[10,51] Other pilot programs that are examining effectiveness include the Junior Reserve Officers Training Corps (JROTC) programs, which use the traditional career academy model,[52] the state of Georgia's intervention program for developing a graduation coach strategy,[53] and the Colorado charter schools act for at-risk for dropouts pilot schools, designed for students in grades 6 to 9 who are defined as being at risk.[54] Each program fulfils its own niche, addresses the at-risk problem in its own unique way, and yet joins in the compelling need to make a difference.

STEPS FOR SUCCESS

The National Education Association (NEA) believes that every child in America should attend a great public school. Well aware of the crisis we face in education, they unite to fulfill this promise. In January 2007, the NEA produced a monograph[55] outlining 12 action steps for reducing the nation's school drop-out rate.

1. It would be necessary to mandate high school graduation or its equivalent as compulsory for everyone below the age of 21 years.
2. High school graduation centers for students 19 to 21 years old need to be established to provide specialized instruction and counseling to all students in this older age group.
3. It will be necessary to make sure that students receive individual attention. Schools are to be safe, have smaller learning communities, and have smaller classes of 18 or fewer students. Auxiliary programs will need to be established to have before-school, after-school, summer, and weekend tutoring available when needed.
4. Graduation options for students need to be expanded. Partnerships with community colleges and in career and technical fields need to be developed to make the curriculum real and relevant. Alternative schools should be provided so that students have another way to earn a high school diploma. Incarcerated students need to have the appropriate resources for instruction and have high school graduation required as a factor of their release at the end of their sentence.
5. Programs must be developed to increase career education and workforce readiness. Students need to be able to see the connection between school and career. We must ensure that the skills for these careers are integrated into the curriculum. We need to increase all students access to and use of 21st-century technology.
6. We need to intervene early to prevent dropout. Developing high-quality, universal preschools, full-day kindergarten, and strong elementary school programs is vital. Students must be well prepared to enter middle school. Middle school programs that address the causes of drop out must be created. The school system must ensure that each child has a secure foundation for success in high school: algebra, science, and other courses must be provided. A secure foundation for studies beyond high school must be provided regardless of whether vocational or academic goals are considered.
7. A system must be created to ensure the involvement of families in their child's learning at school and at home. Families and single parents from poverty and minority communities all need support to enable them to help their children achieve academically, engage in healthy behaviors, and stay

actively involved in their child's education process from preschool through high school graduation and beyond.
8. Student academic progress must be monitored adequately. To monitor students' progress, the educational system should be required to provide a full picture of students' learning. Help must be provided by teachers to help students so that they do not fall behind academically.
9. A system of accurate reporting is necessary to monitor progress, intervene, and, therefore, work to reduce drop-out rates. Accurate data collection with common calculation formulas must be initiated and take into account the racial, ethnic, and economic makeup of the student body. Benchmarks in each state for eliminating dropouts should be realistic and standard. States should adopt the standardized reporting method developed by the National Governors Association.
10. The entire community should be involved in drop-out prevention. Family-friendly policies should be developed so that parents will have release time to attend parent-teacher conferences. Work schedules for high school students should be such that they can attend classes on time and be ready to learn. Adopt-a-school programs should encourage volunteers to link school and community. Projects should be designed to give students real-world learning experiences in the community.
11. Educators need to be provided the training and resources they need to prevent students from dropping out. Professional development should focus on the needs of a diverse student population. Techniques should be provided that addresses the needs of the students who are at risk of dropping out. Up-to-date textbooks and materials should be provided to everyone along with computers and access to information technology. We need to have safe, modern schools.
12. To make high school graduation a federal priority, it will be necessary to invest $10 billion over the next 10 years to support drop-out–prevention programs. We need to ensure that states make high school graduation compulsory and to enlist the services and support of Congress and the President of the United States to make sure this happens.[55]

INVESTING IN THE FUTURE

In review of the evidence already presented, the position of the NEA is strong: making high school graduation a national priority is long overdue. In addressing the plight of the million high school students who fail to graduate from high school every year, they call for a national priority to invest $10 billion within the next 10 years, with the first $1-billion appropriation beginning in fiscal year 2008.

Supporters of the plan have remarked:

> "Just as we established compulsory attendance to the age of 16 or 17 at the beginning of the 20th century, we must now eradicate the idea of

'dropping out' before you achieve your diploma," Reg Weaver, NEA President.[56]

Bruce S. Gordon, National Association for the Advancement of Colored People president, insists that "the plan ensures that educators have the training, tools and resources needed to provide a high-quality education and prevent students from dropping out."[56]

"We can't call high school reform successful if only half of the students benefit from increased rigor, because the other half don't graduate." Rep. Ruben Hinojosa, D-TX (NEA; www.nea.org).[56]

Work has begun, but we are far from the completion of a renovated and restructured educational system. We are still beset by this silent epidemic. Students dropping out of high school affect us all, socioemotionally and economically. It is time to put our money on the line and our energy in action and begin to make significant difference; only by working together for a common cause can we succeed.

REFERENCES

1. Bennett A, Bridglall BL, Cauce AM, et al. *All Students Reaching the Top: Strategies for Closing the Academic Achievement Gaps—A Report of the National Study Group for the Affirmative Development of Academic Ability* [monograph]. Naperville, IL: North Central Regional Educational Lab; 2004
2. Lloyd SC. States notch slow, steady progress toward consistent graduation goals [monograph]. Diplomas Count 2008: school to college. *Educ Week.* 2008;23(40):28–36
3. Hightower MM. State councils vary in form and focus [monograph]. Diplomas Count 2008: school to college. *Educ Week.* 2008;27(40):16–21
4. Callan PM, Kirst MW. Righting a troublesome "disjuncture": a push-pull strategy for P-16 cooperation [monograph]. Diplomas Count 2008: school to college. *Educ Week.* 2008;27(40): 3–4
5. Young MW. Countdown: the goals 2000—Educate America Act. *Phi Kappa Phi J.* 1993;73(4): 3–4
6. No Child Left Behind Act of 2001, Pub L No. 107-110 (2002), 115 stat 1425, 107th Congress, 1–670. Available at: www.ed.gov/policy/elsec/leg/esea02/107-110.pdf. Accessed February 11, 2009
7. American Council on Education. GED 2008. Available at: www.acenet.edu/AM/Template.cfm?Section=GEDTS&Template=/TaggedPage/TaggedPageDisplay.cfm&TPLID=58&ContentID=25659. Accessed August 1, 2008
8. Whitney-Thomas J, Hanley-Maxwell C. Packing the parachute: parents' experiences as their children prepare to leave high school. *Except Child.* 1996;63(1):75–87
9. Diploma Stakeholder recommendations: report to the Commissioner of Education, November 25, 2008. Available at: http://maine.gov/education/diploma/112508finalreport.pdf. Accessed February 11, 2009
10. Jimerson S, Egeland B, Sroufe L, Carlson. B. A prospective longitudinal study of high school dropouts examining multiple predictors across development. *J Sch Psychol.* 2000; 58(6):525–549
11. Doll B, Hess RS. Through a new lens: contemporary psychological perspectives on school completion and dropping out of high school. *Sch Psychol Q.* 2001;16(4):351–356

12. Orfield G. Race and schools: the need for action. UCLA research brief from the NEA Research Visiting Scholars Series. Spring 2008;1B. Available at: www.nea.org/home/ns/13054.htm. Accessed January 29, 2009
13. Gándara P. The crisis in the education of Latino students. UCLA research brief from the NEA Research Visiting Scholars Series. Spring 2008;1A. Available at: www.nea.org/home/17404.htm. Accessed January 29, 2009
14. Gándara P. *The Latino Education Crisis: The Consequences of Failed Social Policies*. Cambridge, MA: Harvard University Press; 2006
15. Morningstar MD, Turnbull AP, Turnbull III HR. What do students with disabilities tell us about the importance of family involvement in the transition from school to adult life? *Except Child.* 1995;62(3):249–260
16. Morrison GM, Cosden MA. Risk, resilience, and adjustment of individuals with learning disabilities. *Learn Disabil Q.* 1997;20(1):43–60
17. Rojewski JW. Educational and occupational aspirations of high school seniors with learning disabilities. *Except Child.* 1996;62(5):463–476
18. Zentall SS. Research on the educational effects of attention deficit hyperactivity disorder. *Except Child.* 1993;60(2):143–153
19. Cech SJ. P-16 councils bring all tiers of education to the table [monograph]. Diplomas Count 2008: school to college. *Educ Week.* 2008;27(40):6–9
20. Individuals With Disabilities Education Act, Pub L No. 94-142. Available at: www.scn.org/~bk269/94-142.html. Accessed June 8, 2008
21. DiClemente RJ, Wingood GM, Crosby R, et al. Parental monitoring: association with adolescents' risk behaviors. *Pediatrics.* 2001;107(6):1363–1368
22. Cheadle B. PL-94-142: what does it really say? Available at: www.nfb.org/images/nfb/Publications/fr/fr6/Issue1/f060113.html. Accessed June 8, 2008
23. Lapointe JM, Legault F, Batiste SJ. Teacher interpersonal behavior and adolescents' motivation in mathematics: a comparison of learning disabled, average, and talented students. *Int J Educ Res.* 2005;41(3):39–54
24. Dembo MJ, Eaton MJ. School learning and motivation. In: *Handbook of Academic Learning*. New York, NY: Academic Press; 1997:65–103
25. Schunk DH, Pajares F. The development of academic self-efficacy. In: *The Development of Achievement Motivation*. New York, NY: Academic Press: 2002:15–3
26. Skinner EA, Belmont MJ. Motivation in the classroom: reciprocal effects of teacher behavior and student engagement across the school year. *J Educ Psychol.* 1993;85(4):571–581
27. Glascoe FP. Evidence based approach to developmental and behavioral surveillance using parents' concerns. *Child Care Health Dev.* 1999;26(2):137–149
28. Wachelka D, Katz RC. Reducing test anxiety and improving academic self-esteem in high school and college students with learning disabilities. *J Behav Ther Exp Psychiatry.* 1999;30(3):191–198
29. Zeidner M. Test anxiety and aptitude test performance in an actual college admissions testing situation: temporal considerations. *Pers Individ Dif.* 1991;12(2):101–109
30. Thurlow ML, Johnson DR. High stake testing of students with disabilities. *J Teach Educ.* 2000;51(4):305–314
31. Jimerson SR. Meta-analysis of grade retention research: implications for practice in the 21st century. *School Psych Rev.* 2001;30(3):420–437
32. Jimerson SR, Anderson GE, Whipple AD. Winning the battle and losing the war: examining the relation between grade retention and dropping out of high school. *Psychol Sch.* 2002;39(4):441–457
33. Roderick M. Grade retention and school dropout: investigating the association. *Am Educ Res J.* 1994;31(4):729–759
34. Hammond C, Smink J, Drew S. *Dropout Risk Factors and Exemplary Programs: A Technical Report*. Clemson, NC: National Dropout Prevention Center; 2007. Available at: http://eric.ed.gov/ERICDocs/data/ericdocs2sql/content_storage_01/0000019b/80/29/91/0b.pdf. Accessed January 29, 2009

35. Hinshaw SP. Externalizing behavior problems and academic underachievement in childhood and adolescence: Causal relationships and underlying mechanisms. *Psychol Bull Am Psychol Assoc.* 1992;111(1):127–155
36. Stoep AV, Weiss NS, Kno ES, Cheney D, Cohen P. What proportion of failure to complete secondary school in the US population is attributable to adolescent psychiatric disorder? *J Behav Health Serv Res.* 2003;30(1):119–124
37. Garnier HE, Stein JA, Jacobs JK. The process of dropping out of high school: a 19-year perspective. *Am Educ Res J.* 1997;34(2):395–419
38. Boyer CB, Shafer MA, Shaffer RA, et al. Evaluation of a cognitive-behavioral, group, randomized controlled intervention trial to prevent sexually transmitted infections and unintended pregnancies in young women. *Prev Med.* 2005;40(4):420–431
39. American Medical Association. A GAPS approach to screening and health guidance for suicide and depression: Guidelines for Adolescent Preventive Services (GAPS). Available at: www.ama-assn.org/ama/pub/category/1980.html. Accessed July 28, 2008
40. Greenberg MT, Weissberg RP, O'Brien MU, et al. Enhancing school-based prevention and youth development through coordinated social, emotional, and academic learning. *Am Psychol.* 2003;58(6–7):466–474
41. Benz MR, Yavanoff P, Doren B. School to work components that predict post-school success for students with and without disabilities. *Except Child.* 1997;63(2):151–165
42. Vallerand RJ, Rortier MD, Guay F. Self-determination and persistence in a real-life setting: toward a motivational model of high school dropout. *J Pers Soc Psychol.* 1997;72(5):1161–1176
43. Preston C. Charity works to transform lives by transforming youth-correctional facilities. *Chron Philanthropy.* 2008;20(15). Available at: www.mysiconsulting.org/news/Chronicle%20of%20Philanthropy.pdf. Accessed January 29, 2009
44. Stern D, Dayton C, Paik IW, Weisberg A. Benefits and costs of dropout prevention in a high school program combining academic and vocational education: third-year results from replications of the California Peninsula Academies. *Educ Eval Policy Anal.* 1989;11(4):405–416
45. Supovitz J. *Building System Capacity for Improving High School Graduation Rates in California.* Santa Barbara, CA: UC Santa Barbara, Gevirtz Graduate School of Education; 2008. California Dropout Research Project report 9. Available at: www.lmri.ucsb.edu/dropouts/pubs_reports.htm. Accessed January 29, 2009
46. Reynolds AJ, Temple JA, Robertson DL, Mann EA. Long-term effects of an early childhood intervention on educational achievement and juvenile arrest: a 15-year follow-up of low-income children in public schools [published correction appears in *JAMA.* 2001;286(9):1026]. *JAMA.* 2001;285(18):2339–2346
47. Temple JA, Reynolds AJ, Miedel WT. Can early intervention prevent high school dropout? Evidence from the Chicago child-parent centers. *Urban Educ.* 2000;35(1):31–56
48. Lehr CA, Hansen A, Sinclair MF, Christenson SL. Moving beyond dropout towards school completion: An integrative review of data-based interventions. *School Psych Rev.* 2003;32(3):342–364
49. Clark P, Dayton C, Stern D, Tidyman S, Weisberg A. *Can Combining Academic and Career-Technical Education Improve High School Outcomes in California?* Santa Barbara, CA: UC Santa Barbara, Gevirtz Graduate School of Education; 2008. California Dropout Research Project report 4. Available at: www.lmri.ucsb.edu/dropouts/pubs_reports.htm. Accessed January 29, 2009
50. Belfield CR, Levin HM. *The Return on Investment for Improving California's High School Graduation Rate.* Santa Barbara, CA: UC Santa Barbara, Gevirtz Graduate School of Education; 2008. California Dropout Research Project report 2. Available at: www.lmri.ucsb.edu/dropouts/pubs_reports.htm. Accessed January 29, 2009
51. Lamb S. *Alternative Pathways to High School Graduation: An International Comparison.* Santa Barbara, CA: UC Santa Barbara, Gevirtz Graduate School of Education; 2008. California Dropout Research Project report 7. Available at: www.lmri.ucsb.edu/dropouts/pubs_reports.htm. Accessed January 29, 2009

52. Lehr CA, Hansen A, Sinclair MF, Christenson SL. Moving beyond dropout towards school completion: an integrative review of data-based interventions. *School Psych Rev.* 2003;22(1): 342–364
53. Jacox M. High school intervention program at Risley Learning Center, Performance Learning Center. Available at: http://helpdesk.glynn.k12.ga.us/goals/2007/rlcintervention.pdf. Accessed February 11, 2009
54. Marsh J, Hamilton L, Gill B. Assistance and accountability in externally managed schools: the case of Edison Schools, Inc. *Peabody J Educ.* 2008;83(3):423–458
55. National Education Association. NEA's 12-Point Action Plan for Reducing the School Dropout Rate. NEA monograph January 2007. Available at: www.nea.org/home/18106.htm. Accessed February 11, 2009
56. Jehlen A. The Dropout Directive NEATODAY, January 2007. Available at: www.nea.org/home/10586.htm. Accessed February 11, 2009

Adolescent Contraceptive Care for the Practicing Pediatrician

Kaiyti Duffy, MPH*[a], Yolanda Wimberly, MD, MSc[b], Chevon Brooks, MD[a]

[a]Physicians for Reproductive Choice and Health, 55 W. 39th Street, Suite 1001, New York, NY 10018

[b]Department of Pediatrics, Morehouse School of Medicine, 720 Westview Drive, SW, Atlanta, GA 30314

Adolescence is a time of many physical, mental, and emotional changes. Adolescents frequently experience new challenges as they develop their identities. In early adolescence, an interest in sexuality emerges. Although this is a normal part of human development, sexual behaviors place young people at risk for unintended pregnancy and sexually transmitted infections (STIs). Indeed, the United States maintains some of the highest teenaged pregnancy and STI rates in the industrialized world.[1] Currently, 750 000 teenagers become pregnant every year,[2] and 82% of these pregnancies are unintended.[3]

Although these numbers are still high, there have been significant declines in teenaged pregnancy rates in the past 2 decades. Between 1990 and 2004, the pregnancy rate for 15- to 19-year-olds dropped 38%, reaching a historic low of 72.2 per 1000. The most dramatic decrease (46%) occurred in pregnancy rates for 15- to 17-year-olds. Overall, pregnancy rates for black and white non-Hispanic teenagers declined 45% and 48%, respectively.[4]

In recent years, there has been much debate about how to address teenaged pregnancy. Most adolescent health experts agree that abstinence from sexual behavior is the most effective way to avert unintended reproductive health outcomes. However, data from the 2007 Youth Risk Behavior Survey demonstrate that by the 12th grade, 65% of US high school students have had sexual intercourse. Because a sexually active teenager who is not using contraception has a 90% chance of becoming pregnant within 1 year,[5] sexually active teenagers need contraceptive counseling and access to appropriate methods. There are data to show that contraception can play a pivotal role in preventing teenaged

*Corresponding author.
E-mail address: kaiyti@prch.org (K. Duffy).

pregnancy. A 2007 study showed that 86% of the decline in teenaged pregnancies was primarily a result of improved contraceptive use.[6]

MINORS' ABILITY TO CONSENT TO CONFIDENTIAL CONTRACEPTIVE CARE

Providers may have concerns about the laws surrounding contraception in their state and whether young patients need parental consent to initiate a method. Currently, 21 states[7] and the District of Columbia have laws that explicitly allow minors to consent to contraceptive services. Twenty-five[7] states permit minors to consent to contraceptive services under certain conditions such as a physician determining that contraception is in the best interest of the patient. Other conditions include being or having ever been pregnant or being married. Four states[7] have no explicit laws addressing minors and contraception. Therefore, the decision to administer contraception to a minor is left to the discretion of the provider and/or the institution.

Regardless of the state of residence, all minors can consent to confidential contraceptive care at Title X–funded clinics. The Title X program was established by Congress in 1970 to ensure affordable access to family planning and preventive health screening services for "all people desiring the service."[8] In 1978, Congress amended Title X to place "a special emphasis on preventing unwanted pregnancies among sexually active adolescents," adding services specifically for teenagers.[9]

DISCUSSING CONTRACEPTION WITH ADOLESCENTS

There are several factors to consider when helping a patient choose a contraceptive method. First, a provider must assess the readiness of the patient. Is she ready to start on birth control? How committed is she to staying with a birth control regimen? Other considerations include the frequency of administration. Does she prefer daily, weekly, or quarterly administration? Does she have personal preferences and biases toward certain methods? Does she have an aversion to pills or shots? A provider must also take into account the patient's health history and whether certain methods would hinder or help her current conditions. Does she have any contraindications to estrogen or progesterone? Will she benefit from methods with estrogen? Finally, when counseling a patient on contraception, providers need to consider efficacy, convenience, cost, ease of use, confidentiality, noncontraceptive benefits, and the adverse-effect profile in relation to the teenager.

Because a sexually active young woman's risk of pregnancy is so great, providers should make every attempt to facilitate contraceptive initiation. A full gynecologic examination may deter a young woman from seeking contraception, therefore increasing her risk of pregnancy. Recent protocols assert that asymptomatic adolescents need not receive a pelvic examination before initiating a hormonal contraception method.[10] In most cases, an inspection of the external genitalia and either a urine screen or a vaginal swab for STIs may be substituted for a pelvic examination.[11]

Before initiating any form of hormonal contraception, adolescents should be counseled that these agents do not protect against STIs. Consistent condom contraceptive use is necessary for preventing disease. Providers can use models to ensure that their teenaged patients are able to correctly put on and take off a condom. There is some evidence that these messages are getting across. According to the National Survey of Family Growth, 1.6% of females who had their first sex before 1980 used both a condom and another method. Seventeen percent of females whose first sex was between 1999 and 2002 reported dual use.[12]

Conventional hormonal contraception initiation instructions require waiting until after menses to begin the method. Although there is no clinical evidence that any hormonal contraception adversely affects a developing fetus,[13] this measure is intended to rule out an existing pregnancy. However, stipulating that initiation can only occur within this small window requires a young woman to return for another appointment and to abstain from sexual intercourse or to use barrier methods of contraception in the interim. For a substantial number of women, this increases her risk of unintended pregnancy.[14] Increasingly in recent years, providers have been starting young women on contraception on the day of their visit. Commonly referred to as "quick start," this method has been shown to improve compliance while maintaining a good safety and adverse-effect profile.[15,16] In a recent randomized study of young women aged 14 to 26 years, receiving the first injection of Depo-Provera (DMPA) (Pfizer, New York, NY) at the conclusion of their first visit (known as Depo Now) was associated with improved adherence to DMPA continuation and fewer pregnancies.[17]

If a young woman's menses occurred more than 5 days before the day of the visit, providers should assess the last time that unprotected sex occurred and obtain a pregnancy test. If unprotected sex occurred within 5 days, patients should be given emergency contraception (EC). In previous studies, ~3% of patients were found to be pregnant after their DMPA injection was started as a quick start.[18-20] These data support the need for a 21-day follow-up after quick-start initiation with any contraceptive method. Therefore, providers must discuss the risk of pregnancy and the necessity of the return visit with all patients. To increase the likelihood that young women will return for this visit, providers can develop internal office protocols to facilitate a 21-day return visit such as follow-up telephone calls or text-message reminders.

EMERGENCY CONTRACEPTION

Regardless of the method chosen, all patients should be counseled about the availability of EC and given advanced prescription with refills.[21] Contrary to common misconception, research shows that advanced prescription of EC does not increase sexual or contraceptive risk-taking behavior.[22,23] EC provides women with a second chance to prevent pregnancy after contraceptive delay or failure. Although most effective the sooner it is taken, EC can prevent pregnancy within 5 days of unprotected sex.[24] EC is not an abortifacient and will not disrupt an existing pregnancy, and it will not have any adverse affect on the fetus. Currently, the only designated product is Plan B (Barr Pharmaceuticals, Montvale, NJ), a levonorgestrel-only regimen consisting of 2 doses of 0.75 mg of levonorgestrel. Providers should advise patients to take both doses at the same time to improve compliance. Several other brands of oral contraceptive pills (OCPs) can be used successfully as EC, but dosing depends on the specific formulation.

When discussing EC with patients, providers should stress that the regimen must be taken after each act of unprotected sex. Taking EC once in a month does not provide protection for the entire month. EC can also be obtained over the counter at most major pharmacies to persons aged 18 and older. Prices vary between $38 and $50. Because cost can be a deterrent to EC use, providers should discuss with patients how they will pay for the pills and, if possible, direct them to a location that dispenses EC for free.

ORAL CONTRACEPTIVE PILLS

OCPs are the most frequent choice for adolescent girls. Of the 3.1 million teenaged girls who use contraceptives, more than half (53%) use the pill.[25] In the past several decades, many changes have occurred in OCPs, increasing their noncontraceptive benefits and reducing adverse effects, making this option more appealing to all women, especially teenagers. There are 3 main types of OCPs currently available: monophasic formulations, in which each pill contains same dose of estrogen and progestin; multiphasic formulations, which vary the dosages of estrogen and progestin; and progestin-only pills. In combined pills, ethinyl estradiol is most commonly the estrogenic compound, with doses ranging from 20 to 50 μg per pill, although a few of the newer pills contain >35 μg of estrogen. There are 8 types of progestins used in OCPs that are classified according to pharmacology and generation. The estrane family, also called first-generation progestins, includes norethindrone and other progestin drugs that metabolize to norethindrone. The gonane family consists of second- and third-generation progestins. The second-generation progestins include levonorgestrel and norgestrel and possess varying degrees of androgenic and estrogenic properties. The third-generation progestins have the least androgenic effects and include desogestrel and norgestimate.[26] Dropirenone is a fourth-generation progestin. Unlike the others, this progestin is derived from 17a-spirolactone, not from 19-nortetosterone.[27]

In May 2001, the US Food and Drug Administration (FDA) approved the first OCP to use the fourth-generation progestin drospirenone (Yasmin 28 [Bayer

HealthCare Pharmaceuticals, Montville, NJ]).[28] This is a monophasic formulation containing 30 μg of ethinyl estradiol and 3 mg of drospirenone. A little more than 5 years later, the FDA approved a contraceptive pill (Yaz [Bayer HealthCare Pharmaceuticals]) containing 20 μg of ethinyl estradiol and 3 mg of drospirenone.[29] Yaz includes 24 active pills and only 4 placebo pills to offer patients fewer hormonal fluctuations. This drug regimen has also been approved by the FDA for treatment of premenstrual dysphoric disorder[30] and acne.[31] Another 24-day active hormonal regimen containing 0.02 mg of norethindrone acetate and 1 mg of ethinyl estradiol plus 4 iron-containing placebo pills was approved in 2006 (Loestrin 24 Fe [Warner Chilcott Pharmaceuticals, Rockaway, NJ]).[32] The advantage of having 24 days of active pills and 3 days of placebo is the decrease in the number of days for menses and the alleviation of symptoms associated with premenstrual syndrome. This method will also eliminate symptoms related to estrogen withdrawal (such as headaches) during the placebo phase of the 28-day regimen.

In 2003, the FDA approved the first 91-day (84 days of active pills followed by 7 days of placebo) oral-contraceptive regimen that reduces or eliminates a monthly withdrawal bleed (Seasonale [Barr Pharmaceuticals]).[33] This regimen contains 0.15 mg of levonorgestrel and 0.03 mg of ethinyl estradiol. Under the dosing regimen, the number of expected menstrual periods that a woman usually experiences is reduced from once per month to approximately once every 3 months. As with the conventional 28-day regimen, women will have their period while taking the placebo tablets. Although users of this method report fewer scheduled menstrual cycles, data from clinical trials have shown that many women, especially in the first few cycles of use, had more unplanned bleeding and spotting between the expected menstrual periods than women taking a conventional 28-day cycle oral contraceptive.[34] To lessen the frequency of breakthrough bleeding, another extended-cycle pill was developed that replaced the week of placebo with 7 days of low-dose ethinyl estradiol. Approved by the FDA in May 2006 (Seasonique [Barr Pharmaceuticals]), this regimen consists of 84 levonorgestrel (0.15-mg) and ethinyl estradiol (0.03-mg) pills and 7 ethinyl estradiol (0.01-mg) pills. The latest extended-cycle pill was approved by the FDA in May 2007 (Lybrel [Wyeth Pharmaceuticals, Madison, NJ]).[35] Containing 90 μg of levonorgestrel and 20 μg of ethinyl estradiol, this regimen is designed to have no placebo interval in an effort to stop menses completely.

Primarily, combined oral contraceptives (COCs) prevent pregnancy by suppressing ovulation. They do this by inhibiting the production of both follicle-stimulating hormone and luteinizing hormone.[36] The progestins in COCs provide secondary mechanisms that include altering the cervical mucus to prevent sperm penetration.[37] When used correctly and consistently, the failure rate for COCs is less than 1%, but because the pill requires daily maintenance, efficacy rates for typical use are ~3% in adults (Table 1).[27] Failure rates in adolescents range from

Table 1
Percentage of women experiencing an unintended pregnancy during the first year of typical use and first year of perfect use of contraception, and the percentage continuing use at the end of the first year. United States

Method	Women Experiencing an Unintended Pregnancy Within the First Year Use, % Typical Use	Perfect Use	Women Continuing Use at 1 y, %	Cost, $
None	85	85	NA	NA
Spermicides	29	18	42	7.00–18.00 per container; 0.25 per use
Withdrawal	27	4	43	NA
Fertility awareness based	25	NA	51	NA
Standard-days method	NA	5	NA	
2-d method	NA	4	NA	
Ovulation method	NA	3	NA	
Sponge				2.00–5.00 each
Parous women	32	20	46	
Nulliparous women	16	9	57	
Diaphragm	16	6	57	25.00–45.00
Condom				
Female (Reality)	21	5	49	2.50–5.00 each
Male	15	2	53	0.20–2.50 each
Combined pill and progestin only pill	8	0.3	68	30.00–50.00/mo
Ortho-Evra patch	8	0.3	68	50.00/mo
NuvaRing	8	0.3	68	50.00/mo
DMPA	3	0.3	56	60.00–75.00 for quarterly injection plus the cost of the visit
IUD				
ParaGard	0.8	0.6	78	250.00–300.00 every 10 y
Mirena	0.2	0.2	80	300.00–400.00 every 5 y
Implanon	0.05	0.05	84	300.00–350.00 every 3 y

NA indicates not applicable
Data source: Trussell J. Contraceptive Efficacy, Safety, and Personal Considerations. In: Hatcher RA, Trussell J, Nelson A, Cates W, Stewart F, Kowal D, eds. *Contraceptive Technology*. 19th revised ed. New York, NY: Ardent Media; 2007:24

5% to 25%, mainly because of noncompliance.[38,39] Research indicates that only 33% of adolescents are still adherent after 1 year of use.[40]

Most healthy women are potential candidates for COCs. There are a few World Health Organization (WHO) category 3 conditions[41] for which COCs are usually not used unless there are no other contraceptive methods available and/or acceptable because of the increased risk of complications. Women with these complications include those who are <21 days' postpartum or lactating (6 weeks to 6 months), have gallbladder disease, are on medications that may interfere with OCP efficacy, or have undiagnosed abnormal vaginal/uterine bleeding.

Women who have WHO category 4 conditions are advised against COC use. These conditions include a current or past history of deep vein thrombosis or pulmonary embolism, cerebrovascular accident, or coronary (or ischemic) heart disease, complicated structural heart disease (eg, pulmonary hypertension, atrial fibrillation, or history of subacute bacterial endocarditis), pregnancy, lactation <6 weeks' postpartum, complicated diabetes mellitus (eg, retinopathy, neuropathy, nephropathy), breast cancer, headaches (including migraine headaches) with focal neurologic symptoms, liver disease (including liver cancer, benign hepatic adenoma, active viral hepatitis, severe cirrhosis), surgery involving the lower extremities, and/or prolonged immobilization and severe hypertension (≥160/≥100 mm Hg or with vascular complications).

COCs have many noncontraceptive benefits. Primarily, they alleviate menstrual disturbances. Studies have shown COCs to substantially decrease dysmenorrhea, menstrual blood loss,[42] premenstrual syndrome,[43,44] and anovulatory bleeding.[45] In addition, COCs are associated with a reduction in risk for ovarian and endometrial cancer and benign breast conditions. Particularly important for adolescents, COCs can reduce the incidence of acne. Although only 3 formulations (Yaz, Ortho Tri-Cylcen [Ortho-McNeil-Janssen Pharmaceuticals, Inc, Raritan, NJ], and Estrostep [Warner Chilcott Pharmaceuticals]) were specifically approved by the FDA for this purpose, many other formulations have also been shown to improve acne.[46]

When discussing contraception options with teenagers, it is important to address some of the disadvantages of COCs, including the need for daily maintenance, a monthly prescription, and the possibility of having a pill pack discovered by a parent or partner. The high cost of birth control pills may also be a deterrent to some youth. Trade-name pills cost approximately $50, and generic pills cost approximately $30 for those without insurance or prescription coverage for pills. In addition, providers should discuss all possible adverse effects and adverse events associated with COCs, because these are often listed as reasons for discontinuation. During the first 3 months of use, some women may experience menstrual irregularities, nausea, mood swings, breast tenderness, and/or headache.[47] It is important to discuss these possible adverse effects before initiation to increase compliance. Although often a concern for adolescents, well-controlled studies have not associated weight gain with COC use.[48] Very rare but serious adverse effects are also possible with COC use, although they are even rarer in healthy, younger women. These effects include venous thromboembolism (this risk is greatest for women with clotting disorders and a family history of thrombosis), myocardial infarction, breast cancer, and stroke.[27]

When providing counseling, health care professionals should stress that adverse effects are often transient and may last for ~2 to 3 months. If they persist, there are many other formulations and hormonal methods from which to choose. Providers can also help young women develop a schedule to facilitate daily adherence. Setting a daily alarm on a cell phone is an effective mean as a reminder for some. Patients should be counseled that missed pills are most risky in the beginning and at the end of a hormonal cycle and, if >2 consecutive pills are missed in any cycle, an additional method should be used.

TRANSDERMAL PATCH

The transdermal patch (Ortho Evra [Ortho-McNeil-Janssen Pharmaceuticals, Inc]) is a thin, beige, 20-cm^2 plastic patch that includes an outer protective layer, a middle medicated adhesive layer, and a clear liner. Each patch contains 6.00 mg of norelgestromin and 0.75 mg of ethinyl estradiol and releases 159 μg of norelgestromin and 20 μg of ethinyl estradiol daily. The patch can be applied to the buttocks, upper arm, lower abdomen, or upper torso but not to the breasts. A new patch is applied once per week followed by 1 week off.

In clinical trials, failure rates for the patch were similar to those of COCs: 0.3% with perfect use and 8% with typical use.[49] Because the patch requires weekly, not daily, maintenance, compliance rates with younger women are higher. One study of 50 adolescents found that 87.1% of the participants reported perfect compliance.[50] In addition, the method is forgiving of delayed patch reapplication. Hormone levels remain active for at least 9 days after application of a second patch, suggesting that ovulation would be inhibited with a delay of at least 2 days.[51] Data regarding the noncontraceptive benefits of the patch are not yet available. Yet, because the patch has similar mechanisms of action and hormonal levels as COCs, this suggests that the noncontraceptive benefits will also be similar.[49]

Although clinical data have shown that the patch adheres to the skin well in the general population, detachment rates are much higher for adolescents. One 3-month study of adolescents revealed that participants experienced a 35.5% rate of complete or partial detachment of at least 1 patch.[51] Teenagers may also have concerns about lack of privacy because partners or parents can discover the patch. Additional disadvantages of this method include skin irritation or rash at the site of application, breast tenderness, headache, and nausea. Limited evidence also suggests that the patch may be less effective for women who weigh >198 lb.[52] Although data are limited, patch users may also face some of the rare but serious health complications associated with COCs.[49]

Concerns have arisen about the safety of the transdermal patch, because this method contains 60% more estrogen than 35-μg pills.[53] On September 20, 2006, the FDA announced that the Ortho Evra patch was getting new labeling with more information on the risk of nonfatal blood clots associated with the patch. The label change added information from 2 conflicting observational studies about clotting risk in women using the patch versus OCPs containing 35 µg of estrogen. The first study examined a database of 200 000 women and looked at the risk of heart attack, stroke, and venous thromboembolic events in first-time users of the patch. The authors concluded that the risk of nonfatal venous thromboembolic events for women taking the contraceptive patch is similar to the risk for those taking oral contraceptives containing 35 µg of ethinyl estradiol and norgestimate.[54] The second study compared the combined risk of heart attack, stroke, and blood clots in the legs or lungs in women using the patch and women taking COCs. The study found that the risk for heart attack and stroke in women using the patch occurred too rarely to ascertain precise risk estimates, but users had approximately double the risk of blood clots as the woman taking the pills.[55]

When counseling young people about this method, it is essential to place these risks within context. Although given tremendous media attention in recent years, these adverse events are extremely rare, especially for young, healthy women. If, however, a patient has lingering concerns about these risks, other methods are available.

VAGINAL CONTRACEPTIVE RING

The vaginal contraceptive ring (NuvaRing [Schering-Plough, Kenilworth, NJ]) is a soft, flexible ring made of ethylene vinyl acetate copolymer with an outer diameter measuring 54 mm and the cross-sectional diameter measuring 4 mm. Approved by the FDA in 2001,[56] the ring releases 120 µg of etonogestrel and 15 µg of ethinyl estradiol directly into the vaginal wall. It is designed to emulate the cycle of the 28-day pill packs. Each ring is inserted into the vagina for 21 days and removed for 7 days to allow for a withdrawal bleed.[57]

With perfect use in adult women, the ring has similar efficacy rates as COCs.[58] Because the ring is so new, there have been no studies completed to assess failure rates with typical use in the adolescent population. A recent trial did show that compliance rates for ring use are high (91%),[59] which could suggest that typical-use failure rates will be lower than those of COCs.[27]

In addition to being low maintenance and private, this method has several other advantages. The ring is easy to insert, comfortable to use, and easy to remove. Although 28% of women and 42% of partners reported being able to feel the ring at times, this did not affect its acceptability with users.[59] In addition, this method is forgiving of delayed ring replacement and may remain effective for up to 2 weeks if a woman forgets to remove or replace the device. Noncontraceptive benefits of the ring are most likely similar to COCs. Adverse effects are also similar to other low-dose combined hormonal methods and include breast tenderness, headaches, nausea, and some breakthrough bleeding/spotting and an increased risk of the more serious condition of thrombotic events. Method-specific adverse effects may include vaginal symptoms of discharge, discomfort, and device problems.[49]

The vaginal ring may be an excellent choice for adolescents who are initiating contraception. Providers should assess a young woman's comfort with self-removal and insertion and stress that it will become more comfortable with time.

INJECTABLE CONTRACEPTION

DMPA is a progestin-only injectable contraceptive containing depot medroxyprogesterone and administered in a deep intramuscular injection of 150 mg every 12 weeks. This method prevents pregnancy by acting at the level of the pituitary and the hypothalamus.[60] Primarily, DMPA inhibits ovulation by suppressing the level of follicle-stimulating hormone and luteinizing hormone, ultimately preventing the luteinizing-hormone surge.[61] DMPA also decreases the quality of the cervical mucus, thereby preventing sperm penetration.[62]

DMPA is a safe, highly efficacious method, with rates ranging from 0.3% with correct and consistent use to 3% with actual use.[63] Because DMPA does not require daily maintenance, efficacy rates for typical use are much higher than those for oral contraceptives. DMPA is reversible (although return to fertility may take as long as 10 months[64]) and affords young users a certain level of privacy because the method is not visible to partners or parents. In addition, because effective plasma concentration is sustained for at least 14 weeks and ovulation is suppressed, on average, for 18 weeks,[65] the method is forgiving of delayed injections. For these reasons, teenager use has increased over the last several years. According to the National Survey of Family Growth, 10% of young women aged 15 to 19 reported using DMPA in 1995. By 2002, this usage had grown to 21%.[12]

Almost all adolescents are potential candidates for DMPA, because there are few contraindications for its use. In fact, according to the WHO,[41] the only absolute contraindication category 4 condition to DMPA use is current breast cancer. There are several category 3 conditions, including current cardiovascular disease, abnormal liver function or liver tumors, and history of breast cancer or unexplained vaginal bleeding. DMPA is also an alternative for patients who have contraindications to estrogen use (including deep vein thrombosis or recent pulmonary embolism) and for women who are breastfeeding.[66]

Importantly, DMPA has several noncontraceptive benefits. Because DMPA does not contain estrogen, the method does not seem to carry the rare but serious risks of complications attributable to exogenous estrogen.[67] DMPA has also been shown to decrease menstrual disturbances including ovulation pain, dysmenorrhea, mood changes, headaches, breast tenderness, and nausea.[68] The thickened cervical mucus caused by DMPA may prevent pathogens from entering the upper genital tract, therefore decreasing the risk of pelvic inflammatory disease in DMPA users.[69] DMPA use may also help young women with some chronic illnesses. For instance, possibly because of the sedative properties of progestins, research indicates that DMPA can decrease the frequency of grand mal seizures.[70,71] DMPA use is associated with greater reduction in the frequency of sickle cell crises when compared with combined oral contraception or no intervention.[72] There are also minimal drug interactions between DMPA and antibiotics or enzyme-inducing drugs. The only drug that decreases the effectiveness of DMPA is aminoglutethimide, which is generally indicated for suppression of adrenal function in selected cases of Cushing disease.[73]

Because women who initiate DMPA must deal with adverse effects and adverse effects for 3 months, it is important to consider these factors when counseling. Primarily, women taking DMPA will experience menstrual irregularities. In the first several months after initiating the method, many women experience unpredictable and prolonged spotting. After 1 year of DMPA use, 40% to 50% of women experience amenorrhea and, after 5 years, up to 80% no longer menstruate.[74] Research indicates that menstrual disturbances are the most frequent cause of dissatisfaction with this method, causing 20% to 25% of patients to discontinue use.[75,76] Therefore, providers must candidly discuss a patient's comfort with initial spotting and the eventual lack of periods to ascertain whether DMPA is an appropriate contraceptive choice. If, after the first 3 months, a young woman has serious concerns about these menstrual irregularities, providers may try to offer her a short course of exogenous estrogen[77] or a prostaglandin synthetase inhibitor.[77,78] These regimens have been shown to decrease bleeding in the short-term, but menstrual irregularities most likely will return after discontinuation.[77]

Weight gain is another adverse effect that should be considered before initiating young women on DMPA, because in 1 study, 18% of the adolescents reported discontinuing the method for this reason.[75] Although weight gain is frequently reported, observational and randomized studies have not shown consistent results in this regard. The authors of 2 recent retrospective analyses that compared DMPA use to intrauterine device (IUDs)[79] and COCs[80] similarly reported that DMPA was associated with an ~9-lb weight increase, whereas participants who received IUDs or COCs gained an average of 5 lb. However, the only randomized trial to investigate the effect of DMPA on weight concluded that DMPA did not cause weight gain in normal-weight young women over a 3-month period and that there was also no effect of DMPA on energy intake or expenditure.[81]

There have been conflicting reports on the effect of DMPA on women with depression. Although a history of depression is not a contraindication (the WHO medical eligibility rates DMPA use in women with a history of depression as category 2),[41] a 2000 study found that DMPA users had elevated depressive symptoms before and immediately after discontinuation relative to nonusers.[82]

However, 2 later studies found no such effect.[83,84] Because individual young women may experience an increase in depression while taking DMPA and discontinuation is not possible for 3 months, access to mental health care should be discussed during preadministration counseling.

DMPA, like all hormonal methods, does not protect against STIs, and young women must be counseled to use condoms at every act of intercourse. This is even more essential, because in several observational studies, DMPA use was associated with a chlamydia diagnosis[69,85,86] and inconsistently associated with gonorrhea.[69,86] It is unclear if this association is a result of inherent bias in the studies[87] or because of the effects that progestins may have on the growth of chlamydia.[69] To date, there have been no randomized, controlled trials to examine this issue. Therefore, providers should strongly urge women who use DMPA (or any other hormonal method) to use condoms during every act of sexual intercourse.

In recent years, concerns have arisen over the effect of DMPA on bone mineral density (BMD) in adolescent girls. Research has demonstrated that after DMPA initiation, women lose from 1% to 3% of their BMD per year.[88,89] This results from DMPA's suppression of gonadotropin secretions, which in turn suppresses ovarian estradiol production and creates a hypoestrogenic state.[90] Bone resorption in women in this state exceeds bone formation, which results in declines in BMD.[91]

This is of particular concern with adolescent girls who are accruing BMD during this period. Four studies that evaluated the specific effect of DMPA on bone density in adolescent girls found that BMD at the lumbar spine decreased a grand average of −3.1%, compared with +7.2% in adolescents not using the method.[92–94] In response to these data, in November 2004 the FDA added a black-box warning to the label for DMPA raising concerns about the effect of DMPA on peak BMD and questioning the risk for osteoporotic fracture in later life.[95]

Recent research, however, has suggested that the effect of DMPA on BMD is temporary and reversible. A 2005 study followed 80 DMPA users and 90 controls aged 14 to 18 years with BMD testing every 6 months for 23 to 36 months. Although the authors found a −5.0% loss at the spine among new DMPA users after 24 months, adjusted BMD values for discontinuers were at least as high as those of nonusers after 12 months after discontinuation.[96]

This research is encouraging, but there remain many uncertainties about the effect of DMPA use on bone health in adolescents. It is still unclear whether young women who use DMPA ultimately reach the same peak bone mass as they would have had they not used this method. Ultimately, there is concern that DMPA use may increase the risk of future fracture, but no studies that investigated DMPA use and fracture risk in adolescents have been published, and few studies have considered fracture risk in young women. A study of female military recruits that evaluated risk factors for stress fractures during basic training found an increased risk of fractures in white women using DMPA, but after adjustment for baseline bone density, the association was no longer statistically significant.[97]

A new formulation of DMPA was approved by the FDA in March 2005.[98] Administered subcutaneously instead of intramuscularly, this formulation contains 104 mg of medroxyprogesterone acetate (Depo-Subq Provera [Pfizer]) and follows the same dosing schedule as its predecessor. Although this route makes home administration possible (possibly eliminating a barrier to compliance), there has been no research to assess home use in adolescents. Although the subcutaneous formulation contains a lower dose of hormones, research has indicated that the irregular uterine bleeding patterns found in intramuscular users is also evident with the subcutaneous formulation.[99]

INTRAUTERINE CONTRACEPTION

Increasingly, adolescent providers are considering intrauterine contraception (IUC) as viable options for their young patients. IUC provides superior contraceptive ability with virtually no physical or financial maintenance. Because there are many wide-spread myths about IUDs, such as a supposed increase in pelvic inflammatory disease, providers have been reluctant to discuss IUDs with adolescents.

Currently, there are 2 IUDs available in the United States: the copper T 380A (ParaGard [Barr Pharmaceuticals]) and the levonorgestrel intrauterine system (IUS) (Mirena [Bayer HealthCare Pharmaceuticals]). The copper T 380A IUD was introduced in the United States in 1998 and is currently approved by the FDA for up to 10 years of use (although data indicate effectiveness as long as 12 years[100]). Consisting of a T-shaped polyethylene frame with barium sulfate added to create radiograph visibility, the device measures 3 mm tall and 32 mm wide and includes 380 mm^2 of exposed surface. Fine copper wire is wrapped around the vertical stem and each of the horizontal arms. To facilitate removal of the device, a monofilament polyethylene string is tied to a 3-mm bulb on the bottom of the vertical stem.

The levonorgestrel IUS consists of a polyethylene T-frame surrounded by a cylinder containing 52 mg of levonorgestrel in polydimethylsiloxane attached to the vertical stem. The system initially releases 20 μg of levonorgestrel per day directly into the endometrial cavity. To minimize hormonal adverse effects, this rate declines to 14 μg per day after 5 years. This IUS was approved by the FDA for use in the United States in 2000. Current guidelines stipulate a life span of 5 years, although research has indicated effectiveness of at least 7 years.[101]

IUC prevents fertilization by interfering with the sperm's ability to reach the ova. Specifically, the copper IUD functions by creating an environment toxic to sperm. Because this device is a foreign body, its presence in the uterus stimulates an inflammatory reaction, causing the endometrium to release white blood cells, enzymes, prostaglandins, and copper ions.[102] These biochemical changes may interfere with the migration of sperm.[102] This is supported by recent studies that demonstrated reduced capacity of the sperm found in IUD users when compared with other women.[103]

The levonorgestrel IUS functions similarly to other progestin methods. Primarily, it prevents pregnancy by thickening cervical mucus, thus preventing sperm from entering the uterus. The system also suppresses the endometrium. In some women, the low-dose levonorgestrel suppresses ovulation.[104]

IUC is one of the most effective forms of birth control available to women today.[105] The annual failure rate for the copper T 380A device is 0.6 per 100 women for perfect use and 0.8 per 100 for actual use.[63,106] The levonorgestrel system is slightly more efficacious, with failure rates for perfect and actual use at 0.2 per 100 women.[63]

In addition to being long-acting, reversible methods of contraception, the copper T 380A and levonorgestrel IUS have been shown to decrease a woman's risk of ectopic pregnancy.[101,107] In the long run, IUC is also more cost-effective than other forms of contraception. Because the copper T 380A contains no hormones, it therefore is an optimal method for those young women who want a highly efficacious method but do not want to take hormones.

The levonorgestrel IUS provides several noncontraceptive benefits resulting from decreased menstrual blood loss, which is associated with increased hemoglobulin concentrations and effective treatment of menorrhagia.[108,109] Another important noncontraceptive benefit of the levonorgestrel IUS is its efficacy in treating pain associated with endometriosis.[110]

Although it is an excellent form of contraception, mild-to-moderate discomfort is common during IUD insertion. In addition, many women experience bleeding abnormalities in the first few months of use with both the copper IUD and the levonorgestrel IUS. Women using the copper IUD normally experience heavier menses and dysmenorrhea. These are the most frequently cited reasons for removing the device.[111] After the initial few months, irregular bleeding in levonorgestrel IUS users will subside, and a marked decrease in menses will occur. In addition, IUD expulsion is more common with adolescents because of null parity and the presence of a smaller uterus.[106]

Contrary to common misperception, IUC does not increase the risk of pelvic inflammatory disease.[112] The insertion process, not the device or the long-term usage of the device, increases the risk of infection.[113] Research also refutes any association between IUC and tubal infertility.[114]

To help facilitate the use of IUC, providers should give each woman an identification card with the name and picture of the IUC, date of insertion, and date of removal. Also, include instructions on what to do in the event that the device comes out.

IMPLANTABLE CONTRACEPTION

The only implantable contraceptive currently available in the United States is a single rod implant containing 68 mg of etonogestrel (Implanon [Schering-Plough]). Approved by the FDA in the United States in 2006,[115] this method has been used in Europe since 1998. The etonogestrel implant is highly efficacious and provides 3 years of uninterrupted pregnancy prevention. In prospective follow-up studies of more than 2467 woman-years of exposure, no pregnancies occurred.[116]

In addition to being easy to use, private, and highly efficacious, the etonogestrel implant is associated with a reduction in dysmenorrhea[116] and endometriosis.[117] However, the initial cost of insertion is fairly high, which may turn off some young people. In addition, like all progestin-only methods, young women using this method will experience bleeding abnormalities.[116] Other possible adverse effects include rare insertion complications, ovarian cysts, weight gain, and possible increased risk of thromboembolic conditions.[118] As with DMPA, it is essential to discuss these possible adverse effects with patients who are considering the implant.

CONCLUSIONS

Adolescent girls have a wide array of contraceptive options to help them successfully prevent pregnancy. In recent years, there have been many innovations in hormonal contraception, particularly in advances in long-acting reversible methods, which make it easier for younger women to adhere to a birth control regimen. To further facilitate this process, health care providers can play a unique role in helping their young patients understand the options available, selecting the most appropriate method, and providing anticipatory guidance to ensure compliance.

REFERENCES

1. Singh S, Darroch J. Adolescent pregnancy and childbearing: levels and trends in developed countries. *Fam Plann Perspect.* 2000;32(1):14–23
2. Guttmacher Institute. US teenage pregnancy statistics: national and state trends and trends by race and ethnicity. Available at: www.guttmacher.org/pubs/2006/09/12/USTPstats.pdf. Accessed October 1, 2008
3. Finer LB, Henshaw SK. Disparities in rates of unintended pregnancy in the United States, 1994 and 2001. *Perspect Sex Reprod Health.* 2006;38(2):90–96

4. Ventura SJ, Abma JC, Mosher WD, Henshaw SK. Estimated pregnancy rates by outcome for the United States, 1990–2004. *Natl Vital Stat Rep.* 2008;56(15):1–25, 28
5. Harlap S, Kost K, Forrest JD. *Preventing Pregnancy, Protecting Health: A New Look at Birth Control Choices in the United States.* New York, NY: AGI; 1991
6. Santelli JS, Lindberg LD, Finer LB, Singh S. Explaining recent declines in adolescent pregnancy in the United States: the contribution of abstinence and improved contraceptive use. *Am J Public Health.* 2007;97(1):150–156
7. Guttmacher Institute. *State Policies in Brief: Minors' Access to Contraceptive Services.* New York, NY: Guttachmer Institute; 2008. Available at: www.guttmacher.org/statecenter/spibs/spib_MACS.pdf. Accessed October 9, 2008
8. Family Planning Services & Population Research Act of 1970, Pub L. No. 91-572, 84 Stat 1504 (1970) (codified as amended at 42 USC §§300 et seq (1991 and Supp. 2000)
9. S. Rep. No. 95–822 at 24 (1978)
10. Stewart FH, Harper CC, Ellertson CE, Grimes DA, Sawaya GF, Trussell J. Clinical breast and pelvic examination requirements for hormonal contraception: current practice vs evidence. *JAMA.* 2001;285(17):2232–2239
11. American Academy of Pediatrics, Committee on Adolescents. Contraception and adolescents. *Pediatrics.* 2007;120(5):1135–1148
12. Abma JC, Martinez GM, Mosher WD, Dawson BS. Teenagers in the United States: sexual activity, contraceptive use, and childbearing, 2002. *Vital Health Stat 23.* 2004;(24):1–48
13. Bracken MB. Oral contraception and congenital malformations in offspring: a review and meta-analysis of prospective studies. *Obstet Gynecol.* 1990;76(3 pt 2):552–557
14. Ohlemeyer CL. Adolescents' compliance with return visits for depot medroxyprogesterone initiation. *J Pediatr Adolesc Gynecol.* 2003;16(5):297–299
15. Lara-Torre E, Schroeder B. Adolescent compliance and side effects with Quick Start initiation of oral contraceptive pills. *Contraception.* 2002;66(2):81–85
16. Westhoff C, Kerns J, Morroni C, Cushman LF, Tiezzi L, Murphy PA. Quick Start: a novel oral contraceptive initiation method. *Contraception.* 2002;66(3):141–145
17. Rickert VI, Tiezzi L, Lipshutz J, León J, Vaughan RD, Westhoff C. Depo Now: preventing unintended pregnancies among adolescents and young adults. *J Adolesc Health.* 2007;40(1):22–28
18. Polaneczky M, Slap G, Forke C, Rappaport A, Sondheimer S. The use of levonorgestrel implants for contraception in adolescent mothers. *N Engl J Med.* 1994;331(18):1201–1206
19. Morroni C, Grams M, Tiezzi L, Westhoff C. Immediate monthly combination contraception to facilitate initiation of the depot medroxyprogesterone acetate contraceptive injection. *Contraception.* 2004;70(1):19–23
20. Sneed R, Westhoff C, Morrni C, Tiezzi L. A prospective study of immediate initiation of depo medroxyprogesterone acetate contraceptive injection. *Contraception.* 2005;71(2):99–103
21. American Academy of Pediatrics, Committee on Adolescence. Emergency contraception. *Pediatrics.* 2005;116(4):1026–1103
22. Gold MA, Wolford JE, Smith KA, Parker AM. The effects of advance provision of emergency contraception on adolescent women's sexual and contraceptive behaviors. *J Pediatr Adolesc Gynecol.* 2004;17(2):87–96
23. Raine T, Harper C, Leon K, Darney P. Emergency contraception: advance provision in a young, high-risk clinic population. *Obstet Gynecol.* 2000;96(1):1–7
24. Rodrigues I, Grou F, Joly J. Effectiveness of emergency contraceptive pills between 72 and 120 hours after unprotected sexual intercourse. *Am J Obstet Gynecol.* 2001;184(4):531–553
25. Mosher WD, Martinez GM, Chandra A, Abma JC, Willson SJ. Use of contraception and use of family planning services in the United States: 1982–2002. *Adv Data.* 2004;(350):1–36
26. Speroff L, DeCherney A. Evaluation of a new generation of oral contraceptives. The Advisory Board for the New Progestins. *Obstet Gynecol.* 1993;81:1034–1047
27. Nelson A. Combined oral contraceptives. In: Hatcher RA, Trussell J, Nelson A, Cates W, Stewart F, Kowal D, eds. *Contraceptive Technology.* 19th revised ed. New York, NY: Ardent Media; 2007:193–257

28. US Food and Drug Administration, Center for Drug Evaluation and Research. Yasmin 28 (application 21-098) approval letter, May 11, 2001
29. US Food and Drug Administration, Center for Drug Evaluation and Research. Yaz (application 21-873) approval letter, March 16, 2006
30. US Food and Drug Administration, Center for Drug Evaluation and Research. Yaz (application 21-676) approval letter, October 4, 2006
31. US Food and Drug Administration, Center for Drug Evaluation and Research. Yaz (application 22-045) approval letter, January 6, 2007
32. US Food and Drug Administration, Center for Drug Evaluation and Research. Loestrin FE (application 21-871) approval letter, February 17, 2006
33. US Food and Drug Administration, Center for Drug Evaluation and Research. Seasonale (application 21-544) approval letter, September 5, 2003
34. Anderson FD, Hait H. A multicenter randomized study of an extended cycle oral contraceptive. *Contraception*. 2003;68(2):89–96
35. US Food and Drug Administration, Center for Drug Evaluation and Research. Lybrel (application 21-864) approval letter, May 22, 2007
36. Goldzieher JW. The hypothalamo-pituitary-ovarian system. In: Goldzieher JW, Fotherby K, eds. *Pharmacology of the Contraceptive Steroids*. New York, NY: Raven Press; 1994:185–198
37. Moghissi KS. Effects of microdose progestogens on endogenous gonadotrophic and steroid hormones, cervical mucus properties, vaginal cytology and endometrium. *Fertil Steril*. 1971; 22(7):424–434
38. Berenson AB, Wiemann CM. Use of levonorgestrel implants versus oral contraceptives in adolescents: a case-control study. *Am J Obstet Gynecol*. 1995;172(4 pt 1):1128–1137
39. Burke AE, Blumenthal PD. Successful use of oral contraceptives. *Semin Reprod Med*. 2001; 19(4):313–321
40. Clark LR. Will the pill make me sterile? Addressing the reproductive health concerns and strategies to improve adherence to hormonal contraceptive regimens in adolescent girls. *J Pediatr Adolesc Gynecol*. 2001;14(4):153–162
41. World Health Organization. *Improving Access to Quality Care in Family Planning: Medical Eligibility Criteria for Contraceptive Use*. 2nd ed. Geneva, Switzerland: World Health Organization: 2000
42. Larsson G, Milsom I, Lindstedt G, Rybo G. The influence of a low-dose combined oral contraceptive on menstrual blood loss and iron status. *Contraception*. 1992;46(4):327–334
43. Parsey KS, Pong A. An open-label, multi-center study to evaluate Yasmin, a low-dose combination oral contraceptive containing drospirenone, a new progestogen. *Contraception*. 2000; 61(2):105–111
44. Freeman EW, Borisute H, Deal L, Smith L, et al. A continuous-use regimen of levonorhestrel/ethinyl estradiol significantly alleviates cycle-related symptoms: results of a phase 3 study. *Fertil Steril*. 2005;84:S25
45. Davis A, Godwin A, Lippman J, Olson W, Kafrissen M. Triphasic norgestimate ethinyl estradiol for treating dysfunctional dysphoric disorder. *Obstet Gynecol*. 2000;96:913–920
46. Palatsi R, Hirvensalo E, Liukko P, et al. Serum total and unbound testosterone and sex hormone binding globulin in female acne patients treated with two different types of oral contraceptives. *Acta Derm Venereol*. 1984;64(6):517–523
47. Rosenberg MJ, Waugh MS. Oral contraceptive discontinuation: a prospective evaluation of frequency and reasons. *Am J Obstet Gynecol*. 1998;179(3 pt 1):577–582
48. Reubinoff BE, Grubstein A, Meirow D, Berry E, Schenker JG, Brzezinski A. Effects of low-dose estrogen oral contraceptives on weight, body composition, and fat distribution in young women. *Fertil Steril*. 1995;63(3):516–521
49. Nanda K. Contraceptive patch and vaginal contraceptive ring. In: Hatcher RA, Trussell J, Nelson A, Cates W, Stewart F, Kowal D, eds. *Contraceptive Technology*. 19th revised ed. New York, NY: Ardent Media; 2007:271–292
50. Rubinstein ML, Halpern-Felsher BL, Irwin CE. An evaluation of the use of the transdermal contraceptive patch in adolescents. *J Adolesc Health*. 2004;34(5):395–401

51. Abrams LS, Skee D, Natarajan J, Wong FA. Pharmacokinetic overview of Ortho Evra/Evra. *Fertil Steril.* 2002;77(2 suppl 2):S3–S12
52. Zieman M, Guillebaud J, Weisberg E, Shangold GA, Fisher AC, Creasy GW. Contraceptive efficacy and cycle control with the Ortho Evra/Evra transdermal system: the analysis of pooled data. *Fertil Steril.* 2002;77(2 suppl 2):S13–S18
53. Ortho Evra [Prescribing Information]. Raritan, NJ: Ortho-McNeil-Janssen Pharmaceuticals; 2008. Available at: www.myortho360.com/myortho360/shared/pi/OrthoEvraPI.pdf#zoom=100. Accessed February 25, 2009
54. Jick SS, Kaye JA, Russmann S, Jick H. Risk of nonfatal venous thromboembolism with oral contraceptives containing norgestimate or desogestrel compared with oral contraceptives containing levonorgestrel. *Contraception.* 2006;73(6):566–570
55. Cole JA, Norman H, Doherty M, Walker AM. Venous thromboembolism, myocardial infarction, and stroke among transdermal contraceptive system users [published correction appears in *Obstet Gynecol.* 2008;111(6):1449]. *Obstet Gynecol.* 2007;109(2 pt 1):339–346
56. US Food and Drug Administration, Center for Drug Evaluation and Research. NuvaRing (application 21-87) approval letter, October 3, 2001
57. NuvaRing [prescribing information]. Roseland, NJ: Organon USA; 2005
58. Oddsson K, Leifels-Fischer B, de Melo NR, et al. Efficacy and safety of a contraceptive vaginal ring (NuvaRing) compared with a combined oral contraceptive: a 1-year randomized trial. *Contraception.* 2005;71(3):176–182
59. Roumen FJ, Apter D, Mulders TM, Dieben TO. Efficacy, tolerability and acceptability of a novel contraceptive vaginal ring releasing etonogestrel and ethinyl oestradiol. *Hum Reprod.* 2001;16(3):469–475
60. Ismail AA, el-Faras A, Rocca M, el-Sibai FA, Toppozada M. Pituitary response to LHRH in long-term users of injectable contraceptives. *Contraception.* 1987;35(5):487–495
61. Petta CA, Faúndes A, Dunson TR Timing of onset of contraceptive effectiveness in Depo-Provera users: II. Effects on ovarian function. *Fertil Steril.* 1998;70(5):817–820
62. Petta CA, Faúndes A, Dunson TR, et al. Timing of onset of contraceptive effectiveness in Depo-Provera users: Part I. Changes in cervical mucus. *Fertil Steril.* 1998;69(2):252–257
63. Trussell J. Contraceptive failure in the United States. *Contraception.* 2004;70(2):89–96
64. Mishell DR. Pharmacokinetics of depot medroxyprogesterone acetate contraception. *J Reprod Med.* 1997;41(5 suppl):381–390
65. Kaunitz AM. Long-acting injectable contraception with depot medroxyprogesterone acetate. *Am J Obstet Gynecol.* 1994;170(5 Pt 2):1543–1549
66. Halderman LD, Nelson AL. Impact of early postpartum administration of progestin-only hormonal contraceptives compared with nonhormonal contraceptives on short-term breastfeeding patterns. *Am J Obstet Gynecol.* 2002;186(6):1250–1256; discussion 1256–1258
67. McCann MF, Potter LS. Progestin-only oral contraception: a comprehensive review. *Contraception.* 1994;50(6 suppl 1):S1–S195
68. Kaunitz AM. Injectable depot medroxyprogesterone acetate contraception: an update for US clinicians. *Int J Fertil Womens Med.* 1998;43(2):73–83
69. Baeten J, Nyange P, Richardson B, et al. Hormonal contraception and risk of sexually transmitted disease acquisition: results from a prospective study. *Am J Obstet Gynecol.* 2001;185(2):380–385
70. Mattson RH, Cramer JA, Darney PD, Naftolin F. Use of oral contraceptives by women with epilepsy. *JAMA.* 1986;256(2):238–240
71. Mattson RH, Rebar RW. Contraceptive methods for women with neurologic disorders. *Am J Obstet Gynecol.* 1993;168(6 pt 2):2027–2032
72. de Abood M, de Castilo Z, Guerrero F, Austin KL. Effect of Depo-Provera or Microgynon on the painful crises of sickle cell anemia patients. *Contraception.* 1997;56(5):313–316
73. Hatcher RA, Schare S. Ask the experts: progestin-only contraceptives. *Contracept Technol Update.* 1993;14(7):114–115
74. Belsey EM. Vaginal bleeding patterns among women using one natural and eight hormonal methods of contraception. *Contraception.* 1988;38(2):181–206

75. Polaneczky M, Liblanc M. Long-term depot medroxyprogesterone acetate (Depo-Provider) use in inner-city adolescents. *J Adolesc Health.* 1998;23(2):81–88
76. Paul C, Skegg DC, Williams S. Depot medroxyprogesterone acetate: patterns of use and reasons for discontinuation. *Contraception.* 1997;56(4):209–214
77. Said S, Sadek W, Rocca M, et al. Clinical evaluation of the therapeutic effectiveness of ethinyl oestradiol and oestrone sulphate on prolonged bleeding in women using depot medroxyprogesterone acetate for contraception. World Health Organization, Special Programme of Research, Development and Research Training in Human Reproduction, Task Force on Long-acting Systemic Agents for Fertility Regulation. *Hum Reprod.* 1996;11(suppl 2):1–13
78. Tantiwattanakul P, Taneepanichskul S. Effect of mefenamic acid on controlling irregular uterine bleeding in DMPA users. *Contraception.* 2004;70(4):277–279
79. Bahamondes L, Del Castillo S, Tabares G, Arce XE, Perrotti C. Comparison of weight increase in users of depot medroxyprogesterone acetate and copper IUD up to 5 years. *Contraception.* 2001;64(4):223–225
80. Mangan SA, Larsen PG, Hudson S. Overweight teens at increased risk for weight gain while using depot medroxyprogesterone acetate. *J Pediatr Adolesc Gynecol.* 2002;15(2):79–82
81. Pelkman CL, Chow M, Heinbach R, Rolls BJ. Short-term effects of a progestational contraceptive drug on food intake, resting energy expenditure, and body weight in young women. *Am J Clin Nutr.* 2001;73(1):19–26
82. Civic D, Scholes D, Ichikawa L, et al. Depressive symptoms in users and non-users of depot medroxyprogesterone acetate. *Contraception.* 2000;61(6):385–390
83. Gupta N, O'Brien R, Jacobsen LJ, et al. Mood changes in adolescents using depot-medroxyprogesterone acetate for contraception: a prospective study. *J Pediatr Adolesc Gynecol.* 2001; 14(2):71–76
84. Westhoff C, Truman C, Kalmuss D, et al. Depressive symptoms and Depo-Provera. *Contraception.* 1998;57(4):237–240
85. Jacobson DL, Peralta L, Farmer M, Graham NM, Gaydos C, Zenilman J. Relationship of hormonal contraception and cervical ectopy as measured by computerized planimetry to chlamydial infection in adolescents. *Sex Transm Dis.* 2000;27(6):313–319
86. Morrison C, Bright P, Wong E, et al. Hormonal contraceptive use, cervical ectopy, and the acquisition of cervical infections. *Sex Transm Dis.* 2004;31(9):561–567
87. Dayan L, Donovan B. Chlamydia, gonorrhea, and injectable progesterone. *Lancet.* 2004; 364(9443):1387–1388
88. Berenson AB, Radecki CM, Grady JJ, Rickert VI, Thomas A. A prospective, controlled study of the effects of hormonal contraception on bone mineral density. *Obstet Gynecol.* 2001;98(4): 576–582
89. Clark MK, Sowers MF, Nichols S, Levy B. Bone mineral density changes over two years in first-time users of depot medroxyprogesterone acetate. *Fertil Steril.* 2004;82(6):1580–1586
90. Clark MK, Sowers M, Levy BT, Tenhundfeld P. Magnitude and variability of sequential estradiol and progesterone concentrations in women using depot medroxyprogesterone acetate for contraception. *Fertil Steril.* 2001;75(5):871–877
91. Gbolade BA. Depo-Provera and bone density. *J Fam Plann Reprod Health Care.* 2002;28(1): 7–11; quiz 11, 50
92. Cromer BA, Blair JM, Mahan JD, Zibners L, Naumovski Z. A prospective comparison of bone density in adolescent girls on depot medroxyprogesterone acetate, levonorgestrel, or oral contraceptives. *J Pediatr.* 1996;129(5):671–676
93. Busen NH, Britt RB, Rianon N. Bone mineral density in a cohort of adolescent women using depot medroxyprogesterone acetate for one to two years. *J Adolesc Health.* 2003;32(4):257–259
94. Cromer BA, Stager M, Bonny A, et al. Depot medroxyprogesterone acetate, oral contraceptives and bone mineral density in a cohort of adolescent girls. *J Adolesc Health.* 2004;35(6):434–441
95. US Food and Drug Administration. Black Box Warning Added Concerning Long-Term Use of Depo-Provera Contraceptive Injection, November 17, 2004. Available at: www.fda.gov/bbs/topics/ANSWERS/2004/ANS01325.html. Accessed February 24, 2009

96. Scholes D, LaCroix AZ, Ichikawa LE, Barlow WE, Ott SM. Change in bone mineral density among adolescent women using and discontinuing depot medroxyprogesterone acetate contraception. *Arch Pediatr Adolesc Med.* 2005;159(2):139–144
97. Lappe JM, Stegman MR, Recker RR. The impact of lifestyle factors on stress fractures in female Army recruits. *Osteoporos Int.* 2001;12(1):35–42
98. US Food and Drug Administration, Center for Drug Evaluation and Research. DepoSub Q (application 21-584) approval letter, March 5, 2005
99. Jain J, Jakimiuk AJ, Bode FR, Ross D, Kaunitz AM. Contraceptive efficacy and safety of DMPA-SC. *Contraception.* 2004;70(4):269–227
100. World Health Organization. Long-term reversible contraception: twelve years of experience with the TCu380 A and TCu220C. *Contraception.* 1997;56(6):341–352
101. Sivin I, Stern J, Coutinho E, et al. Prolonged intrauterine contraception: a seven-year randomized study of the levonorgestrel 20 mcg/day (LNg 20) and the copper T380 Ag IUDs. *Contraception.* 1991;44(5):473–480
102. Ortiz ME, Croxatto H. The mode of action of IUDs. *Contraception.* 1987;36(1):37–53
103. Ortiz ME, Croxatto HB, Bardin CW. Mechanisms of action of intrauterine devices. *Obstet Gynecol Surv.* 1996;51(12 suppl):S42–S51
104. Barbosa I, Olsson SE, Odlind V, Goncalves T, Coutinho E. Ovarian function after seven year's use of levonorgestrel IUD. *Adv Contracept.* 1995;11(2):85–95
105. Steiner MJ, Dalebout S, Condon S, Dominik R, Trussell J. Understanding the risk: a randomized controlled trial of communicating contraceptive effectiveness. *Obstet Gynecol.* 2003;102(4):709–717
106. Tolaymat LL, Kaunitz AM. Long acting contraceptives in adolescents. *Curr Opin Obstet Gynecol.* 2007;19(5):453–460
107. Pakarinen P, Toivonen J, Luukainen T. Therapeuatic use of the LNG IUS, and counseling. *Semin Reprod Med.* 2001;19(4):365–372
108. American College of Obstetricians and Gynecologists, Committee on Gynecologic Practice. ACOG committee opinion. No. 337: noncontraceptive uses of the levonorgestrel intrauterine system. *Obstet Gynecol.* 2006;107(6):1479–1482
109. Xiao B, Wu SC, Chong J, Zeng T, Han LH, Luukkainen T. Therapeutic effects of the levonorgestrel-releasing intrauterine system in the treatment of idiopathic menorrhagia. *Fertil Steril.* 2003;79(4):963–969
110. Bahamondes L, Petta CA, Fernandes A, Monteiro I. Use of the levonorgestrel-releasing intrauterine system in women with endometriosis, chronic pelvic pain and dysmenorrhea. *Contraception.* 2007;75(6 suppl):S134–S139
111. Rivera R, Chen-Mok M, McMullen S. Analysis of client characteristics that may affect early discontinuation of the TCu-380A IUD. *Contraception.* 1999;60(3):155–160
112. Grimes DA. Intrauterine device and upper-genital tract infection. *Lancet.* 2000;356(9234):1013–1019
113. Lee NC, Rubin GL, Ory HW, Burkman RT. Type of intrauterine device and the risk of pelvic inflammatory disease. *Obstet Gynecol.* 1983;62(1):1–6
114. Skjeldestad F, Bratt H. Fertility after complicated and non-complicated use of IUDs: a controlled prospective study. *Adv Contracept.* 1988;4(3):179–184
115. US Food and Drug Administration, Center for Drug Evaluation and Research. Implanon (application 21-529) approval letter, July 17, 2006
116. Funk S, Miller MM, Mishell DR Jr, et al. Safety and efficacy of Implanon, a single-rod implantable contraceptive containing etonogestrel. *Contraception.* 2005;71(5):319–326
117. Yisa SB, Okenwa AA, Husemeyer RP. Treatment of pelvic endometriosis with etonogestrel subdermal implant. *J Fam Plann Reprod Health Care.* 2005;31(1):67–70
118. Raymond E. Contraceptive implants. In: Hatcher RA, Trussell J, Nelson A, Cates W, Stewart F, Kowal D, eds. *Contraceptive Technology.* 19th revised ed. New York, NY: Ardent Media; 2007

Anxiety and Anxiety-Related Disorders in the Adolescent Population: An Overview of Diagnosis and Treatment

Carol L. Rizzolo, RPA-C, MA[*,a], John E. Taylor, MA[b], Robert L. Cerciello, MD, FAAP[c]

[a]476 Wood Hill Road, Cheshire, CT 06410, USA

[b]Child and Youth Mental Health, Ministry of Children and Family Development, Victoria, British Columbia, Canada V8W 9S1

[c]Departments of Neurology and Pediatrics, University of Connecticut School of Medicine, 263 Farmington Road, Farmington, CT 06030; Connecticut Children's Medical Center, 60 Hartland Street, East Hartford, CT 06108

Anxiety is a common component of visits to the doctor's office by adolescents; however, it is often overlooked as a possible causative agent of the presenting complaint. With a high index of suspicion and proper questioning, a clinician can analyze the contribution that anxiety plays in the life of an adolescent patient. Behavioral and pharmacologic interventions exist for this group of disorders, and with proper diagnosis and treatment the symptoms of these disorders can possibly be ameliorated. The following provides a concise guide to the diagnosis and treatment of anxiety and anxiety-related disorders including hyperventilation syndrome, syncope, sleep disorders, panic disorder, and obsessive compulsive disorder (OCD).

ANXIETY

Anxiety is one of the most common causes of symptomatology resulting in an office visit. When an adolescent presents with loss of consciousness, mental status change, cardiac problems, stomachaches, headaches, or any set of symptoms that seem to be disparate, a diagnosis of anxiety disorder should be considered. Anxiety ought to be treated as a piece of diagnostic information that may or may not require treatment and should be considered as a possible cause, or at the very least a component, of any chronic medical condition.

---

*Corresponding author.
E-mail address: Carol.Rizzolo@gmail.com (C. L. Rizzolo).

Approaching the history of the presenting problem, it is the responsibility of the clinician to maintain an awareness of the differing perspectives that will be offered as the patient or family describes the problem. In the case of anxiety, it is likely that the level of anxiety in the family will affect the adolescent, but the adolescent will have his or her own perspective on the extent of the disability. In the interest of eliciting candid answers from an adolescent patient, we encourage the clinician to try to interview the patient without the adult present.

History

The clinician should consider the possibilities of metabolic disturbances (eg, thyroid disease), substance abuse or substance exposure, or psychiatric conditions as part of the differential diagnosis when evaluating for anxiety disorder. As always, the clinician ought to question how long this symptom has been present. Was the onset associated with any other occurrence (eg, illness, emotional or physical trauma)? Questions such as "When and in what situation does anxiety usually occur?" and "Is anxiety more likely to occur at home, school, or other social situations?" will help to further focus the evaluation. It is important for the clinician to explore whether anxiety is more likely to occur in social situations that are peer related or in family situations. It is our experience that school is the most likely setting for the adolescent experiencing anxiety.

Next, the clinician can try to discern what patients actually experience when they say they are feeling "anxious." One can attempt to elicit an explanation of symptomatology as well as what the patient can do to "make it better" or "prevent" the feeling. To discern the chronicity of the problem, one may ask, "Is the anxiety there all the time for you, or is it episodic?" If it is episodic, one should elicit a description of the last 2 to 3 times that anxiety occurred.

Frequently, a precipitating factor in adolescent anxiety is the stress of school. To discern whether the stress is academic or social, it is important that the clinician ask about grades, family expectations, and personal expectations. Commonly, one might hear single-syllable answers to these queries. Regardless of the answer, the clinician can question more deeply (eg, by asking questions such as "What are your grades like?" "How do you do on tests?" and "Do you think you study more or less than your peers?") Exploring social stress, the clinician can ask questions such as, "Is the teacher picking on you?" "Are peers making fun of you?" "Have you had any recent altercations with any peer(s) at school?" "Are you being ostracized?" "Are you getting into trouble in school because of misbehavior?" and "Are your parents pressuring you to do better in school?" There are a plethora of questions that can be asked to shed light on the source of the anxiety. It is our hope that the above-listed questions give the clinician several tools to aid in eliciting a more precise history of the condition.

Last, in obtaining a history from the adolescent it may be important to ask the patient to describe recent episodes that occurred in interactions with peers. With this style of questioning, the clinician is attempting to get every bit of information, because one may never know what piece of information will provide an important clue. As we have all experienced, the most important piece of data might not seem important to the patient and may not be offered without directed history questions.

Treatment

Depending on the level of anxiety, one may wish to consider helping a patient get the nonpharmacologic help they need to cope with anxiety levels. Although counseling can be quite effective in dealing with disabling levels of anxiety, it is often rejected by family or patients for many different reasons (eg, unobtainable for financial reasons or the social stigma associated with counseling). Relaxation techniques including meditation and yoga have been shown to reduce stress in adolescents.[1,2] Nonpharmacologic modalities can aid the adolescent in developing coping skills. In this way, he or she is not merely a passive victim of anxiety; rather, these skills allow the patient to actively engage in treatment.

If nonpharmacologic therapies are not an option or are not successful, one can consider using pharmaceuticals to ease the symptoms of anxiety.[3,4] Treatment may vary depending on whether the anxiety is chronic or acute and recurring.

One of the significant concerns in a patient who suffers from anxiety is that the patient will self-medicate if anxiety is significant enough. This should be taken into account when considering pharmaceutical treatment. The most beneficial treatments for acute anxiety are the benzodiazepines, but this class of drug also carries a significant risk of abuse. That said, for episodic anxiety, the benzodiazepines are the best choice because of the quick-acting nature of the chemical. Unfortunately, with chronic use, a patient may develop a tolerance, and the dose will need to be increased periodically to remain effective. Suggested benzodiazepines include alprazolam (Xanax [Pfizer, New York, New York]) and lorazepam (Ativan [Biovail, Bridgewater, NJ]). Alprazolam (0.25–1 mg orally three times per day), which has a half-life of 6 to 20 hours, is the most effective and quick acting. Lorazepam (0.5–2 mg PO orally three times per day) has a half-life of 10 to 20 hours and is also helpful but not as quick acting as alprazolam. Again, we need to emphasize the need to be extremely cautious with benzodiazepines because of the potential for abuse. These drugs can cause physical and psychological dependence. Withdrawal can occur, especially if benzodiazepines are used for 3 to 6 months at relatively high doses. When used intermittently, the dose can remain the same, and addiction and tolerance issues are less likely to occur.

Note that in the case of an adolescent with a comorbid seizure disorder, one should consider if this patient is being treated chronically with a benzodiazepine.

If this patient were to have an episode of status epilepticus, benzodiazepines may be less effective, because the patient may have a developed tolerance to this class of medications.

When starting a patient on these medications, we suggest beginning the medication regimen on a non–school day or after school hours to try to avoid the possibility of problematic sedation.

The selective serotonin reuptake inhibitors (SSRIs) have been shown to be effective in treating generalized and social anxiety. There is a black-box warning on SSRI medications[5] concerning an increase in suicidal ideation associated with the use of these medications; however, there are also published reports regarding increased suicide in adolescents caused by decreased prescribing of SSRIs by primary care physicians.[6–9] It is worth noting that a warning is not a contraindication, and SSRIs can be used in adolescents with caution and careful follow-up.[10] SSRIs may take as long as 4 weeks to show some effectiveness and, therefore, are useful for chronic anxiety but not for intermittent acute anxiety. Therefore, these medications are not useful when taken on an as-needed basis. Depending on the severity of the acute symptoms, the clinician might need to begin treatment by providing the patient with dual coverage of a short-acting benzodiazepine in conjunction with an SSRI, with the goal of tapering the benzodiazepine.

One major problem with SSRI medications is that they can decrease sexual libido, which can be a frequent reason for discontinuation. Other adverse effects can include headaches, sweating, abdominal discomfort, and other less common adverse effects (refer to the Physicians' Desk Reference[11] for a full listing of adverse effects). The clinician is encouraged to educate the patient about these possible effects. To some clinicians the question of sexual activity may seem premature for many of these patients; however, it is important to inquire about sexual activity. Compliance with medications has its share of challenges in the best of situations, and if the patient sees decreased sexual libido as problematic, then it should be discussed openly in the clinical setting. In addition, the clinician needs to ask the patient directly about suicidal ideations.

When prescribing an SSRI, the clinician should be attentive to the importance of a slow titration upward and also downward to avoid serotonin syndrome, an adverse drug reaction resulting in excess serotonin. Symptoms of serotonin syndrome include seizures, restlessness, muscle twitches and myoclonus, confusion, exaggerated reflexes, sweating, and gastroenterological symptoms. Due to its long half life, fluoxetine (Prozac) is the only SSRI which is safe to discontinue abruptly. While this is not recommended, fluoxetine should be considered to be the first choice because of the significant risk of noncompliance in the adolescent population. Recommended follow up visits every week for 4 weeks, every other week for 4 weeks, and then again at 12 weeks. After 12 weeks, the clinician can make a judgment concerning follow-up, but monthly visits for the next 2 months and then a minimum of every 3 months may be best. Last, SSRI medications can cause hypomania and behavioral disinhibition.[12,13] Behavioral disinhibition might include doing things that one thought about doing in the past but were not done, such as fighting, destroying property, running away, etc—in short, getting into trouble.[12,13]

If the clinician is going to treat an anxious patient, consideration should be given to placing strong demands on the family to go for psychological counseling so that a trained professional in the behavioral health field is also involved. In the case of mild anxiety, behavioral therapy alone might be sufficient. If a counselor or therapist sees something problematic with a patient, it can be addressed in a timely manner. In addition, the relationship between the mental health provider and the clinician is paramount in the successful treatment of these adolescents, not just for suicidal concerns or hypomania. The goal of treatment is to get the patient off medications. In our opinion, the best way to do that is to get these patients the psychological help they need. Medication is only a temporary treatment that will help to reduce anxiety in the patient and, therefore, improve counseling outcomes.

If the clinician decides to use SSRI medications, one can start adolescents on 10 mg of fluoxetine (Prozac [Eli Lilly and Company, Indianapolis, IN]) orally once per day. Because of its long half-life, abrupt discontinuation of fluoxetine is the least likely of the SSRIs to cause serotonin syndrome. Although abrupt discontinuation is not recommended, fluoxetine should be considered to be a good choice because of the risk of noncompliance in the adolescent population. A recommended follow-up visit schedule is every week for 4 weeks, every other week for 4 weeks, and then again at 12 weeks. After 12 weeks, the clinician can make a judgment concerning follow-up, but monthly visits for the next 2 months and then a minimum of every 3 months may be best. We strongly encourage the clinician to explore the possibility of hypomania as well as any other adverse effects at each follow-up visit.

If the patient is improved, one can stabilize the dose, but it is imperative that the clinician see the patient for follow-up, as per above. If there is no sign of relief in 2 to 4 weeks, the dose can be increased to 20 mg orally once per day. The adult maximum is 80 mg. If fluoxetine does not work, one can switch to a different SSRI medication such as fluvoxamine (Luvox, Jazz Pharmaceuticals, Inc, Palo Alto, CA), sertraline (Zoloft [Pfizer]), or paroxetine (Paxil [GlaxoSmithKline, Philadelphia, PA]).

If the adolescent's condition fails to respond to SSRIs and the patient has been diagnosed with uncomplicated anxiety disorder or determined to have a history of substance abuse, the clinician can consider buspirone (Buspar [Bristol-Myers Squibb, New York, NY]) as a potential treatment. However, it should be noted that buspirone is only recommended for patients older than 18 years. If the clinician decides to use buspirone in adolescents, consider that the starting dose in adults is 5 mg 2 to 3 times per day or 7.5 mg twice per day, and it can be titrated with 5-mg increases per day every 2 to 3 days. The usual adult dose is 20 to 30 mg orally every day in divided doses, with a maximum of 60 mg each day. Buspirone is used in uncomplicated patients with generalized anxiety disorders whose conditions have failed to respond other anxiolytic agents or those who have a history of substance abuse.

Although there are several pharmaceutical treatment options available, the rapid onset of action of the benzodiazepines makes this class of medications the most efficacious for the treatment of acute intermittent anxiety.

HYPERVENTILATION SYNDROME

Hyperventilation is an extremely common problem in the adolescent patient. The chief complaint is usually a loss of consciousness with no apparent or precipitating event. However, most often, hyperventilation syncope will result from an anxiety-provoking event. Before making this diagnosis, there are several conditions that the clinician should rule out, including neurologic, cardiac, or respiratory problems and medications, drugs, or alcohol. In addition, the possibility of an epileptic event having caused the episode(s) should be considered. In the case of hyperventilation syncope, the adolescent may remember feeling light-headed or a sensation of darkening vision before losing consciousness. In the case of an epileptic event, it is unlikely that the patient will report these symptoms. If the patient describes true vertigo, this might be indicative of an epileptic event and should be explored as such. In addition, when exploring a syncopal episode the clinician should discern what the patient means by "black out" or "vision loss" as compared with a true loss of consciousness. Associated symptoms may include darkening of vision, tingling and numbness (especially of hands, feet, and face), stomachache, and increased heart or respiratory rate. The clinician can ask the patient, or one who observed the event, questions such as, "Tell me what you remember about the fall. Did you fall like a log or like a leaf?" Falling like a leaf implies a slower and more controlled fall and is more likely to imply that there was some sense of self-protection during the episode. In the case of hyperventilation syncope, the patient is usually aware that they are blacking out and is more likely to describe falling like a leaf. In the case of a seizure event, the patient is unlikely to remember the fall. Any description of such a fall is usually obtained by questioning an observer, who will commonly answer that the patient fell like a log. This type of fall would imply a true ictal event.

There may be pallor associated with the hyperventilation episode, but there will be no postictal phase. Those patients with hyperventilation syncope will have mental clarity within a few seconds of coming out of the episode. The history should explore where the patient was at the time of the episode (eg, in an emergency department, a dissecting laboratory, a dentist office). The clinician can ask what the patient was doing when the episode occurred (eg, "Did you see blood?" "Were you watching a scary movie?" "Were you dissecting in biology laboratory?"). In what type of situation was the patient and what were the associated symptoms, if any? If the episode was observed by someone else, did the observer think that the patient was mentally clear within a short time after the episode occurred? Continuing to discern if this was an epileptic event, the clinician needs to question if there was any sort of tonic/clonic activity during the episode. Although tonic/clonic activity is possible during hyperventilation syndrome, it is not common.

Ask the patient if he or she was breathing heavily during the episode. Did heart rate increase? Although patients may not be aware of an increase in heart rate and/or of breathing quickly in the moments leading up to the event, when questioned the adolescent may describe that he or she had trouble catching his or her breath. One should also explore the possibilities of heart disease or respiratory problems in the patient or family.

It is important to ascertain if there have been any previous syncopal episodes or any diagnoses made at previous times. If so, was there any follow-up, or were any tests done? Question the patient as to any history of illicit drug use, anxiety, or stress. Be sure to ask what, if any, medications the patient is taking. As always, the clinician should have a healthy suspicion regarding possible drug or alcohol involvement in the episode. The clinician should ask questions about school (eg, "Are there any educational problems?" "Are your grades declining?" "Are you feeling pressure or stress from family or boy/girlfriends?").

Family history questions should include an exploration of epilepsy, cardiac conditions, or fainting. One might ask if there is anyone in the family who blacks out, passes out, or has seizures or "spells."

In the case of hyperventilation syncope, physical and neurologic examination results will be within the normal range. The best test to perform in the office setting is a controlled hyperventilation test to evaluate if one is able to reproduce the symptoms. During this test, patients are asked to hyperventilate and to not speak while they are hyperventilating but to answer all questions with a yes or no nod of the head and then to raise a hand when they are beginning to feel funny. At the time of feeling funny ask, "Are you feeling dizzy?" and "Is your vision darkening?" If yes, stop him or her from further hyperventilation. If no, have him or her continue to hyperventilate until symptoms appear or hyperventilation has gone on for 2 minutes. Afterward, ask the patient if the symptoms have been reproduced. Many patients will say yes, but the symptoms experienced in the office were not as severe as the event itself. Note that the event is short-lived, with a quick recovery.

An explanation to the patient of what is occurring might include the following: "When we breathe normally, the purpose is to increase oxygen and decrease carbon dioxide. When we hyperventilate, we lose excessive amounts of CO_2, and as CO_2 decreases, blood flow also decreases. Less blood flowing to the eyes causes a transient loss of vision, decreased blood flow to the brain causes a feeling of light-headedness, a decrease to the stomach causes a stomachache, and a decrease to the extremities causes a tingling sensation. If we hyperventilate enough, we pass out. In the passed-out state, one can no longer hyperventilate, and so the body auto-corrects."

For treatment, we recommend that the patient hold his or her breath to retain carbon dioxide; a brown paper bag is likely to be socially embarrassing. If the patient is experiencing frequent syncopal episodes and appears to be overly anxious, then we recommend psychological and chemical intervention as a cotreatment until the underlying issues are resolved. For a discussion on medications to be used for anxiety, see "Anxiety" above.

SYNCOPE

Syncope most often occurs in times of stress or anxiety. Triggers might include seeing blood, visiting a hospital, getting an immunization, going to an emergency department, or perhaps going to a dentist's office. Less commonly, a syncopal episode caused by a vasovagal response can be triggered by hair brushing (thus, "hair-brushing syncope"). The changes in blood flow from cephalad to caudad that occur with micturition can also result in a temporary loss of consciousness.

History questions begin with exploring the symptoms experienced by the patient before the episode. Did the patient feel cold or clammy with sweating? If observed by another, the clinician may question if the patient appeared pale before the syncopal episode. The clinician should discern where the patient was, what activity he or she was doing when the event occurred, and at what time the event occurred. Was the patient in a biology laboratory, say, dissecting at the time? Was there psychic or physical trauma? Was there visual trauma (eg, a gory movie)? The clinician should seek clues as to whether there was any associated anxiety with the syncopal episode. It is imperative that the clinician further explore even the "no" answers to any of these questions with follow-up questions as described above.

If someone else observed the event, the clinician should ask the observer how long the episode lasted and what, if any, changes occurred in the skin color of the patient during the episode. Did the patient go pale? Was the patient mentally okay before and after the event? As described in "Hyperventilation Syncope," the clinician can explore if the patient fell like a log or a leaf. The observer might respond that the patient seemed confused and did not know what had happened. The clinician should clarify what the observer means by confused. Importantly, the clinician should ask the same questions of the observer to further delineate and clarify the episode. It is completely within the range of normal responses for a patient to have felt slightly disoriented at the time of the event. If questioned, the patient will usually report being aware of who was present at the time and any subsequent events. It is common for the patient to say, "What happened to me?" However, the clinician should discern the length and extent of the postepisode confusion.

In the case of complex syncope, the patient may have some motor or tonic-clonic activity during the episode and thus appear to be having a true seizure. This type of syncope is triggered most frequently when the patient receives an immunization or has a dental procedure. Complex syncope appears epileptic in presentation, but the preceding and following events will usually delineate or define whether the loss of consciousness was an electrical episode (seizure) or an anoxic episode (syncope). We strongly encourage the clinician to rule out a seizure disorder before making the diagnosis of complex syncope if the history of the event is not clear-cut.

In the differential diagnosis of an episode of loss of consciousness, the clinician should consider the possible presence of orthostatic hypotension. The diagnosis is in the history, and in almost all instances, the patient will report that symptoms occur when he or she goes from a lower to higher body positioning. In simple syncope, there will be no change in body position before the syncopal episode. In the case of simple or complex syncope or orthostatic hypotension, there should be no neurologic findings. On physical examination, particular attention should be given to cardiac, pulmonary, and vascular conditions that might exacerbate or induce the problem. It is our experience that orthostatic hypotension is not uncommon in the depressed adolescent. We strongly encourage the clinician to question the patient at length regarding any depressive symptoms that he or she might be experiencing.

There is no pharmacologic treatment for simple or complex syncope. The adolescent should either try to avoid trigger situations or learn techniques to deal with the problem.

SLEEP DISORDERS

Insomnia is defined as difficulty in maintaining or initiating sleep or have nonrestorative sleep for 1 month.[14] In all patients who suffer with insomnia, studies have shown that 40.5% have concomitant psychiatric disorders, and more than 50% of those will have anxiety disorders.[15] An adolescent who presents with a sleep problem should be questioned as to what exactly he or she is describing regarding difficulties sleeping. Is the patient having difficulty falling asleep? Does he or she describe falling asleep easily but is unable to stay asleep? Or perhaps the patient is having difficulty waking up after a night's sleep. As we have highlighted, it is important that the clinician explore exactly what is meant by difficulty sleeping or sleep problems. Patients with brain damage such as cerebral palsy may often present with sleep disorders. Unfortunately, insomnia in those individuals with structural brain damage can be quite difficult to treat. The clinician should inquire about brain damage or recent brain trauma as a possible causative factor when an adolescent presents with sleep problems. It is important for the clinician to maintain a high index of suspicion regarding abuse of medications, drugs, and alcohol[16] or the consumption of caffeinated high-energy drinks such as Red Bull[17] or 5-Hour Energy.[18]

In the general population of those with insomnia, 8.6% are reported to have dysthymia, 14.0% have major depression, and 23.9% have anxiety.[15] With numbers as high as these, we encourage the clinician to screen for these psychiatric comorbidities. Of those with nonpsychiatric disorders, one should consider physical illness, restless leg syndrome, iron-deficiency anemia, and appropriate or inappropriate use of medications as possible contributing factors in sleep disorders.

After clarifying the actual problem, the clinician should take a thorough sleep history and question what times the adolescent goes to sleep at night and what time he or she awakens. Does the patient nap during the day (hypersomnia), and if so, at what times? Included in the causes of hypersomnias are physical illnesses such as mononucleosis, chronic fatigue syndrome, etc, sleep apnea, and medication use. It is important for the clinician to explore if the adolescent experiences night terrors, sleep walking, or sleep talking (parasomnias). Inquire as to any sources of stress that might be affecting the patient: Would the patient describe his or her family situation as a stable one? Is he or she in a new school? Is the patient experiencing trouble in school or with friends? External stressors are a common source of sleep disorders in the adolescent patient. The primary clinician needs to thoroughly explore the possibility of anxiety or depression to better discern the cause of the problem.[19] A sleep diary can be quite helpful in attempting to ascertain the causative factors of sleep disturbance in the adolescent patient.

The patient who has difficulty falling asleep can consider using a white-noise machine or bright-light therapy (2000–2500 lux for 2–3 hours starting from 6 AM) to induce somnolence and relaxation in the evening. Alternatively, the adolescent can be taught relaxation techniques that might assist with the problem. However, some patients experience a sleep-phase disorder with which it seems that their individual circadian rhythm is dysfunctional (circadian rhythm disorder). If behavioral therapies are not successful, the clinician may consider giving melatonin to the patient to help induce somnolence. Melatonin 1 to 3 mg orally 1 to 2 hours before sleep time has been shown to affect the circadian rhythm in adult patients, thereby inducing sleep.[20–22] Other medications may be used that cause sedation as an adverse effect (eg, diphenhydramine [Benadryl (McNeil PPC, Fort Washington, PA)] or chlorpheniramine [Chlor-Trimeton (Schering-Plough,

Kenilworth, NJ)]). Although clonidine (Catapres [Boehringer Ingelheim, Ingelheim, Germany]) is not recommended for the treatment of insomnia, it can be prescribed for those patients whose sleep problems are recalcitrant to over-the-counter medications.[23] Used as a sleep aid, the starting dose of clonidine is 0.025 to 0.05 mg orally, given 30 minutes before bedtime. This dose is given for 3 to 5 days. If results are not sufficient in this time, the clinician can increase the dosage by 0.05 mg every 3 to 5 days up to a maximum dosage of 0.3 mg each day. Clonidine and the antihistamines can cause the patient to feel tired or a little foggy, so the clinician should assess the daily routines of the patient, particularly as regards driving, when considering prescribing clonidine or other sedation-inducing medications. The patient should be instructed not to abruptly discontinue clonidine, because it may result in rebound hypertension. When a clinician is discontinuing this medication, it is suggested that it be tapered in a stepwise fashion to avoid this potential complication.[23] Although clonidine is a hypotensive agent, it is the experience of the authors that it rarely causes hypotension in normotensive adolescents. However, it is important that the clinician and the patient be aware of the possibility of an increase in hypotensive episodes while taking clonidine. Consideration should be given to pretesting the dose during the day to evaluate for any signs or symptoms of hypotension. When a patient is on clonidine, it is recommended that pulse and blood pressure be monitored every 2 weeks for the first 2 months and at 3-month intervals thereafter.[23]

The patient who is able to fall asleep but unable to stay asleep could be suffering from depression or a parasomnia. Although insomnia may trigger depression, it is also true that depression may trigger insomnia.[24] We strongly encourage any clinician who is evaluating an adolescent for sleep disorder to evaluate the patient for depression. One helpful piece of information regarding depression and sleep disorders is that depression usually causes awakening between 12 AM and 2 AM. Parasomnias are most likely to occur 90 to 120 minutes after the patient has fallen asleep.[25] The patient is likely to have no recall of an event of parasomnia, and the event does not usually interfere with a feeling of restfulness. With this in mind, it is clear that a diagnosis of a parasomnia can only come from an observer rather than from the patient. However, if a parent of the patient describes "something funny" occurring just after the adolescent has fallen asleep, the clinician should probe further and consider the possibility of an epileptic event. If the initial parasomnia presents after the age of 10 years, the differential should include the possibility of a complex partial seizure having occurred.

The patient who has difficulty waking up in the morning is usually going to sleep too late at night and, therefore, is not getting the necessary amount of sleep required to wake up fully refreshed in the morning. With appropriate history taking the clinician can likely rule in or out other illnesses that cause somnolence. A particularly common reason for difficulty waking up is that the adolescent is on the computer or telephone late into the night. Other common reason for this problem are a dislike of school or depression.

Table 1
Panic attack symptoms

- Palpitations, tachycardia
- Shortness of breath
- Chest pain or discomfort
- Nausea or abdominal distress
- Sweating
- Trembling and shaking
- Feeling of choking
- Dizziness, lightheadedness, or faintness
- Paresthesias
- Chills or hot flashes
- Derealization and depersonalization
- Fear of losing control or "going crazy"
- Fear of dying

Data source: "Psychopharmacology" course booklet. September 30–October 2, 2005. Boston, MA. Massachusetts General Hospital, Department of Psychiatry, Harvard Med-CME, PO Box 825, Boston, MA 02117:565

If the parent is trying to wake the adolescent and the youngster has trouble waking or is speaking gibberish or nonsense, the clinician should consider other possibilities, such as atypical migraine or seizure in the differential diagnosis. Headache on waking could be a resultant symptom of an ictal event or of migraine. If the patient went to bed with a headache, then migraine, as opposed to an ictal event, is the more likely cause of difficulty awakening. In the case of an ictal event, the clinician can explore the nature of the event itself and the seizure history of the patient and family and can proceed accordingly to evaluate the youngster for an epileptic disorder.

We strongly encourage any clinician to explore the possibility of a comorbid depression or a history of drug use in an adolescent patient who presents with a history of sleep disorder, because this may help to avert a serious crisis in the life of the patient.

PANIC

Panic disorder is a syndrome characterized by recurrent panic attacks (ie, discreet episodes of intense anxiety associated with at least 4 other symptoms of autonomic arousal and anxiety that develop rapidly and typically peak within 10 minutes)[26] (see Table 1).

Some patients have limited symptom attacks. Rather than experiencing 4 symptoms, these patients may experience 1 or 2 symptoms such as tachycardia, dyspnea, and/or light-headedness. These symptoms cause distress and disability and respond to the same treatments as those for a full-blown panic attack. Panic can have comorbid symptoms such as agoraphobia or claustrophobia, which can function as triggers to an attack. Again, it is important to ascertain details regarding place of occurrence, situation, precipitating factors, and symptomatology when taking the history. If the patient describes an episode of panic that includes tachycardia or tachypnea, the clinician needs to explore if this was an isolated episode of panic or if a preexisting condition was reactivated.

Use of dietary and nutritional supplements should be explored, given that several supplements can be the cause of autonomic symptoms. Consider if the child is on a weight-loss regimen and perhaps using over-the-counter diet supplements that might contain stimulant-type medications. In the workup for panic disorder, consideration should be given to an electrocardiogram, resting blood pressure and pulse, and a thyroid screen, if indicated. If these test results are normal and the clinician is confident that there are no other metabolic causes, then therapy for panic disorder should be considered.

Treatment includes cognitive-behavioral therapy, benzodiazepines, and SSRI medications. For sporadic, longer-lasting but infrequent attacks, benzodiazepines are a good first choice. For chronic frequent episodes, either the benzodiazepines or SSRIs are helpful, although the latter are considered safer. For a fuller discussion of benzodiazepines and SSRIs please see the discussion on use of SSRIs in the adolescent population in "Anxiety."

OBSESSIVE COMPULSIVE DISORDER

Defined as pathologic levels of fears, phobias, and obsessions, OCD is reported to occur in 2% to 3% of all children and adolescents.[27] Many people have fears and phobias that do not impair their quality of life. However, adolescents who suffer from OCD have pathologic levels of fears, phobias, or obsessions that can impair their quality of life.

Diagnosing OCD requires a careful history, particularly because of the difficulty of detecting subtle differences between so-called normal obsessions or compulsions and those that cause impairment. An example would be the adolescent girl who might take 30 to 40 minutes to get dressed in the morning. It is easy to see that this example could well be considered typical behavior in an adolescent girl. However, on further questioning, one might find that this child has to have her hair absolutely perfect or she will not leave the house. The clinician is encouraged to explore if a particular behavior is rooted in fears and phobias. Another example is a child who does not want to leave for school. Is this because the patient is afraid that no one will be home when he arrives home, or is he worried that the bus will crash or perhaps that he will get on the wrong bus and get lost?

OCD in adolescents can present as a sleep problem. One might find that a patient is afraid to go to sleep because of a fear that he or she, or a family member, will not live through the night; or perhaps he or she is afraid of ghosts or thieves. Such patients often experience teasing by family members because the fears and phobias seem to make no rational sense. Clinicians are encouraged to interview the patient separately from the family. Pathologic levels of fear and phobia can cause deep embarrassment for young people, and patients may or may not be forthcoming about the levels of terror they experience.

Although screening tools can be helpful in delineating OCD, it is important that the clinician consider the subjectivity of the person who fills out the diagnostic tools. The clinician is encouraged to screen the family for a history of fears, phobias, obsessions, and tics. As with many other disorders, the diagnosis of OCD is made largely on the history of the patient as well as the family history. The family history can be quite helpful, because OCD is generally an inherited condition. Adolescents who suffer with OCD have a greater chance of having comorbid tic disorder and attention-deficit/hyperactivity disorder (ADHD) than the general population. Given a high rate of comorbidities between these conditions, the clinician might wish to consider the possibility of a diagnosis of OCD in any adolescent diagnosed with ADHD or tic disorder and a diagnosis of ADHD in any adolescent diagnosed with OCD and tic disorder.[23]

Cognitive-behavioral therapy has been shown to be as effective, or more effective, than SSRI medications for patients with OCD. When using SSRI medication, the clinician should be aware of the black-box warning, as discussed earlier, regarding the possible increase in suicidal ideation. For the patient on SSRI medications, it is imperative that the clinician see the patient frequently for follow-up visits to assess for the presence of suicidal ideation. Fluoxetine (Prozac), sertraline (Zoloft), and fluvoxamine (Luvox) have all been approved by the US Food and Drug Administration (FDA) for treatment of OCD in adolescents. Non–FDA-approved treatments for OCD in adolescents include paroxetine (Paxil), citalopram (Celexa [Forest Pharmaceuticals, Inc, New York, NY]), escitalopram (Lexapro [Forest Pharmaceuticals, Inc], the levo-isomer of citalopram), and clomipramine (Anafranil [Patheon Inc. Whitby, Ontario, Canada]).[9]

CONCLUSIONS

It is common for the internist or general practitioner to be on the front lines of treatment for anxiety and anxiety-related disorders. This article is intended to impart a basic working knowledge of the manifestations of anxiety as well as available treatments, thus providing the clinician with useful information and pointing out some of the pitfalls in making diagnoses.

REFERENCES

1. Larun L, Nordheim LV, Ekeland E, Hagen KB, Heian F. Exercise in prevention and treatment of anxiety and depression among children and young people. *Cochrane Database Syst Rev.* 2006;(3):CD004691

2. Smith C, Hancock H, Blake-Mortimer J, Eckert K. A randomised comparative trial of yoga and relaxation to reduce stress and anxiety. *Complement Ther Med.* 2007;15(2):77–83
3. Connolly SD, Bernstein GA; Work Group on Quality Issues. Practice parameter for the assessment and treatment of children and adolescents with anxiety disorders. *J Am Acad Child Adolesc Psychiatry.* 2007;46(2):267–283
4. Winerip M. Child anxiety that goes beyond the norm. *New York Times.* July 20, 2008. Available at: www.nytimes.com/2008/07/20/nyregion/nyregionspecial2/20Rparent.html. Accessed October 1, 2008
5. Food and Drug Administration. FDA public health advisory: suicidality in children and adolescents being treated with antidepressant medications—October 15, 2004. Available at: www.fda.gov/cder/drug/antidepressants/SSRIPHA200410.htm. Accessed August 13, 2008
6. Gibbons RD, Hur K, Bhaumik DK, Mann JJ. The relationship between antidepressant prescription rates and rate of early adolescent suicide. *Am J Psychiatry.* 2006;163(11):1898–1904
7. Are SSRIs safe for children? *Med Lett Drugs Ther.* 2003;45(1160):53–54
8. Which SSRI? *Med Lett Drugs Ther.* 2003;45(1170):93–95
9. Green WH. *Child and Adolescent Clinical Psychopharmacology.* 4th ed. Philadelphia, PA: Lippincott, Williams & Wilkins; 2007
10. Bolfek A, Jankowski JJ, Waslick B, Summergrad P. Adolescent psychopharmacology: drugs for mood disorders. *Adolesc Med Clin.* 2006;17(3):789–808; abstract xiii–xiv
11. *Physicians' Desk Reference.* Montvale, NJ: Thompson PDR; 2009
12. Ramasubbu R. Antidepressant treatment-associated behavioural expression of hypomania: a case series. *Prog Neuropsychopharmacol Biol Psychiatry.* 2004;28(7):1201–1207
13. Akiskal HS, Hantouche EG, Allilaire JF, et al. Validating antidepressant-associated hypomania (bipolar III): a systematic comparison with spontaneous hypomania (bipolar II). *J Affect Disord.* 2003;73(1–2):65–74
14. American Psychiatric Association. *Diagnostic and Statistical Manual of Mental Disorders.* 4th ed. Primary Care Version. Washington, DC: American Psychiatric Association; 1994
15. Ford DE, Kamerow DB. Epidemiologic study of sleep disturbances and psychiatric disorders. An opportunity for prevention? *JAMA.* 1989;262(11):1479–1484
16. Shibley HL, Malcolm RJ, Veatch LM. Adolescents with insomnia and substance abuse: consequences and comorbidities. *J Psychiatr Pract.* 2008;14(3):146–153
17. Red Bull Energy Drink. Ingredients. Available at: www.redbullusa.com/#page=ProductPage.Ingredients. Accessed August 8, 2008
18. 5-Hour Energy Drink. Home page. Available at: www.5hourenergy.com. Accessed August 8, 2008
19. Breslau N, Roth T, Rosenthal L, Andreski P. Sleep disturbance and psychiatric disorders: a longitudinal epidemiological study of young adults. *Biol Psychiatry.* 1996;39(6):411–418
20. Mindell JA, Emslie G, Blumer J, et al. Pharmacologic management of insomnia in children and adolescents: consensus statement. *Pediatrics.* 2006;117(6). Available at: www.pediatrics.org/cgi/content/full/117/6/e1223
21. Owens JA, Rosen CL, Mindell JA. Medication use in the treatment of pediatric insomnia: results of a survey of community-based pediatricians. *Pediatrics.* 2003;111(5 pt 1). Available at: www.pediatrics.org/cgi/content/full/111/5/e628
22. Shneerson JP. *Handbook of Sleep Medicine.* Oxford, United Kingdom: Blackwell Science; 2000
23. Leckman JF, Cohen DJ. *Tourette's Syndrome—Tics, Obsessions, Compulsions: Developmental Psychopathology and Clinical Care.* New York, NY: John Wiley & Sons; 1999
24. Riemann D, Voderholzer U. Primary insomnia: a risk factor to develop depression? *J Affect Disord.* 2003;76(1–3):255–259
25. Deray M. Management of parasomnias. *Int Pediatr.* 1997;12(3):161–163
26. American Psychiatric Association. *Diagnostic and Statistical Manual of Mental Disorders.* 4th ed. Primary Care Version. Washington, DC: American Psychiatric Association; 1994:47–63
27. Stewart SE. Questions & answers about OCD in children and adolescents. Available at: www.ocfoundation.org/UserFiles/File/Questions-Answers-OCD-In-Children-Adolescents.pdf. Accessed August 18, 2008

Helping Adolescents With Attention-Deficit/ Hyperactivity Disorder Transition Toward Adulthood

Edward M. Gotlieb, MD, FAAP, FSAM*, Jaquelin S. Gotlieb, MD, FAAP

The Pediatric Center of Stone Mountain LLC, 5405 Memorial Drive, Building D, Stone Mountain, GA 30083-3236, USA

Kids Health First Pediatric Alliance, 2814 New Spring Road, Suite 104, Atlanta, GA 30339, USA

"I would have done it different."

22-year-old patient with ADHD, looking back at his college career

Attention-deficit/hyperactivity disorder (ADHD) is widely discussed in the general medical literature. The transition of adolescents with ADHD into college and into adult roles is much less discussed, with information scattered sparsely through medical literature, government publications, and popular venues. For the adolescent who is trying to navigate through what can be a challenging time of life, getting useful information and help can be a hit-or-miss process. For the pediatrician who wants to assist patients in their journey, locating useful tools during the course of a busy clinical schedule can be difficult. In this article we attempt to accumulate beneficial information related to the issues surrounding transition to adult status for the adolescent with ADHD and identify resources that can help both the pediatrician and his or her patient.

There have been recent general review articles on ADHD in adolescents[1–3] and adults.[4,5] The August 2008 *Adolescent Medicine: State of the Art Reviews* devoted its entire issue to ADHD and learning disorders.[6] Nonetheless, the peer-reviewed medical literature about the transition to adulthood in patients with ADHD is sparse. In this article we review the current milieu in which older adolescents find themselves and list some of the health and life issues confronting older adolescents with ADHD as they move from high school into college or the

---

*Corresponding author.

E-mail address: edward.gotlieb@emory.edu (E. M. Gotlieb).

Copyright © 2009 American Academy of Pediatrics. All rights reserved. ISSN 1934-4287

workplace. Finally, we list resources that may assist with medical management and patient self-care.

THE CHANGING POSTADOLESCENT ENVIRONMENT

Today's adolescents with ADHD are attempting to enter adulthood in a very different world from that experienced by their parents and their physicians years ago. Increasingly, American adults in their 20s are delaying marriage, childbearing, and permanent employment. In 1960, 70% of 30-year-olds had moved away from home, become financially independent, married, and started a family; in 2000, fewer than 40% of 30-year-olds had reached these milestones.[7,8]

Erikson,[9] in his work on the nuclear conflicts of psychosocial development, wrote that, in young adulthood, the individual's focus shifts from the crisis of identity versus identity confusion to the matter of intimacy versus isolation. Young adults still wants to blend their identity with their friends, but now, as they are preparing for a close personal relationship with another, they have to learn to balance this relationship with learning how to be alone with themselves.

Levine[10] has discussed the challenges confronting those he describes as "startup adults." He believes that young people need to develop 4 specific qualities. "Inner direction" is a realistic sense of who they are and what their strengths and weaknesses are. They also need to know where they are headed. "Interpretation" includes their getting to know the world around them and understanding the ideas and expectations of those that they need to deal with in the world of adult relations and the work environment. "Instrumentation" is the development of a tool kit of strategies that develop organizational skills, harness mental energy, and foster creativity. They need to develop a process for making "sound decisions in a systematic manner." "Interaction" denotes developing the ability to use words to convey thought accurately, promote a point of view, and build and maintain relationships.

Barkley[11] suggested that ADHD might well be seen as an executive function problem of intention and self-control rather than merely a problem of inattention and impulsivity. The problem of intention might express itself in the person with ADHD attending to the issues of the moment rather than to what needs to be done to plan for the future. Brown[12] discussed the executive functions necessary for success when entering adulthood, which include "selecting options and working productively, managing a household and finances, managing work while nurturing relationships, and parenting and sustaining partnerships." Adolescents and young adults with ADHD who have problems with strategic planning may find themselves particularly vulnerable in confronting these issues as they move from high school and the family home into the increasingly complex environments ahead.

HEALTH MANAGEMENT CONCERNS

Long-term Monitoring and Adherence to Treatment

An American Academy of Pediatrics clinical practice guideline on treating ADHD,[13] written for a younger patient population, recommended that primary care clinicians establish a management program that recognizes ADHD as a chronic condition and specify appropriate target outcomes to guide management. The American Academy of Child and Adolescent Psychiatry recommended a well-thought-out, comprehensive treatment plan and periodic assessment for patients who are minors.[14] Because of the paucity of literature specific to transitional adolescents with ADHD, much of the following discussion on the health management of these patients is based on our clinical experience. Many pediatricians find that health information is often better provided in small doses repeatedly over time. Because pediatricians who treat the older adolescent will frequently find themselves guiding patients and their families through many issues around transition and growing independence, it may be helpful to develop a tracking method to begin recording medical comments and preparations. Keeping a flowchart of the counseling provided can remind the pediatrician of areas that have been discussed and gaps that need to be addressed and can be useful in monitoring and advancing a long-term view of treatment.

As they begin to anticipate moving past high school, some older adolescents want to stop taking their ADHD medication either because they are tired of taking daily medication or to express their independence from their parents and physician. They may really see no advantage to being on medication. Even those who ostensibly plan to continue on their medication seem to find ways to "forget" doses, especially when life is busy or on weekends and school holidays. It can be useful to encourage quarterly, or at least home-from-school, follow-up visits and to explore with these patients the benefits of adhering to their treatment schedule. It is sometimes useful to agree to a patient's desire to discontinue medication, particularly if it has been an extended time period since the pediatrician has observed him or her off treatment. Such an approach also tends to diffuse the conflict of the patient perceiving the pediatrician as blocking the desire to stop medication. Schedule the trial for the least precarious time in the school schedule, with the stated understanding that the trial calls for no fewer, and possibly more frequent, medical monitoring visits.

Driving

According to Barkley and Cox,[15] adolescents with ADHD are 2 to 4 times more likely to be the driver in an automobile accident than adolescent drivers without ADHD, and these drivers improve their driving performance by use of their stimulant medications. It is important to emphasize the message that effective compliance with medication adherence is critical to preparation for driving.

Starting this discussion early, long before the age at which patients are legally able to drive, ensures that patients begin to consider the long-term nature of their medical condition and the fact that it affects much more than life in the schoolroom. It also ensures that the pediatrician begins the discussion of safe driving habits before the moment at which these patients may try out driving, either with or without their parent's knowledge or consent.

Following American Academy of Pediatrics guidelines,[16] this is also an ideal time to reiterate the need for other highway safety strategies, such as encouraging seatbelt usage and reminding patients of the role of alcohol and drugs in motor vehicle crashes. Nighttime driving should be addressed directly. Driving with multiple or disorderly passengers, or unbelted passengers needs to be discouraged. Katz[17] and Snyder[18] have described contracts between adolescents and their parents to encourage safe driving. Allstate Insurance provides a driving-contract document on its Web site.[19]

Smoking, Alcohol, and Other Drugs

Many older adolescents, and indeed their parents, may attempt to discontinue ADHD medications in the mistaken belief that the use of the stimulant medications will lead to later drug abuse. It is important for the pediatrician to explain that although people with untreated ADHD are more likely than those in the general population to become involved with alcohol and other drug abuse, those who are appropriately treated for ADHD are no more likely to do so. Treatment, at least when looking at the ADHD population as a whole, seems to diminish the likelihood of drug abuse.[20]

Smoking is more common in this older adolescent population,[21] so it makes sense for the pediatrician to be particularly vigilant in discouraging this behavior. He or she should also be ready to assist the adolescent with smoking-cessation information and treatment or referral if the patient is already smoking.

Drug diversion is a real issue for adolescents with access to stimulant medication. According to Wilens et al,[22] a review of 21 studies suggested that 5% to 35% of college-aged individuals have participated in previous-year nonprescribed stimulant usage. Lifetime rates of medication diversion for students with stimulant prescriptions were 16% to 29%. Careful discussion of the need to protect their medication from others is in order. Office monitoring of the number of pills dispensed and the frequency of requests for refills along with fairly frequent in-office patient-recheck visits to monitor clinical progress and dosing adherence would likely limit, or at least help to expose, this problem. Patients who are away from home at school or other venues should be made aware of the potential of their living quarters being targeted for theft so that their medication storage area may be better protected. In some cases, nonstimulant treatments might be considered if the risk or patient concern is high.

Career Planning

The pediatrician can set the stage for discussing career planning by talking to patients from an early age about what they want to be "when they grow up." As they get closer to making real career choices, this can lead to healthy discussions about school performance, access to funding for post–high school training, and reality testing of dreams of sports or military careers.[23] Having co-location with or easy access to consultation with behavioral and vocational counselors can improve the quality of these discussions. Making the patients aware of resource people and testing at their high school or local community college, or through state-sponsored vocational rehabilitation centers, can open options of which they may be unaware. Written materials about careers and ADHD are also available.[24,25]

Friendship and Intimacy

According to Coleman, in his review of social competence and friendship formation in patients with ADHD, "having friends and keeping them, constitutes a critical milestone in adolescence. Successful and gratifying peer interactions, or the lack of them, affect all domains of a teenager's life."[26]

Learning to deal with intimacy is an issue for all adolescents, but there are special challenges for the adolescent with ADHD. Wender, on the basis of his psychiatric clinical experience, observed, "Because of his social obtuseness, the ADHD adolescent may not be shy, but because of his social ineptitude, he stands a good chance of being unsuccessful."[27]

Barkley et al[28] reported on the social and sexual outcomes in a longitudinal study of 149 hyperactive children and 72 controls (mean age: 20 years) in Milwaukee, Wisconsin, who were followed for at least 13 years. The hyperactive group reported the same number of friends but fewer close friends and reported problems keeping friends. There was no difference in current dating or average duration of steady dating. Those in the hyperactive group began intercourse 1 year earlier than those in the control group (15 vs 16 years, respectively) and had twice as many total sex partners. The hyperactive group was significantly more likely to use birth control measures "rarely or never" (25% vs 10%), and 38% vs 4% had been involved with a pregnancy.

Betchen[29] presented his clinical experiences as a marriage and family counselor to describe some of the common obstacles to the development of intimate relationships for individuals with ADHD. Problems with impulsivity, emotional lability, and hypersensitivity can make it difficult to develop relations with others. A tendency to hyperfocus can be misread by friends and potential intimate partners and can lead to a partner feeling either invaded or ignored. Disorganization can cause forgetting of important dates or prearranged appointments, leading friends to feel unappreciated.

Hallowell and Ratey,[30] writing from their clinical perspective as adult psychiatrists, described some of the problems of adults with ADHD in developing and maintaining a sexual relationship. These include "difficulty lingering" (being impatient to get to the "bottom line"), insatiability, and using sex as self-medication.

In our experience, the pediatrician can anticipate, and attempt to influence, issues that may later lead to difficulties with developing relationships. Cueing an adolescent during a medical visit that his or her stimulation-seeking behavior may be annoying to others can begin a useful conversation. The adolescent's craving for stimulation may move him or her to set up fights with others just for the sake of the emotional high. Discussing limit setting and pointing out when a patient is hitting "below the belt" in a confrontation with a parent or friend may help to build an awareness that the adolescent can use. Noticing when an adolescent is hyperfocusing can lead to a discussion of how this can lead to a friend or partner feeling hurt. Pediatrician feedback to such behaviors may ease a referral to psychotherapy.

Confidentiality

One of the pediatrician's concerns in managing care for the transition to adulthood for all adolescents is the need to separate the discussions he or she has with the patient and his or her parents. This is particularly true when addressing mental health issues such as ADHD. The Health Insurance Privacy and Accountability Act of 1996 (HIPAA)[31] gives pediatricians wide discretion in dealing with the emancipated minor who becomes his or her own "personal representative" on a list of topics mandated by state law but which may include, for example, psychiatric care or information about contraception and drugs. It also allows for "informal" arrangements for confidential care to be developed between the pediatrician and the patient and his or her family. Developing a form that spells out the office's policy on these issues, which is signed by all the parties, can offer an opportunity to discuss these issues directly.[32] Pediatricians would be wise to acquaint themselves with the workings of the HIPAA, state statutes, and specific facility interpretations as they apply to adolescents and their parents and in dealing with the school system. Pediatricians should also be aware of another federal program, the Family Educational Rights and Privacy Act (FERPA),[33] which is specifically exempted from the HIPAA and controls confidentiality in schools and colleges. For the patient who has reached majority, establishing with all concerned the need for a confidential relationship between the pediatrician and the patient needs to be stressed. The pediatrician's office staff should be aware of the rules of this new relationship.[34]

Insurance Coverage

Given that the cost of medical care for patients with ADHD has been reported to be substantially higher than that for the general population,[35–37] lack of insurance coverage becomes a real impediment to obtaining medical care for people with ADHD in general, especially for those who are 18 years of age and older. Pediatricians can help patients with ADHD and their families anticipate and prepare for the financial issues they will confront as adolescents reach young adulthood.

The insurance problems associated with patients with ADHD were previously reviewed by Wolraich et al.[1] Seifert and Hollingsworth[38] reported 2005 data from the Substance Abuse and Mental Health Services Administration stating that some 5.7 million adults did not receive needed mental health treatment in the previous year. Of those polled, 46.8% said that lack of insurance or concerns about cost were the primary reasons they did not seek help. Callahan,[39] in a 2007 article, reported that, at any given time, one third of young adults are uninsured and that some 60% will have gaps in insurance coverage some time during their young adulthood.

Medicaid health coverage ends for patients at 18 years of age if they are unmarried and do not have children. The State Children's Health Insurance Program (SCHIP) and other public funds have been used in some communities to supplement coverage, but this funding seems precarious and not generally available. Many commercial policies no longer cover young people under their parents' policy after the student reaches 18 years of age. Policies that do continue coverage typically have requirements that the young adult be enrolled full-time in college or other advanced training. Young adults leaving their parents' insurance after completing college may be eligible for extended health care coverage under the federal Consolidated Omnibus Budget Reconciliation Act (COBRA),[40] but this is frequently at a considerably more expensive rate than their previous policy. In recent years, a number of states have passed legislation mandating the extension of coverage to young adults from their parents' insurance under varying circumstances. There is, however, no uniformity to these various measures.[41]

According to the Friends Committee on National Legislation,[42] The Paul Wellstone and Pete Domenici Mental Health Parity and Addiction Equity Act of 2008,[43] which was included in Troubled Asset Relief Program[44]:
- ensures that private and government health insurance programs include mental health and addiction-related health coverage;
- makes limits on mental health care and addiction treatment similar to limits on all other medical procedures included in insurance plans (thus establishing "parity" among them; for example, the copay for prescriptions would be the same under a given insurance plan, and the number of office visits allowed for various kinds of treatment would be the same); and
- requires the government to regulate criteria that health insurance providers use to determine "medical necessity."

It is currently unclear how this legislation will be implemented and how or whether it will assist the young adult with ADHD. As the system now stands, therefore, young adults are in a real bind. Affording treatment without insurance is quite expensive for someone just entering the job market. Without medication treatment and continuing medical care, however, they are at a real disadvantage compared with their peers in obtaining employment that provides medical insurance.

Anticipating the Change to Adult Medical Models

Assuming they can continue to obtain medical care, adolescents are then confronted with having to negotiate the adult medical system. The literature on transition to adult health care models has been led mainly by pediatricians attempting to continue coverage for special-needs populations of children with chronic medical illness or handicapping conditions and has not focused on an ADHD diagnosis. This literature suggests that patients and their families find it difficult to transit into the adult system, in which care givers may not have the comfort level or familiarity with chronic pediatric medical conditions.[45-49] Referral to psychiatry may provide more familiarity with medication treatment options but complicates the provision of a "medical home" approach and raises the likelihood of noncompliance because of stigmatization and additional costs. The pediatrician may be willing to continue care at least through 21 years of age or until the patient completes formal education, perhaps in cooperation with, or at least available to, college student health services. The pediatrician can become knowledgeable about local community services such as vocational rehabilitation and mental health professionals who work with young adults with ADHD and their issues. The astute pediatrician can help this transition process by having considered these issues and by preparing the patient and his or her family to interview suitable family physicians and internists in the community.

LEGISLATION MANDATING ACCOMMODATIONS AND SPECIAL SERVICES

Accommodations for adolescents with ADHD may be mandated by several federal government programs. A more complete discussion of the Individual Education Plan (IEP) and the 504 plan is available in a recent review by Cohen.[50] The following are some elements of those programs that may be of particular interest to needs of the older adolescent or young adult.

Individual Education Plan

An IEP is mandated for eligible students under the Individuals With Disabilities Education Act (IDEA), which was established in 1975 and updated in 2004. In part, it regulates how states administer their special education services with the goal of providing "free appropriate education" in the "least restrictive environment." The US Department of Education's Office of Special Education Programs monitors state programs to ensure that they are complying with the IDEA. For the purposes of this document, it is useful to review the transitional services requirements of this legislation.[51] According to the Statement of Transition Service Needs—34 CFR §300.347(b)(1),

> "The IEP must include . . . [f]or each student with a disability beginning at age 14 (or younger, if determined appropriate by the IEP team), and updated annually, a statement of the transition service needs of the student under the applicable components of the student's IEP that focuses on the student's courses of study (such as participation in advanced-placement courses or a vocational education program)."

Transition services must be included in a student's IEP when he or she has reached specific age markers and can include developing postsecondary education and career goals, getting work experience while still in school, and setting up linkages with adult service providers such as the vocational rehabilitation agency. For students beginning at age 14 (and sometimes younger), transition planning assists in planning courses of study for, among other possibilities, advanced placement or vocational education so that the classes they take will lead them to their postschool goals. For students by the age of 16 years, transition services provide them with "a coordinated set of services" to help the move from school to adult life. Services focus on the student's needs or interest in such areas as "higher education or training, employment, adult services, independent living, or taking part in the community."

504 Plan

A 504 plan refers to Section 504 of the Rehabilitation Act of 1973.[52,53] This act is a civil rights law, and according to the legislation, no one who has "an impairment that restricts one or more major life activities" can be excluded from participating in federally funded programs or activities, including elementary, secondary, or postsecondary schooling. A 504 plan spells out the modifications and accommodations that will be needed for these students to have an opportunity to perform at the same level as their peers in the public school system or private schools that receive federal funds. In the context of an ADHD diagnosis, accommodations might include dispensing an extra set of textbooks, home instruction, or a tape recorder or keyboard for taking notes. A student's assignments or testing conditions may be allowed extended time or modification of test questions. A student does not need to qualify for special education services under an IEP to qualify for services under the Rehabilitation Act. According to the US Department of Education:

> "Virtually all public school districts are covered by Section 504 because they receive some federal financial assistance. Public colleges

and universities generally receive federal financial assistance, and most private colleges and universities receive such assistance. There are some private colleges that do not receive any federal assistance, and Section 504 does not apply to them."[54]

Requests for establishing a 504 plan should typically be directed to the principal or counselor of the student's school, most helpfully in writing. The request for a plan may be initiated by a teacher, the parent or legal guardian, certain other designated professionals, or by the student. It should be noted, however, that under Section 504, there are fewer procedural safeguards available to children with disabilities and their parents than under the IDEA.[55] 504 plans are monitored by the Office of Civil Rights of the US Department of Education.

Americans With Disabilities Act in Postsecondary Schools

Title II of the Americans With Disabilities Act (ADA) of 1990 prohibits discrimination based on disability by any public entity, including public schools, colleges, and universities.[56] Colleges and universities are required to provide students with appropriate academic adjustments and auxiliary aids and services that are necessary to afford an individual with a disability an equal opportunity to participate in the school's program. Examples of auxiliary aids that may be required are taped texts, note takers, interpreters, readers, and specialized computer equipment. They are not required to supply students with readers for personal use or study or other devices or services of a personal nature.[54]

The ADA in the Workplace

The ADA applies to businesses with 15 or more employees and would, in theory, protect people who have ADHD. The employee must disclose that he or she has a significant disability that, despite treatment, impacts a major life activity or function. The employer would then be required to provide reasonable accommodations. More than 90% of ADA cases are won by employers, often because of the difficulty in proving the "reasonableness" of the requested accommodations.[57] With this diagnosis, if the case went through the courts, the employer could argue that the employee, by being inattentive, could not perform the basic functions of the job. Consequently, generally speaking, the employee would do best to try to work out an informal arrangement with his or her employer to minimize difficulties with the job.[58]

PREPARING FOR POST–HIGH SCHOOL EDUCATION AND WORK

Applications for College Testing and Admission Accommodation

Each college and university has its own process for applying for special accommodations, and it is crucial for the prospective student to understand the program that the school has in place, what is required for application and acceptance, and what is the timeline under which the application must be made. In addition, it would be reasonable for your patient to ascertain the lead time that you and your staff, and other outside professionals, will need to provide the various parts of the application documentation.

Many colleges and universities, as well as the College Board and the ACT, have adopted or adapted the "Guidelines for Documentation of Attention Deficit/ Hyperactivity Disorder in Adolescents and Adults,"[59] published by the Consortium on ADHD Documentation in 1998. This document largely follows the elements of the *Diagnostic and Statistical Manual of Mental Disorders, Fourth Edition* criteria for an ADHD diagnosis. In addition, each of these entities may, and likely will, have other requirements for establishing special accommodations for your patient. These requirements can typically be addressed by the student at the school's department of disabilities services, but he or she should be careful to allow adequate time for the process.

SAT ("College Board")

According to the College Board,[60] a student, to receive test accommodations, must apply for and receive College Board approval.

> "Scores may be canceled if it is determined that a student received accommodations that were not approved by the College Board.... If possible, a student should apply for accommodations before submitting a test registration, preferably in the spring before his first College Board test."[59]

The student must complete a student eligibility form supplied by the Services for Students With Disabilities coordinator at his or her school. An eligibility approval letter stating the granted accommodations will be sent to students who have been approved. Types of accommodations may include 50% extended time, extended breaks, and additional breaks. According to the College Board Web site, the eligibility application dates for requesting testing with accommodations are earlier than the SAT registration deadlines. There is also a 7-week process for documentation review of requests that are made with documentation from other sources than from the school. The Web site offers up-to-date information and additional details.

The ACT

The ACT has published guidelines for applying for accommodations for students with ADHD, describing the available testing options. Information about their services for students with disabilities is available in booklet form on their Web site.[61]

"evidence that the disability substantially limits one or more major life activities. Applicants must also provide information about previous accommodations made in a similar setting, such as academic classes and test taking, for example, in the form of a current Individual Education Plan or Section 504 Plan. If the applicant has not had previous accommodations, full documentation must be submitted. If a particular element of documentation is not provided, the diagnostician must explain why it is not included in the submission."

Graduate Record Examination

Accommodations will be provided for test takers who meet Educational Testing Service (ETS) requirements. Test takers who need accommodations cannot register online or request standby registration. Details for application are on the Web site.[62]

Military Testing

The Armed Forces qualifying test[63] determines whether an applicant is qualified to enlist in the US military and is a part of the Armed Services Vocational Aptitude Battery. The Armed Forces are not required to grant accommodations, such as extended test time, on the qualifying test. In addition, military regulations provide that academic skills deficits that interfere with school or work after the age of 12 may be a cause for rejection for service in the Armed Forces. These regulations also provide that current use of medication, such as Ritalin or Dexedrine, to improve academic skills is disqualifying for military service.[23]

Traveling With Medication

As students take longer to finish college, there is opportunity for a summer abroad or a "gap year," where there is planned or unplanned time away from school. For the person with ADHD, there are special issues if they require a supply of what are, after all, typically controlled substances. Advanced planning between the student, his or her family, and the pediatrician is in order. If the travel is domestic and short, informal arrangements are probably all that are needed. For longer time frames or foreign travel, more formal arrangements are in order. Finding medical support domestically is greatly ameliorated by the pediatrician's help in locating another practitioner or treatment site at the new location. For foreign travel, local drug laws ought to be understood, and medicine to be transported should be properly labeled and stored. If there are to be medications obtained overseas, government advisories should be heeded and availability and medication name variations known in advance.[64,65]

College Disability-Support Services

There are numerous books[66–68] and articles[69,70] that have addressed the issues of colleges and their approaches to students with ADHD, learning strategies, and potentially available accommodations. These issues are beyond the scope of this article. The pediatrician can benefit patients by making them aware of the availability of these resources. He or she can also simplify the task of filling out requests for special educational services by following the format that the specific college requires.

The National Resource Center on AD/HD (NRC) (discussed below) recommends that prospective students contact the Student Disability Support Office at any college or university they are considering. Accommodations can be assessed early in the process, and generally speaking, colleges will not grant accommodations retroactively. The NRC recommends that the student find out, among a number of concerns,[71] if the head of student disability services or another staff member is a specialist in ADHD and learning disability services, whether there is an organized program to educate the school's faculty about ADHD, whether there is staff involvement in freshman orientation, and whether a school physician is available to prescribe medications to treat ADHD.

Community Colleges

Pediatricians working with students with ADHD can benefit their patients by being aware of the relative strengths of programs provided by community colleges in their community. These colleges are an option for students with ADHD because of their relatively low cost and often open admissions policies.[72] Some may also be attuned to the needs of accommodating students with special needs. According to the MDRC, previously the Manpower Demonstration Research Corporation,[73] community colleges "are the gateway to higher ed and better jobs" for many Americans, with almost half of postsecondary students attending. They attract a large number of low-income and first-generation students. However, 36% of community college students fail to earn a degree anywhere within 6 years.[74] Nonetheless, according to the US Census Bureau in 2005, a 2-year associate degree brings, on average, a yearly increased income of more than $8000.[75]

ADHD Scholarship Aid

There are scholarships available for students with ADHD. These are best pursued with the help of school guidance counselors and other counseling professionals. The Internet also has listings, but they need to be evaluated with reasonable caution for unscreened sources. One site that has received some positive media attention[76] is CollegeScholarships.org.

SELF-MANAGEMENT

Because young adults with ADHD may find themselves with diminished external supports, they may need to develop their own strategies to deal with ADHD. Given that adolescents and adults with ADHD may have particular difficulty with self-management skills, the pediatrician may encourage them to develop these skills and point them to self-help resources. However, there does not seem to be relevant medical literature to validate the success of such an effort.

DuPaul and Evans[77] have reviewed the literature on self-management for adolescents with ADHD and reported some success in teaching self-management skills to high school students.[78] There has also been some experience in the adult education literature for a process called "scaffolding," in which the instructor assists the student in learning a task by verbalizing the thought process, offering an expert model, helping with guided practice, and then "fading" back as the student gains mastery.[79]

ADHD Coaching

A treatment approach has emerged called ADHD coaching. ADHD coaching is practiced by coaches who work 1-on-1 with people with ADHD. The Attention Deficit Disorder Association (ADDA) (discussed below), for one, supports ADHD coaching as an adjunct or additional intervention within the range of available methods of treatment. Further discussion of this form of assistance is discussed on the ADDA's Web site (www.add.org).

Time-Management Tools

On the basis of the clinical observation that people with ADHD have difficulty with time management, the NRC has suggested the use of time-management planners.[80] The increasing ubiquity of smart phones and personal digital assistants allows young adults to cue themselves about upcoming appointments and assignments. For example, Google Calendar (www.google.com/intl/en/googlecalendar/overview.html) is a free, Web-based application that allows online access or text messaging to a calendar of upcoming events, plans, and appointments. The program can then send a prescheduled e-mail or a text message to a smart phone to remind the user in advance of the event. Skoach (http://skoach.com) presents itself as a Web-based "life-management" program. This paid-subscription service offers a 1-click autoscheduler that can be accessed from a Web browser. New appointments can be sent to this Web site by telephone or e-mail. Task trees can organize projects into more manageable sequences of steps. Reminders of elements left to be done can be requested to be automatically sent by e-mail to the program user. There are also facilities to help the user pick up a forgotten schedule track.

ADHD Information Sites

There are many ADHD-focused organizations and Web sites. The American Academy of Pediatrics and other specialty societies have considerable resources about ADHD in general and, in varying degrees, about the young adult with ADHD. The following examples represent national programs with information geared to the needs of those in this age group.

Children and Adults With ADHD (CHADD) (www.chadd.org) is a national nonprofit organization that provides education, advocacy, and support for individuals with ADHD. They have a Web site and publish a journal, *Attention Magazine*. They produce printed materials and conferences to keep members and professionals current on research advances, medications, and treatments that affect individuals with ADHD. Many communities have ongoing CHADD support groups for children with ADHD and their parents and, also, for adults with ADHD.

The ADDA (www.add.org) is a not-for-profit international organization founded in 1989. It provides information, resources, and networking to adults with ADHD and to the professionals who work with them. Its resources focus on advocacy for adults with ADHD and diagnoses, treatments, strategies, and techniques for helping adults with ADHD lead better lives. This organization currently has a quarterly publication, *Focus*, guidelines on topics such as ADHD coaching, videos, tapes, and "teleclasses."

The NRC, which is a program of CHADD, is a national clearinghouse for evidence-based information on ADHD. It was developed after a public health perspective conference on ADHD held in Atlanta, Georgia, in 1999, which recommended the establishment of a national resource center to provide accurate and valid information to the public and professionals. Web-based resources include the NRC Web site (www.help4adhd.org) and a library with bibliographic information of >25 000 records (www.help4adhd.org/library.cfm).

Social Networking Web sites

Social networking sites have proliferated on the Internet over the last few years.[81,82] According to Peter Varhol, the executive editor of *Redmond Magazine*, Facebook has 65 million users generating 1000 page hits per user per month: this is not a fad.[83] Despite privacy concerns,[84] they have offered a haven for adolescents and young adults to congregate in a relatively safe environment.[85] A newly discussed Internet-based health care conception, Health 2.0,[86,87] is described as "the use of social software and its ability to promote collaboration between patients, their caregivers, medical professionals, and other stakeholders."[88] Increasingly, sites that present themselves under this rubric of health support networks (eg, Association of Cancer Online Resources [www.acor.org]

and PatientsLikeMe [www.patientslikeme.com]) have arisen, at which people with shared medical conditions can find and offer support; obtain information about care and treatment options; and post health information that, in aggregate, has the potential to produce patterns that might lead to new insights in clinical care. There is little research in this area, and there are concerns about confidentiality and accuracy of information, because such sites are typically self-monitored by their Web community. Nonetheless, some are reported to be well received and beneficial to their members.[89] It seems worth following the development of these sites for possible recommendation to transitional patients with ADHD should sites with this focus develop.

CONCLUSIONS

One of the most rewarding parts of pediatrics is to see our patients grow up and succeed. It is beneficial for the pediatrician to anticipate issues that older adolescents with ADHD are likely to face, to help them deal with the fact that they have what may be a lifelong medical condition, and to help them find ways for developing the skills and resources that will limit the difficulties that entering the adult world may present. We hope that this article will assist practicing pediatricians negotiate the enormous body of information about ADHD so that they may more easily find useful information and tools for helping their patients succeed during their transition toward adulthood.

REFERENCES

1. Wolraich ML, Wibbelsman CJ, Brown TE, et al. Attention-deficit/hyperactivity disorder among adolescents: a review of the diagnosis, treatment, and clinical implications. *Pediatrics.* 2005; 115(6). Available at: www.pediatrics.org/cgi/content/full/115/6/e1734
2. Barkley RA. Global issues related to the impact of untreated attention-deficit/hyperactivity disorder from childhood to young adulthood. *Postgrad Med.* 2008;120(3):48–59
3. Steihoff KW. Special issues in the diagnosis and treatment of ADHD in adolescents. *Postgrad Med.* 2008;120(3):60–68
4. Culpepper L, Mattingly G. A practical guide to recognition and diagnosis of ADHD in adults in the primary care center. *Postgrad Med.* 2008;120(3):16–26
5. Rostain AL. Attention-deficit/hyperactivity disorder in adults: evidence-based recommendations for management. *Postgrad Med.* 2008;120(3):27–38
6. Robin A, Schubiner H, Coleman WL, eds. ADHD/learning disorders. *Adolesc Med State Art Rev.* 2008;19(2):xiii–xv, 209–351
7. Brooks D. The odyssey years. *The New York Times.* October 9, 2007. Available at: www.nytimes.com/2007/10/09/opinion/09brooks.html. Accessed January 1, 2009
8. Galston WA. *The Changing 20s.* Available at: www.brookings.edu/~/media/Files/rc/speeches/2007/1004useconomics_galston/galston20071004.pdf. Accessed January 1, 2009
9. Erikson E. *Identity: Youth and Crisis.* New York, NY: W. W. Norton & Company, Inc; 1968
10. Levine MD. *Ready or Not, Here Life Comes.* New York, NY: Simon & Shuster; 2005
11. Barkley RA. Attention-deficit/hyperactivity disorder and self-regulation: taking an evolutionary perspective on executive functioning. In: Baumeister RF, Vohs KD, eds. *Handbook of Self-regulation.* New York, NY: Guilford Press; 2004:301–323
12. Brown TE. *Attention Deficit Disorder: The Unfocused Mind in Children and Adults.* New Haven, CT: Yale University Press; 2005:165

13. American Academy of Pediatrics, Subcommittee on Attention-Deficit/Hyperactivity Disorder and Committee on Quality improvement. Clinical practice guideline: treatment of the school-age child with attention deficit/hyperactivity disorder. *Pediatrics.* 2001;108(4):1033–1044
14. Pliszka S; AACAP, Work Group on Quality Issues. Practice parameter for the assessment and treatment of children and adolescents with attention-deficit/hyperactivity disorder. *J Am Acad Child Adolesc Psychiatry.* 2007;46(7):894–921
15. Barkley RA, Cox D. A review of driving risks and impairments associated with attention-deficit/hyperactivity disorder and the effects of stimulant medication on driving performance. *J Safety Res.* 2007;38(1):113–128
16. Gardner HG; American Academy of Pediatrics, Committee on Injury, Violence, and Poison Prevention. Office-based counseling for unintentional injury prevention. *Pediatrics.* 2007;119(1):202–206
17. Katz M. Promising practices: AD/HD safe driving program. *Attention.* 2007;14(6):6–7. Available at: http://tinyurl.com/preview.php?num=9yxrxr. Accessed January 1, 2009
18. Snyder M. Keeping licensed teen drivers with AD/HD safe: parent strategies. Available at: www.greatschools.net/cgi-bin/showarticle/2857. Accessed January 1, 2009
19. Allstate Insurance Company. Teen driving tools and resources. Available at: www.allstateteendriver.com/docs/TeenDriver_sheet_contract.pdf. Accessed January 1, 2009
20. Wilens TE. Attention-deficit/hyperactivity disorder and the substance use disorders: the nature of the relationship, subtypes at risk, and treatment issues. *Psychiatr Clin North Am.* 2004;27(2):283–301
21. Rodriguez D, Tercyak KP, Audrain-McGovern J. Effects of inattention and hyperactivity/impulsivity symptoms on development of nicotine dependence from mid adolescence to young adulthood. *J Pediar Psychol.* 2008;33(6):563–575
22. Wilens TE, Adler AA, Adams J, et al. Misuse and diversion of stimulants prescribed for ADHD: a systematic review of the literature. *J Am Acad Child Adolesc Psychiatry.* 2008;47(1):21–31
23. National Resource Center on AD/HD. AD/HD and the military: Can individuals with AD/HD join the military? Available at: www.help4adhd.org/en/living/workplace/military. Accessed January 4, 2009
24. National Resource Center on AD/HD. Succeeding in the workplace (WWK16). Available at: www.help4adhd.org/living/workplace/WWK16. Accessed January 3, 2009
25. Weiss L. *ADD on the Job: Making Your ADD Work for You.* Dallas, TX: Taylor Publishing Company; 1996
26. Coleman RL. Social competence and friendship formation in adolescents with attention-deficit/hyperactivity disorder. *Adolesc Med State Art Rev.* 2008;19(2):278–299, x
27. Wender PH. *ADHD: Attention-Deficit Hyperactivity Disorder in Children and Adults.* New York, NY: Oxford University Press; 2000:60
28. Barkley RA, Fischer M, Smallish L, Fletcher K. Young adult outcome of hyperactive children: adaptive functioning in major life activities. *J Am Acad Child Adolesc Psychiatry.* 2006;45(2):192–202
29. Betchen SJ. Suggestions for improving intimacy in couples in which one partner has attention-deficit/hyperactivity disorder. *J Sex Marital Ther.* 2003;29(2):103–124
30. Hallowell EM, Ratey JJ. *Delivered From Distraction: Getting the Most out of Life With Attention Deficit Disorder.* New York, NY: Ballantine Books; 2006
31. Gotlieb EM. HIPAA and adolescent privacy in a nutshell. In: Aten CB, Gotlieb EM, eds. *Caring for Adolescent Patients.* 2nd ed. Elk Grove Village, IL: American Academy of Pediatrics; 2006:843
32. Gotlieb EM. Privacy rights, HIPAA, and the AAP: about right; about time. *Pediatrics.* 2002;109(1):146–149
33. US Department of Education. Family Educational Rights and Privacy Act (FERPA). Available at: www.ed.gov/policy/gen/guid/fpco/ferpa/index.html. Accessed January 1, 2009
34. Bourgeois FC, Taylor PL, Emans SJ, Nigrin DJ, Mandl KD. Whose personal control? Creating private, personally controlled health records for pediatric and adolescent patients. *J Am Med Inform Assoc.* 2008;15(6):737–743

35. Leibson CL, Katusic SK, Barbaresi WJ, Ransom J, O'Brien PC. Use and cost of medical care for children and adolescents with and without attention-deficit/hyperactivity disorder. *JAMA*. 2001; 285(1):60–66
36. Birnbaum HG, Kessler RC, Lowe SW, et al. Costs of attention deficit-hyperactivity disorder (ADHD) in the US: excess costs of persons with ADHD and their family members in 2000. *Curr Med Res Opin*. 2005;21(2):195–206
37. Pelham WE, Foster EM, Robb JA. The economic impact of attention-deficit/hyperactivity disorder in children and adolescents. *Ambul Pediatr*. 2007;7(1 suppl):121–131
38. Seifert PJ, Hollingsworth PC. Seeking equal coverage for mental health. *Attention*. 2007;14: 23–25
39. Callahan ST. Bridging the gaps in health insurance coverage for young adults. *J Adolesc Health*. 2007;41(4):321–322
40. US Department of Labor. Health plans & benefits: continuation of health coverage—COBRA. Available at: www.dol.gov/dol/topic/health-plans/cobra.htm. Accessed January 1, 2009
41. Kriss JL, Collins SR, Mahato B, Gould E, Schoen C. *Rite of Passage? Why Young Adults Become Uninsured and How New Policies Can Help, 2008 Update*. New York, NY: Commonwealth Fund; 2008. Available at: www.commonwealthfund.org/usr_doc/Kriss_riteofpassage2008_1139_ib.pdf?section=4039. Accessed January 1, 2009
42. Friends Committee on National Legislation. Issues: Domestic Human Needs: The Final Rescue Package: What's Included in the "Troubled Asset Relief Program." Available at: www.fcnl.org/issues/item.php?item_id=3430&issue_id=144. Accessed February 15, 2009
43. Centers for Medicaid and Medicare Services. Paul Wellstone and Pete Domenici Mental Health Parity and Addiction Equity Act of 2008. Available at: www.cms.hhs.gov/HealthInsReformforConsume/Downloads/MHPAEA.pdf. Accessed January 1, 2009
44. US Government Printing Office. H. R. 1424. Available at: http://frwebgate.access.gpo.gov/cgi-bin/getdoc.cgi?dbname=110_cong_bills&docid=f:h1424enr.txt.pdf. Accessed February 15, 2009
45. American Academy of Pediatrics; American Academy of Family Physicians; American College of Physicians-American Society of Internal Medicine. A consensus statement on health care transitions for young adults with special health care needs. *Pediatrics*. 2002;110(6 pt 2):1304–1306
46. Kelly AM, Kratz B, Bielski M, Rinehart PM. Implementing transitions for youth with complex chronic conditions using the medical home model. *Pediatrics*. 2002;110(6 pt 2):1322–1327
47. Reid GJ, Irvine MJ, McCrindle BW, et al. Prevalence and correlates of successful transfer from pediatric to adult health care among a cohort of young adults with complex congenital heart defects. *Pediatrics*. 2004;113(3 pt 1). Available at: www.pediatrics.org/cgi/content/full/113/3/e197
48. Burke RB, Spoerri M, Price A, Cardosi AM, Flanagan P. Survey of primary care pediatricians of the transition and transfer of adolescents to adult health care. *Clin Pediatr (Phila)*. 2008; 47(4):347–354
49. Houtrow AJ, Newachek PW. Understanding transition issues: asthma as an example. *J Pediatr*. 2008;152(4):453–455
50. Cohen MD. Educational rights of children and adolescents with attention-deficit/hyperactivity disorder. *Adolesc Med State Art Rev*. 2008;19(2):327–338, xi
51. US Department of Education. My child's special needs: a guide to the Individualized Education Program. Available at: www.ed.gov/parents/needs/speced/iepguide/index.html. Accessed January 1, 2009
52. Mauro T. What is a 504 plan? Available at: http://specialchildren.about.com/od/504s/f/504faq1.htm. Accessed January 1, 2009
53. Mauro T. How does a 504 plan differ from an IEP? Available at: http://specialchildren.about.com/od/504s/f/504faq2.htm. Accessed January 1, 2009
54. US Department of Education. Questions and answers on disability discrimination under Section 504 and Title II. Available at: www.ed.gov/about/offices/list/ocr/qa-disability.html. Accessed January 1, 2009

55. WrightsLaw. Discrimination: Section 504 and ADA. Available at: www.wrightslaw.com/info/sec504.index.htm. Accessed January 1, 2009
56. US Department of Education. Americans With Disabilities Act (ADA). Available at: www.ed.gov/about/offices/list/ocr/docs/hq9805.html. Accessed January 1, 2009
57. National Resource Center on AD/HD. Dealing with Systems: Legal Rights: Higher Education and the Workplace (WWK14). Available at: www.help4adhd.org/en/systems/legal/WWK14. Accessed February 15, 2009
58. ADDitude. ADDitude Helpful Tips: What You Need to Know About the Americans with Disabilities Act. Available at: www.additudemag.com/adhd-web/article/674.html. Accessed February 15, 2009
59. Consortium on ADHD Documentation. Guidelines for documentation of attention deficit/hyperactivity disorder in adolescents and adults. Available at: www.dartmouth.edu/~accessibility/docs/adhd_guidelines.doc. Accessed January 1, 2009
60. College Board. Test accommodations. Available at: http://professionals.collegeboard.com/testing/sat-reasoning/register/accomodations. Accessed January 1, 2009
61. The ACT. Services for Students with Disabilities. Available at: www.act.org/aap/disab/index.html. Accessed February 15, 2009
62. GRE. Test takers with disabilities (PBT). Available at: http://tinyurl.com/8stvxw. Accessed January 1, 2009
63. Latham, PH. The law after high school. Available at: www.ldonline.org/article/6098. Accessed January 1, 2009
64. Mitchell M. Medications: tips for traveling internationally. Available at: www.miusa.org/ncde/tipsheets/medications. Accessed December 31, 2008
65. US Food and Drug Administration. FDA public health advisory: January 2006—consumers filling U.S. prescriptions abroad may get the wrong active ingredient because of confusing drug names. Available at: www.fda.gov/oc/opacom/reports/confusingnames.html. Accessed January 1, 2009
66. Dendy CAZ. *Teenagers With ADD and ADHD.* 2nd ed. Bethesda, MD: Woodbine House, Inc; 2006
67. Nadeau KG. *Survival Guide for College Students With ADHD or LD.* 2nd ed. Washington, DC: Magination Press; 2006
68. Quinn PO, ed. *ADD and the College Student.* Revised ed. Washington, DC: Magination Press; 2001
69. Gotlieb EM, Teens with AD/HD: transitions from high school to college or career. In: *The NEW CHADD Information and Resource Guide to AD/HD.* Landover, MD: National Resource Center on AD/HD; 2006:84–88
70. Katz LJ. College success: accommodations and strategies that work. In: *The NEW CHADD Information and Resource Guide to AD/HD.* Landover, MD: National Resource Center on AD/HD; 2006:93–97
71. National Resource Center on AD/HD. What we know: succeeding in college (WWK13). Available at: www.help4adhd.org/en/education/college/WWK13. Accessed January 1, 2009
72. MDRC. How much is a college degree worth? Available at: www.mdrc.org/area_fact_33.html. Accessed January 1, 2009
73. MDRC. About MDRC: what is MDRC? Available at: www.mdrc.org/about_what_is_mdrc.htm. Accessed January 1, 2009
74. MDRC. Community colleges. Available at: www.mdrc.org/subarea_index_31.html. Accessed January 1, 2009
75. US Census Bureau. Table 220: mean earnings by highest degree earned—2005. Available at: www.census.gov/compendia/statab/2008/tables/08s0220.pdf. Accessed January 1, 2009
76. Caron C. Blog for scholarship money or tutor online. Available at: http://abcnews.go.com/Business/PersonalFinance/Story?id=5648319. Accessed January 1, 2009
77. DuPaul GJ, Evans SW. School-based interventions for adolescents with attention-deficit/hyperactivity disorder. *Adolesc Med State Art Rev.* 2008;19(2):300–312, x

78. Shapiro ES, DuPaul GJ, Bradley-Klug KL. Self-management as a strategy to improve the classroom behavior of adolescents with ADHD. *J Learn Disabil.* 1998;31(6):545–555
79. Lipscomb L, Swanson J, West A. Scaffolding. In: Orey M, ed. Emerging perspectives on learning, teaching, and technology. 2004. Available at: http://projects.coe.uga.edu/epltt/index.php?title=Scaffolding. Accessed January 1, 2009
80. National Research Center on AD/HD. Time management: learning to use a day planner (WWK11). Available at: www.help4adhd.org/en/living/organdtime/WWK11. Accessed January 1, 2009
81. Wikipedia. List of social networking sites. Available at: http://en.wikipedia.org/wiki/List_of_social_networking_websites. Accessed January 1, 2009
82. Top 10 Reviews. Social networking websites services review. Available at: http://social-networking-websites-review.toptenreviews.com. Accessed January 1, 2009
83. Verbol P. Social networking is no IT fad. *Redmond.* 2008;14(6):9. Available at: http://redmondmag.com/reports/article.asp?EditorialsID=721. Accessed January 1, 2009
84. Ybarra ML, Mitchell KJ. How risky are social networking sites? A comparison of places online where youth solicitation and harassment occurs. *Pediatrics.* 2008;121(2). Available at: www.pediatrics.org/cgi/content/full/121/2/e350–e357
85. Fuld GL. Social networking and adolescents. *Adolesc Med.* 2009;20(1):57–72
86. Health 2.0. *The Economist.* September 6, 2007:103
87. Eysenbach G. Medicine 2.0: social networking, collaboration, apomediation, and openness. *J Med Internet Res.* 2008;10(30):e22. Available at: www.jmir.org/2008/3/e22. Accessed January 1, 2009
88. Sarason-Kahn J. The wisdom of patients: health care meets online social media. Available at: www.chcf.org/documents/chronicdisease/HealthCareSocialMedia.pdf. Accessed February 15, 2009
89. Avitzur O. Finding patient support online. *Consum Rep Health.* 2008;20(07):11

Office-Based Care for Gay, Lesbian, Bisexual, and Questioning Youth

David A. Levine, MD*

Department of Pediatrics, Morehouse School of Medicine, 720 Westview Drive, SW, Atlanta, GA 30310, USA

Robert was a new 16-year-old patient to my teen clinic. He presented as a follow-up from the emergency department after treatment for urethritis. Robert had had unprotected insertive intercourse recently. He was appropriately managed in the emergency department, and his symptoms had resolved with treatment. His gonorrhea test result was positive. Other testing for chlamydia was negative; blood serology tests were negative for syphilis, hepatitis B (he was antibody-positive after immunization), hepatitis C, and HIV. When discussing adolescent risk behaviors, Robert told me that he had been hospitalized briefly at a state mental hospital after a suicide attempt. When asked what may have triggered the suicidal thinking, he answered that he tried to kill himself when his father angrily kicked him out of the house when Robert told him that he was gay. Fortunately, he was able to reside with a maternal aunt after that time, although he did not have limits and came and went as he pleased. Six months later, at follow-up, his HIV test result was positive; he had seroconverted sometime in the previous 6 months.

Fortunately, for Robert, the denouement of his story was that he was transitioned successfully to a great local adolescent HIV program. His HIV was not aggressive, and he was compliant with care. My last contact with him was when he informed me that he was graduating from college. Robert's case illustrates many of the issues and problems that face gay, lesbian, bisexual (GLB), and questioning youth. Although most sexual minority teenagers are quite resilient and emerge from adolescence relatively unscathed, the health disparities in working with this vulnerable population can be significant and daunting.

This review article also is derived from a wonderful curriculum. Physicians for Reproductive Choice and Health, the "voice of the prochoice physician" spon-

---

*Corresponding author.
E-mail address: dlevine@msm.edu (D. A. Levine).

Copyright © 2009 American Academy of Pediatrics. All rights reserved. ISSN 1934-4287

sored the development of a comprehensive curriculum related to adolescent sexuality. The Adolescent Reproductive Health Education Program has been nationally endorsed by the American Academy of Pediatrics, the Society for Adolescent Medicine, and the American College of Obstetrics and Gynecology as a preferred curriculum to use in training medical students and residents and in providing continuing education to physicians, nurses, other allied health personnel, and even the public about the issues facing today's youth. One important module is "Gay, Lesbian, Bisexual, Transgender, and Questioning Youth."[1] More information about the program is available at www.prch.org/arhep.

This review article will update previous, formidable publications by Garofalo and Harper in 2003[2] and Ryan and Futterman in 1997,[3] both of which were published in previous issues of this journal. I will define and attempt to quantify the number of our sexual minority youth, discuss the unique challenges faced by these young people, and suggest some evidence-based interventions that have allowed youth to reduce their risk behaviors. The role of homophobia and heterosexism will be discussed and how the 2 issues affect the developing mind of a GLB teenager. Finally, issues in providing clinical care and modifying our patient care approaches to providing culturally competent care will be discussed. Along the way, there will be illustrative patient cases, all which are based on adolescents I have encountered in my general pediatrics and adolescent medicine clinics for the underserved in Oakland, California, and Atlanta, Georgia.

Although transgendered youth are some of the most underserved and vulnerable youth, their unique needs are beyond the scope of this article. In addition, I have personally had very little experience in working with these adolescents.

THE PARADIGM OF SEXUALITY

Adolescence is characterized as a time of intense physical, emotional, and sexual change. One normative process during this time is sexual discovery, exploration, and experimentation, including sexual fantasies and realities, incorporating sexuality into one's own identity. Adolescents solidify their gender identification and expression by observing the gender roles of their parents and adults, siblings, peers, and others. A young person's sexual orientation often (but not always) emerges in adolescence. In a June 2004 clinical report, Frankowski and the American Academy of Pediatrics Committee on Adolescence published "Sexual Orientation and Adolescents."[4] They wrote, "Sexual orientation refers to an individual's pattern of physical and emotional arousal toward other persons." Individuals who self-identify as heterosexual are attracted to persons of the opposite sex; homosexual individuals self-identify as being attracted to the same sex; and bisexual teenagers report attraction to both genders. In common usage, homosexual self-identified folk are often referred to as "gay" if male and "lesbian" if female. In this review, the term "GLB" (gay, lesbian, or bisexual) will refer to all sexual minority youth.

Gender identity and gender role usually conform to anatomic sex in both homosexual and heterosexual teenagers. Exceptions are transgendered persons; their gender identity does not match their anatomic and chromosomal sex. More information and resources about these children can be found on the World Professional Association for Transgender Health Web site (www.wpath.org). The organization also publishes *The International Journal of Transgenderism*.

As a society, our culture tries to force people to "pigeon-hole" individuals into a sexual identity. It is assumed that men or women who self-identify as gay or lesbian will only have attraction or sexual activity with the same gender. The following case illustrates that the paradigm of sexuality is much more complex.

> *Thomas was a 17-year-old gay high school junior in Oakland. He was quite comfortable with his sexual orientation at a very early age and "came out" to his friends and classmates when he was in middle school. He was well liked by his classmates, who by and large accepted his sexuality. During the summer between his junior and senior year, he decided to have sex with a woman "to see if he was a real man." Thomas Jr was born in February of his senior year.*

It should not be surprising that human men and women are more complex than expected according to sexual identification. Many adolescents who self-report as lesbian will still occasionally have sex with males, and gay men have sex with females. Behavior does not always equal identity. Sexual orientation and gender identity are not always synonymous with sexual activity or even gender orientation. Some men who have sex with men or women who have sex with women actively resist being identified as gay or lesbian. Further complicating the issue is that someone does not have to be sexually active to self-identify as GLB. Many adolescents are still struggling with their sexual identities; often these teenagers are referred to as "questioning" youth. Dr Robert Winn, medical director of the Mazzoni Center in Philadelphia, Pennsylvania, developed a pictorial representation of the "revolutionary gender model" (Fig 1) for the Adolescent Reproductive Health Education Program curriculum.[1]

Today's pediatricians and adolescent medicine physicians may have a role in helping teenagers sort through their feelings and behaviors. As will be discussed, with proper support and guidance, the majority of GLB and questioning youth emerge with a strong adult identity and little or no significant increase in risk behaviors compared with other youth. Of course, parental and other adult reaction to "coming out" will vary, and adolescents will need support from health care providers.

While adolescents and young adults are developing their sexual identity and self-identified sexual orientation, it may be difficult for health care providers to understand where the adolescent fits along the spectrum. It is essential that we

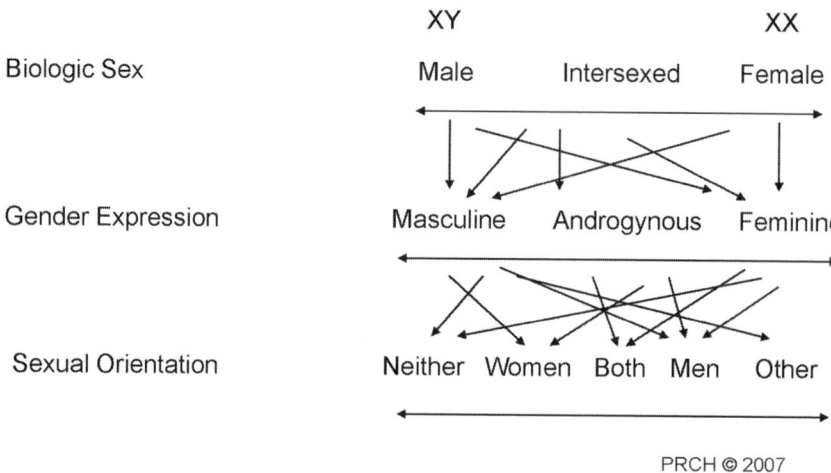

Fig 1. Revolutionary gender model.

obtain a comprehensive sexual history from all adolescents, asking about attraction and activity. Later in this review, clinical approaches to obtaining full, useful information from teenagers will be discussed. As illustrated in the case above, just because a young man self-identifies as gay, it does not mean that he will never have sex with women. Young people need information about healthy positive expressions of sexuality, and health providers should assist adolescents as they develop their identity and help them to avoid the pitfalls of teenage pregnancy and sexually transmitted infections (STIs) regardless of their sexual orientation.

Of course, there are many providers across this country who have powerful feelings about the issue of GLB youth. Many providers have come from traditional religious backgrounds, from faiths that do not accept other than a heterosexual orientation. Our American culture has many "taboos" about sexuality, often forcing our teenagers to hide their feelings and activities. As will be discussed later, "staying in the closet" and hiding sexuality is maladaptive and may lead to a negative self-image and even depression and substance abuse.

You yourself may not feel that you can address this issue for your teenagers. Like any other clinical issue in medicine, if you do not feel comfortable evaluating or treating a patient, it is the provider's responsibility to refer to another provider who can provide the service. Physicians certainly do not agree with patients or parents on every issue or concern, but we still can provide culturally competent care even if we do not agree. Supporting and working with GLB teenagers is no different.

PREVALENCE OF GLB AND QUESTIONING YOUTH

There are inherent difficulties in obtaining accurate data about our sexual minority youth. Of course, virtually all of our information is from self-reporting on survey instruments. Although some adolescents are comfortable enough to reveal their sexuality on these instruments, many may not trust that their information will truly be protected. And, of course, many adolescents are still struggling with developing their sexual identities and may not be ready to even "come out" to themselves, let alone to family, friends, or others. Also, unfortunately, some of the best data are state specific, such as the Minnesota, Massachusetts, and Vermont adaptations of the Centers for Disease Control and Prevention (CDC) Youth Risk Behavior Surveillance System, asking specific questions related to same-gender sexual activity.

For Vermont, in the 2007 administration, 3% of students had reported having engaged in same-sex sexual intercourse. Overall, 1% self-identified as gay or lesbian, 3% described themselves as "bisexual," and an additional 3% said they were not sure.[5] It is an interesting cultural phenomenon that currently in the US adolescent culture it is more comfortable and accepted for teenagers to say they are bisexual than to self-identify as gay or lesbian. In the 2007 Massachusetts survey, 5.4% described themselves as GLB; 9.2% of all students described themselves as GLB and reported same-sex sexual contact.[6] In the 2007 Minnesota survey, only 9th- and 12th-graders were surveyed, and they were only asked about sexual behavior, not orientation. They found that 2% of 9th-grade boys and 4% of 12th-grade boys had had sex with another male. Similarly, they found that 1% of 9th-grade girls and 2% of 12th-grade girls had had sex with another female.

Data that are more nationally representative are more difficult to obtain. It is estimated that between 2% and 4.5% of high school students self-identify as GLB.[1] In the 2002 National Survey of Family Growth, in the 15- to 44-year age group, 10.6% of females and 4.5% of males reported having sexual contact with a member of the same sex.[7]

THE RESILIENCE OF GAY YOUTH

> *Cheryl was a 16-year- old who presented to a primary care office. Interviewed originally by a medical student as part of the pediatrics clerkship, Cheryl stated that she was dating a 17-year-old girl. She had come out to her family and friends within the last year. After some processing time, they accepted her sexuality and continued to support Cheryl emotionally. She later earned a "Hope" scholarship from the State of Georgia and attended Georgia Tech, majoring in chemical engineering. She denied fights, violence, mental health issues, substance abuse, or risky sexuality. She always uses a condom with a male*

> *partner or with sex toys and uses a dental dam with her partner, even if they are in a relationship.*

As will be discussed below, the unique challenges faced by sexual minority youth may lead to increased risk behaviors: mental health issues, substance abuse, and sexual risks. However, the majority of GLB youth emerge from adolescence unscathed. Most grow up healthy and lead happy, productive lives. Adolescence for GLB youth, like their heterosexual peers, is a developmental phase in which many physical, emotional, social, and sexual changes take place. For many gay youth, these struggles are made more difficult by the pervasive disapproval they may receive from family, peers, and society. Yet, in overcoming the stress created by stigmatization, many GLB youth develop and possess remarkable strength and self-determination. These teenagers often develop quite resilient adaptations to social biases and mistreatment.[1] In 2004, Eccles et al[8] performed a qualitative study of gay male youth aged 16 to 22 and concluded that "general developmental dysfunction is not inevitable for gay adolescents, nor is identifiable personal or family pathology directly related to sexual identity."

Being GLB, therefore, is not a "problem" or "risk behavior" in itself. These teenagers, like all teenagers, should be assessed individually as to challenges and opportunities. Positive behaviors should be reinforced; teenagers can be engaged in targeted behavior interventions to reduce existing risk behaviors. As with all adolescents, it is part of the responsibility of a physician to help young people identify their strengths and build on their existing talents.

HEALTH DISPARITIES FOR GLB YOUTH

> *Khalil was 17-year-old boy who presented initially to the emergency department with urethritis that later turned out to be chlamydia. Unfortunately, as well, his HIV test result was positive. I had the unenviable task of informing a new patient that he was HIV-positive. Fortunately, Dr Bande Virgil, a wonderful medical student who is now a pediatric resident at Morehouse, spent 2 hours with him that first evening. He revealed that he had been on his own since about age 16. In his case, he was out to his mother, who accepted his sexuality. Unfortunately, his mother was also homeless and also has a toddler to care for; when Khalil was able to stay with friends, she did not object. Khalil told me that he made extra money "dancing" for older men. At least for him, his HIV was not aggressive, and he continued to have a normal immune system. He decided that he would move to San Francisco, California, when he turned 18. Fortunately, he was able to be engaged at the wonderful Larkin Street Youth Services. He was able to get into a subsidized apartment, get into medical care to maintain his immune system, and is about reenter school in a program that will grant him a diploma and transition him to degree programs at San Francisco State University.*

Unfortunately, the prevailing homophobia and heterosexism found in homes, neighborhoods, and schools can alter a developing adolescent's self-image. Struggles with this negative self-image and with self-esteem often put sexual minority youth at greater risk. Like other adolescents who are struggling with developmental issues, conflicts can result in adolescents "acting out" and increasing risk behaviors, including high-risk sexuality, substance abuse, and violence. Certainly depression and other mental health issues may be manifest as these teenagers struggle with developing their stable identity. Clearly, there are no biological or genetic factors that make a GLB or questioning adolescent more susceptible to behavioral risk factors and disease.

Although overt homophobia may damage the emerging self-image of an adolescent, often heterosexism is more insidious and damaging. The questioning adolescent who is sitting at the dinner table with parents and family or at lunch with his or her friends, expecting that their child/friend is "straight," may have conversations that suggest to the teenager that he or she should hide their sexuality. Homophobia refers to an irrational fear of homosexuality and homosexual individuals. Homophobia unfortunately is based in hate, in this case an irrational hatred of GLB individuals and so-called lifestyle. Pervasive in our culture, homophobia is institutionalized in stereotypes promoted in the media and in casual conversation. Heterosexism is the societal expectation that heterosexuality is the expected norm and that somehow GLB teenagers are "abnormal." Although it is rather easy for the majority of sexual minority youth to hide their sexuality from family and friends, using heterosexism to their advantage, it may ultimately be damaging to the developing psyche.

Unfortunately, many adolescents in school are being taught that "abstinence only until heterosexual marriage" is the norm, based on curricula developed by religious conservatives. This only serves to further isolate and alienate many students.

MENTAL HEALTH DISPARITIES

Although most GLB teenagers do emerge from adolescence relatively unscathed, there are health disparities related to depression and suicidality, substance abuse, altered body image, and other mental health issues.

GLB youth do have more mental health difficulties. They are approximately twice as likely to report depression and 2 to 7 times more likely to attempt suicide.[1] Even for these teenagers, however, protective factors come into play. Data from the 2004 Minnesota student survey of 9th- and 12th-graders were examined. There were 2255 respondents who reported a same-sex experience. Over half of the GLB students had thought about suicide, and 37.4% had reported a suicide attempt. Just like other teenagers, there were protective factors discovered as well. Family connectedness, adult caring, and school safety were significantly protective against suicidal ideation and attempts.[9] In another study that sought risk factors that might correlate with suicide attempts, D'Augelli et al[10] discovered that suicide attempts were positively correlated with parental psychological abuse, being considered gender-atypical in childhood by parents, and with parental efforts to discourage gender-atypical behavior. Not surprisingly, GLB teenagers who runaway or are put out by family after acknowledging their sexuality are often victimized. Homeless teenagers were more likely to have been physically and sexually abuse by caretakers, were more likely to engage in risky survival strategies, including unprotected "survival sex." Homeless teenagers were more likely to meet criteria for each of 4 mental disorders (conduct disorder, major depressive disorder, posttraumatic stress disorder, and substance abuse).[11] Of course, general pediatricians and adolescent medicine providers have developed skills in elucidating adolescent mental health concerns through the adolescent psychosocial interview. These skills would also serve quite well in evaluating the mental health of GLB teenagers.

Social anxiety is another important disorder faced by many GLB adolescents. In a study that compared 87 heterosexual and gay undergraduates at the State University of New York at Stonybrook, it was discovered that gay men reported greater fear of negative evaluation and social interaction anxiety and lower self-esteem than heterosexual men.[12] This places young gay men and women at higher risk, including sexual risks. Hart and Heimberg[13] studied 100 young gay men in a 3-state area of the US east coast. They discovered that social anxiety predicted an increased probability of having engaged in unprotected anal intercourse in the previous 6 months.

Not surprisingly, as well, when GLB teenagers are victimized, they have increased mental health disorders. When teenagers come out and acknowledge their sexuality as adolescents, there are often repercussions. As many as 25% to 40% of homeless youth may be GLB. In 1 study, 84% of "out" adolescents reported verbal harassment, 30% reported being punched, kicked, or injured, and 28% dropped out of school because of harassment.[1] Friedman et al[14] established a strong association between victimization and suicidality among sexual minority adolescents recruited from gay youth community or university-based organizations.

Gay and bisexual men also may face eating disorders more than heterosexual male teenagers. There is a significant body of knowledge that has documented more altered body-image issues than in heterosexually self-identified boys. Although 10% to 15% of all cases of eating disorders are in men, as many as 42% of these men may be gay or bisexual. The authors of 1 study performed regression analysis to establish whether there was a strong association. After controlling for depression, self-esteem, and comfort with sexual orientation, the authors found that self-identifying as gay accounted for a significant amount of the variance.[15] In addition, a major risk factor for altered body image in gay men is a history of childhood sexual abuse.[16]

SUBSTANCE ABUSE

Eric began smoking marijuana by 11 years of age. Known in the community as "Dozier," a common slang term for marijuana, he grew up in a small housing project in Oakland. He saw the effects of cocaine, especially crack cocaine; he pledged that he would never fall into the trap of significant substance abuse. After moving to Nevada, he realized that he was bisexual. Like many young African-American men, he kept his sexuality hidden or "on the down-low." In his new circle of acquaintances, a few smoked "crystal meth" (methamphetamine). Eric had no previous knowledge of this drug growing up. He noted that many of his new friends who smoked were professionals and did not seem to have a "problem" with methamphetamine. After starting, he was addicted within a month. He lost his relationship, became estranged to family and friends, and finally, in a drug-induced rage, fought back when in an altercation, severely injuring his assailant. He was incarcerated for 4 years; when he was released, he pledged to live a substance-free lifestyle.

Substance abuse is another risk behavior often faced by the GLB adolescent. Not surprisingly, with psychosocial stress, the escape of getting high may be addictive and lead to increasing use of substances. Even our so-called least major substance, tobacco, is overrepresented among gay youth.[17] Fortunately, research into the best ways to prevent tobacco use and reduce existing use is underway. Remafedi and Carol[18] published their needs assessment in working with sexual minority youth to engineer an effective prevention/intervention program.

For more significant substances, especially today's "club drugs," the data are difficult to obtain. Underreporting of both sexuality and substance abuse makes estimating the numbers very difficult. Physicians for Reproductive Choice and Health analyzed the literature. Studies showed that in the previous 30 days, gay teenagers were more likely to have used alcohol (89.4% vs 35.2 of heterosexual identified youth) and cocaine (25.3% vs 2.7%). Alarmingly, the percentage of GLB teenagers beginning before the age of 13 is double for alcohol (59.1% vs 30.5%) and markedly increased for cocaine (17.3% vs 1.2%). Of course, these early adolescents are at greater risks, because they have not developed the strengths necessary to resist substances. Substance abuse treatment facilities are filled with teenagers who began early and with multiple drug abuse patterns.[1] Not surprisingly, substance-abusing gay or lesbian teenagers also have other risk behaviors, leading to higher rates of HIV seropositivity. Young men who worked in service or sales positions were overrepresented compared with young men who worked in "professional" occupations.[19] Even college students, presumably headed toward professional occupations, were at higher risk. At a major Louisville, Kentucky, university, lesbian/bisexual women were 4.9 times more likely to smoke, 10.7 times more likely to drink, and 4.9 times more likely to smoke marijuana. Interestingly, in this study, gay/bisexual men did not differ from heterosexual men.[20] Homeless sexual minority youth were at even greater risk.[21] Of course, we are most concerned about the use of more significant drugs such as ecstasy, methamphetamine, and other so-called club drugs (γ-butyrolactone [GHB], ketamine, lysergic acid diethylamide [LSD], and cocaine). Methamphetamine specifically has become a significant problem and is markedly associated with other risky behaviors, especially unprotected intercourse. Young sexual minorities that "PNP" or "party and play" are advertised every day on Internet Web sites that attract GLB youth and young adults. Recent studies have focused on how young people are initiated into methamphetamine use. Interestingly, in 1 qualitative study of 54 young gay and bisexual men in New York City, it was discovered that initiation was usually in a social, nonsexual setting. One of the major recurrent themes was that the users admitted to limited knowledge of methamphetamine use, just like Eric.[22] This finding that initiation correlates with experiencing "gay-related activities" was also supported by another study. The authors noted that as young men were more involved in going to gay clubs and other gay-related activities, their risk of alcohol and marijuana use increased. The authors felt that this would be a great potential area for intervention to prevent or decrease substance use.[23]

SEXUAL HEALTH DISPARITIES

Although the majority of GLB teenagers emerge from adolescence unscathed—not pregnant, never had an STI, and remained HIV-negative—there continue to be health disparities in all of these areas. The CDC has developed specific screening recommendations for men who have sex with men (also noted in their literature as MSM). This is also designed to reduce the perceived stigma of identifying as gay or bisexual, focusing instead on sexual behavior. Women who have sex with women (WSW) also have increased risks. Although the specific topic of working with sexual minority youth on these issues may seem daunting, it is really the same as providing standard of care for all adolescents. The newly released version of *Bright Futures*, in collaboration with the American Academy of Pediatrics "Recommendations for Preventive Pediatric Health Care," continues to emphasize STI screening and risk reduction and cervical dysplasia screening (the latter now 3 years after the start of sexual intercourse or age 21).[24] The adolescent psychosocial history is the standard tool for us to use in obtaining relevant sexual history information. The HEEADSSS (home, education/employment, eating, peer-group activities, drugs, sexuality, suicide/depression, and safety) interview will be discussed in a later section on "Making the Office Teen-Friendly for GLB Adolescents." The bottom line is that every preteenager (after age 11 at the latest) and adolescent should have some private time with the physician to talk about personal and sensitive issues. A comprehensive sexual history is part of that process.

Another source for data related to sexual behaviors is the National Study of Family Growth. In the 2002 administration, reported in 2005, it was noted that

10.6% of females and 4.5% of males had engaged in any sexual contact with someone of the same sex.[7] GLB youth were more likely to have had sexual intercourse, to have more partners, and to have experienced sexual contact before the age of 13. Of course, all of these behaviors increase the risk of STIs, HIV, and teenage pregnancy.[1] Although, in general, during the last 15 years, rates of gonorrhea, chlamydia, and syphilis have trended downward for adolescents, common reportable bacterial STIs have increased among men who are having sex with men.[25] Recent widespread media reports have analyzed new data from the CDC; unfortunately, HIV rates have continued to rise among young men and in the African-American population. For men of all ages, the annual increase between 2001 and 2006 was a low 1.5%. Yet, males who had sex with other males between the ages of 13 and 24 had an annual increase of 12.4%, and young African-American men who had sex with men showed a 15% increase.[26] It is very difficult to get good information about women who have sex with women. Until recently, little research was devoted to lesbian health, and many clinicians incorrectly assumed that lesbians were at minimal risk for STIs and HIV. Data to drive clinical practice are difficult to obtain. However, given the high rates of self-identified lesbians and bisexual women who have had sexual contact with men and the documented transmission of STIs, including human papillomavirus (HPV), via exclusively female-to-female sexual intercourse, it is prudent to screen these young ladies with the same general recommendations as other adolescent girls.[25] In a 1999 self-reported survey of 6935 self-identified lesbians, 17.2% reported a history of an STI.[1] Unfortunately, GLB youth are less likely to report contraceptive use at last sex. Young women who identified themselves as "unsure" of their sexual orientation were almost twice as likely to report not using contraception at the last sex.[1] Of course, when sexual minority youth are taught about sexuality through abstinence-only-until-heterosexual-marriage curricula, they realize that the information does not apply to them, which may make these youth less likely to consider using contraception. Given high rates of earlier sexual initiation, the paradigm of sexuality that predicts that teenagers will at least at sometime have sexual behaviors that are not consistent with orientation, a greater number of partners, and less contraceptive use, it should not be surprising that young women who have sex with women are at higher risk for teenage pregnancy.

> *Carly was 15 years old when she realized that her primary sexual attraction was to other women. She had her first same-sex encounter when she was 16 years old. After her parents questioned her repeatedly about her frequent visits and tight "friendship" with Monica, she felt that she needed to show her family that she was "straight." At this time in her life, Carly felt she was "bisexual," although she had never felt attraction to men. After a summer party when she was intoxicated, she had sexual intercourse with a childhood friend. Her parents were pleased when Carly told them about her new relationship, especially considering that they had known him and his family for a long time.*

They were, however, not pleased at all when Carly told them that she was pregnant 3 months later, and they were even more distraught when Carly finally revealed her sexual orientation and attraction to her parents. Fortunately, with family counseling, the family was able to get back to being supportive of Carly. Her son was born very healthy, and Carly and Monica coparented Carly's son.

Having known about the paradigm of human sexuality, it should not have been surprising that young women who have sex with women would have a greater risk of STIs, HIV, and teenage pregnancy. Data, however, are very difficult to obtain. An older study from the 1999 Minnesota Adolescent Health Survey documented that when compared with heterosexual-identified youth, lesbian and bisexual women were about as likely to have had intercourse (33% vs 29%). However, they had twice the rate of pregnancy (12% vs 6%) and were more likely to have had 2 or more pregnancies (23.5% vs 9.8%). Women who have sex with women also reported high rates of physical and sexual abuse (19%–22%). Clearly, we need to provide better reproductive care to young sexual minority women.[26] Providing quality care for sexual minority youth is paramount, and we must acknowledge the potential range of human sexuality in our clinical encounters with teenagers.

PROVIDING "CULTURALLY COMPETENT" CARE FOR SEXUAL MINORITY YOUTH

When thinking through the overall theme of this section, it is clear that providing excellent clinical care to sexual minority youth is really nothing that should be surprising to the general pediatrician or adolescent medicine specialist. Providing care for these young people is entirely consistent with providing quality care to any adolescent.

The term "culturally competent health care" has been quite popular lately as more and more agencies and think tanks document that a potential solution for eliminating health disparities is to meet the patient at his or her cultural level. Asking questions about beliefs and communicating effectively are part of this care. Of course, most of our sexual minority youth are not of another culture; they are part of their own ethnic group, neighborhood group, family identification, and religious affiliation. Good communication with sexual minority youth is paramount, but, as will be discussed, is really no different from working with any teenager in a clinical encounter.

MAKING THE OFFICE "TEEN-FRIENDLY" FOR GLB ADOLESCENTS

One of the challenges in providing care and lowering barriers is the fact that it is not the pediatrician alone who cares for our kids in the office. Before seeing the physician, the teenager will encounter, at a minimum, a front office clerk and a back office nurse or medical assistant. It is important to work with these important members of the health care team so that they do not inadvertently offend or create additional barriers. Heterosexism that is internalized by staff members may inadvertently interfere. Asking a young lady who is in a relationship with another woman if she has a boyfriend may be interpreted by the young lady as unwillingness to consider her relationship seriously. This then may hamper the physician-client interaction; the client may feel that the attitude of the provider is the same as the staff member and discourage her from disclosing her sexuality and prevent her from receiving the proper care in the office. Likewise, we must watch for assumptions on intake forms and questionnaires. Gay teenagers are used to the heterosexism of our society and will likely not challenge any staff or forms, but there are some gentle and effective strategies to use by both staff and pediatricians and adolescent medicine specialists.

Of course, like all adolescents, confidentiality should be assured. Many GLB clients may hear you pledge confidentiality, but other negative experiences may not allow them to disclose their sexuality or to discuss any risk behaviors.

> Derrick was a 17-year-old boy who presented to the teen clinic with a complaint of "bumps" in the perineum. Physical examination revealed these to be genital warts. When obtaining a sexual history, using gender-neutral terms and giving permission for a teenager to reveal sexuality, Derrick affirmed that he had only previously had sex with females. Because it was not out of the realm of possible, his explanation of having "grinded" with women as the causal activity was accepted. He was referred for removal and had an excellent outcome. On his next visit 3 months later, Derrick apologized for not being frank at the time of the first encounter about his sexuality. He said that he had been treated very poorly at a previous clinician's office who had suggested that he enter "reparative" therapy to "fix" his sexuality. He recognized the gender-neutral terms used to elicit history but still wanted to "test it" to make sure that his family had not been notified about his sexuality or his STI.

When a GLB teenager does not feel that the provider has any sensitivity, or if there is no trust in the office or provider, the teenager will likely not challenge the provider. Instead these teenagers will hide their sexuality or deny any sexuality, creating a barrier to receiving optimal clinical care. Because of homophobia and heterosexism, it is unlikely that adolescents will disclose their sexuality without the provider using excellent communication strategies. In 1 study of a biased sample of teenagers who were very comfortable with their sexuality, attending an empowerment conference, only 35% reported that their physician knew that they were GLB.[27] GLB adolescents who are hiding their sexuality become quite adept at using gender-neutral terms to describe their relationships

Table 1
Using gender-neutral terms

Heterosexist question	Instead ask...
"Do you have a girlfriend?"	"Are you seeing anybody?"
	"Are you in a relationship?"
"What do you and your boyfriend do together?"	"What do the two of you do together?"
	"Tell me about your partner"
"Are you and your girlfriend sexually active?"	"Are you having sex?"
	"Are the two of you in a sexual relationship?"
"Are you using birth control?"	"Are the two of you using protection?"
	"When was the last time you had sex without using protection?"

and sexual behaviors or may instead substitute gender to remain "in the closet." These teenagers immediately recognize when a provider uses gender-neutral terms in obtaining history. That does not mean that the teenager will immediately trust the provider to not disclose their sexual history to others. Just like Derrick's case, trust in the health care system is earned and not just immediately granted, especially if there were negative experiences in the past. Of course, adolescent communication is facilitated by using the HEEADSSS social history.[28] Experienced clinicians recognize that bridging questions between sections and going from open-ended to closed questions assists in obtaining full information from the client. One effective strategy when starting to obtain a sexual history is to ask, "How is your social life?" Some teenagers may interpret that as what they do with their friends, but most will recognize that you are talking about relationships. Of course, how the teenager responds will dictate whether we need to clarify that we are talking about relationships and sexual partners and not just peer-group activities. After getting the teenager on the same page, using gender-neutral terms will maximize the information you are able to obtain from a teenager who is just starting to build a trusting relationship with a provider. Table 1 offers suggestions for discrete questions that may be asked as we introduce this section of the psychosocial interview and get to the important sexual behavior of the adolescent.

ACKNOWLEDGING AND NORMALIZING SEXUALITY

As discussed earlier, just because a teenager acknowledges being heterosexual does not mean that the teenager is not having same-sex fantasies or activities. Similarly, women who have sex with women still may have fantasies about or sexual behavior with men. For pediatricians to provide optimal clinical care, it must be contingent on obtaining full information about sexual activities and fantasies, then working with the teenagers to promote healthy, protected sexuality for those who have begun to have sex. Of course, those teenagers who are abstinent should have their abstinence acknowledged and reinforced as a preferred method of prevention.

Table 2
Examples of questions in the sexual history

- Have you ever had oral sex? Has a partner ever "gone down" on you or have you ever "gone down" on a partner.
- Have you ever had vaginal sex?
- Have you ever had anal sex? Was this insertive or receptive?
- Have you ever done anything else sexually with a partner?

One classic suggested question is, "Are you having sex with guys, girls, or both?" Although not a bad question, it may be difficult for the teenager to answer when they have not yet established trust in the provider. Normalize it by a bridging statement such as, "Many teenagers your age have had sexual activities with members of the same sex." Then, go onto the question about the gender of partners. One suggested question is, "Have you ever had a sexual relationship with a guy or a girl?" Of course, behavior does not always equal orientation, so asking about fantasies and attractions gives additional insights. Ask, "When you think of people to whom you are attracted, are they male, female, or both? Are you unsure?"[1]

Often when asking these questions of heterosexual and even somewhat homophobic teenagers, they may respond curtly or even angrily, "No! Why are you asking?" You can get them past that simply by noting that "many teens don't feel comfortable bringing up their sexuality, so that if I ask the question this way, it allows that teens who are having sex with the same sex to answer." I have had no further resistance with normalizing the experience.

Having a full picture of the teenager's sexuality is important for providing optimal preventive care and reproductive health care. Fortunately, sexual practices, for the most part, are not dissimilar between heterosexual and gay teenagers. Many heterosexual youth engage in oral intercourse, and some engage in anal intercourse. Sometimes for gay teenagers who are not able to trust the provider to reveal their sexuality, focusing on types of sexual behaviors rather than the gender of the partner may allow him or her to disclose risk behaviors. Table 2 has suggested questions to politely and nonintrusively ask about discrete sexual behaviors. Of course, you may need to break down the questions to more understandable terms when asking the questions. For example, when you ask about vaginal intercourse, if you get a blank or confused look, then respond, "Have you ever had penis-vagina sex?"

Once you have obtained this important information, in the context of the remainder of the psychosocial history, then important preventive activities can be encouraged. Of course, if the teenager is abusing substances, it places him or her at higher sexual risk because of lack of judgment in using condoms or contraception. Likewise, depressed or suicidal teenagers must be carefully evaluated for any risk of self-injury.[29] Most GLB teenagers are quite resilient, as discussed

Table 3
Screening recommendations for men who have sex with men (MSM)

- HIV serology, if HIV-negative or not tested within the previous year
- Syphilis serology
- Test for urethral infection with *Neisseria gonorrhoeae* and *Chlamydia trachomatis* in men who have had insertive intercourse during the preceding year
- Test for rectal infection with *N gonorrhoeae* and *C trachomatis* in men who have had receptive anal intercourse during the preceding year
- Test for pharyngeal infection with *N gonorrhoeae* in men who have acknowledged participation in receptive oral intercourse during the preceding year; testing for *C trachomatis* pharyngeal infection is not recommended[32]

above. Although as a group there may be higher risks of mental health issues, substance abuse, and sexuality, just because a teenager self-identifies as gay does not mean that the teenager is at high risk as in individual. However, if he or she is abusing substances or has mental health issues, it is important to address these issues to reduce risks. And, of course, there is a growing body of evidence that demonstrates that positive youth development is an outstanding way to reduce risks in teenagers.[30]

There are discrete, evidence-based recommendations for testing men who have had sex with men that are well documented in the latest version of "Sexually Transmitted Diseases Treatment Guidelines, 2006," published by the CDC in 2006.[31] Interestingly, for heterosexual teenagers there are well-established screening recommendations for girls, whereas the recommendations for boys are less clear and established. This is exactly opposite for same-sex–loving teenagers and adults. The CDC has excellent, discrete recommendations for males but few or no recommendations for women who have sex with women. Of course, we should base our recommended STI testing on the sexual behaviors that we learned from obtaining a quality sexual history. Screening recommendations for men who have sex with men are listed in Table 3.

Which test should be used? The one that you have that is approved by the US Food and Drug Administration for use. For example, the local system in my teen clinic uses a ligase chain reaction nucleic acid–amplification test; chlamydia and gonorrhea testing is approved only for urine specimen or urethral or cervical swab specimens. We would use chlamydia and gonorrhea culture for rectal testing and gonorrhea culture for pharyngeal testing. As the technology advances, more nucleic acid amplification testing undoubtedly will be validated for screening in the rectum and pharynx. The documentation that is provided with whatever test or laboratory that is used should have the information for you.

There are also a growing number of experts who consider type-specific testing for herpes simplex virus 2 (HSV-2) if infection status is unknown. Routine testing for anal cytological abnormalities and HPV testing is not recommended currently until more reliable data are available.[31] In HIV-infected adults who have engaged in receptive anal intercourse, there is a growing body of evidence that should encourage testing for this even-higher-risk population. One study was performed in Atlanta that examined cytology reports from HIV-positive patients, with significant rates (47%) of anal dysplasia shown.[32]

Similar to other populations of adolescents, if adolescents are having healthy, protected intercourse (monogamous relationship, using condoms 100% of the time and correctly), it is reasonable to test them once per year. However, those who have multiple or anonymous partners, have substance abuse issues, or other risk factors should be tested at 3- to 6-month intervals. Of course, if not vaccinated already against hepatitis B or A, all men who have sex with men should receive these important vaccines.[31]

The CDC's sexually transmitted diseases treatment recommendations[31] for women who have sex with women are based largely on expert opinion and translation of information from other populations. Few data are available on the risk of transmission of STIs between women who have sex with women. Sexual behaviors that involve digital-vaginal or -anal contact or with "shared penetrative devices" may transmit infected cervicovaginal secretions. Evidence is based on specific metronidazole-resistant trichomonas strains and genotype-concordant HIV transmission found in sexual partners. HPV may be transmitted with skin-to-skin or skin-to-mucosa contact. The CDC's sexually transmitted diseases treatment guidelines also emphasize that 53% to 99% of women who have sex with women have had sex with men, so these women should continue to receive routine recommended screening tests for HPV and cervical dysplasia regardless of identified orientation. HSV-2 transmission is actually inefficient in women who have sex with women, but orogenital contact might be anticipated to cause genital herpes with higher rates of HSV-1. Transmission of syphilis by female partners, probably through oral sex, has been reported.[31] Women should, again, have a complete sexual history, and on the basis of the activities in which they have participated, testing should be targeted to the likely STIs.

Also, because so many women have had sex with men or may have sex again with men in the future, a discussion of contraception, in the context of the patient's life, should also take place in the clinical setting when a same-sex–loving woman is in the office. Emergency contraception must be discussed, because many young women who have sex with women do not identify the need for contraception because they do not have sex with men "often." Of course, providers should also provide the context that many teenagers who are self-identifying as GLB may have sexual encounters that may not be predicted by their orientation, necessitating the important conversation about birth control.

CONCLUSIONS

Pediatricians and adolescent medicine providers are skilled at providing culturally competent, developmentally appropriate care for teenagers. GLB teenagers represent a very underserved population, many of whom struggle with acceptance of their sexuality at the same time that they are managing the other rigors of adolescence. Too many fall into the path of substance abuse. Many have chronic dysthymia or even major depression, and some fall prey to suicidal thoughts. Many teenagers who are depressed have low self-esteem and may be preyed on by older partners or feel unempowered to insist that their partners remain monogamous or even to negotiate condom use. Gay, bisexual, and even lesbian teenagers are at higher risk from most STIs, largely because of them having more risky intercourse: multiple partners, substance abuse, and not consistently using condoms. Of course, orientation does not equal behavior, because most men who are self-identified as gay and most women who are self-identified as lesbian have had sex with the opposite sex. Many do not identify at all as bisexual. It is paramount that we establish a caring, trusting relationship with these vulnerable children, allowing for full communication of risk behaviors and drafting testing and targeted behavioral interventions to allow the teenagers to lower their risk. Not surprisingly, positive youth development is an effective strategy, as it is with all teenagers.

Knowledge of local resources can also be quite helpful. In Atlanta we have a wonderful multiservice organization known as YouthPride (www.youthpride.org). There is also transitional housing for homeless and runaway GLB or transgendered kids, known as Rainbow House, a special program in a network of group homes known as Chris Homes (www.chriskids.org/programsRainbow.htm). Finding local resources in your community may help your teenagers. Because most of its members are nonprofit organizations, the United Way is a great place to start, as well as looking for adult GLB advocacy organizations that may know of youth-serving agencies.

We must care for and protect this group of vulnerable youth. Every teenager is valuable, and we must continue to work with teenagers to allow them to achieve their potential. Sexual orientation and sexual behaviors are part of the puzzle, but like all teenagers, they need our help, our caring, and our compassion. We need the talents of every young person if we are to address the growing issues that face our country and our world. Every time that we lose a teenager, we all lose.

REFERENCES

1. Physicians for Reproductive Choice and Health. *Gay, Lesbian, Bisexual, Transgender, and Questioning Youth.* 2nd ed. New York, NY: Adolescent Reproductive Health Education Program; 2007. Available at: www.prch.org/gay-lesbian-bisexual-transgender-and-questioning-youth. Accessed February 12, 2009

2. Garofalo R, Harper G. Not all adolescents are the same: Addressing the unique needs of gay and bisexual male youth. *Adolesc Med.* 2003;14(3):595–611, vi
3. Ryan C, Futterman D. Lesbian and gay youth: care and counseling. *Adolesc Med.* 1997;8(2): 207–374
4. Frankowski BL; American Academy of Pediatrics, Committee on Adolescence. Sexual orientation and adolescents. *Pediatrics.* 2004;113(6):1827–1832
5. Moffat S, Cate R. *The 2007 Vermont Youth Risk Behavior Survey.* Burlington, VT: Vermont Department of Health, Division of Health Surveillance; 2007
6. Massachusetts Department of Education. *Massachusetts High School Students and Sexual Orientation: Results of the 2007 Youth Risk Behavior Survey.* 2007. Available at: www.mass.gov/Eeohhs2/docs/dph/com_health/violence/youth_risk_behavior_survey07.pdf. Accessed February 4, 2009
7. Mosher W, Chandra A, Jones J. Sexual behavior and selected health measures: men and women 15–44 years of age. *Adv Data.* 2005;(362):1–55
8. Eccles TA, Sayegh MA, Fortenberry JD, Zimet GD. More normal than not: a qualitative assessment of the developmental experiences of gay male youth. *J Adolesc Health.* 2004;35(5): 425.e11–425.e18
9. Eisenberg ME, Resnick MD. Suicidality among gay, lesbian, and bisexual youth: the role of protective factors. *J Adolesc Health.* 2006;39(5):662–668
10. D'Augelli AR, Grossman AH, Salter NP, Vasey JJ, Starks MT, Sinclair KO. Predicting the suicide attempts of lesbian, gay, and bisexual youth. *Suicide Life Threat Behav.* 2005;35(6): 646–660
11. Whitbeck LB, Chen X, Hoyt DR, Tyler KA, Johnson KD. Mental disorder, subsistence strategies, and victimization among gay, lesbian, and bisexual homeless and runaway adolescents. *J Sex Res.* 2004;41(4):329–342
12. Pachankis JE, Goldfried MR. Social anxiety in young gay men. *J Anxiety Disord.* 2006;20(8): 996–1015
13. Hart TA, Heimberg RG. Social anxiety as a risk factor for unprotected intercourse among gay and bisexual male youth. *AIDS Behav.* 2005;9(4):505–512
14. Friedman MS, Koeske GF, Silvestre AJ, Korr SS, Sites EW. The impact of gender-role conforming behavior, bullying, and social support on suicidality among gay male youth. *J Adolesc Health.* 2006;38(5):621–623
15. Russell CJ, Keel PK. Homosexuality as a specific risk factor for eating disorders in men. *Int J Eat Disord.* 2002;31(3):300–306
16. Feldman MB, Meyer IH. Childhood abuse and eating disorders in gay and bisexual men. *Int J Eat Disord.* 2007;40(5):418–423
17. D'Augelli AR. High tobacco use among lesbian, gay, and bisexual youth. *Arch Pediatr Adolesc Med.* 2004;158(4):309–310
18. Remafedi G, Carol H. Preventing tobacco use among lesbian, gay, bisexual, and transgender youths. *Nicotine Tob Res.* 2005;7(2):249–256
19. Greenwood GL, White EW, Page-Shafer K, et al. Correlates of heavy substance use among young gay and bisexual men: the San Francisco Young Men's Health Study. *Drug Alcohol Depend.* 2001;61(2):105–112
20. Ridner SL, Frost K, LaJoie AS. Health information and risk behaviors among lesbian, gay, and bisexual college students. *J Am Acad Nurse Pract.* 2006;18(8):374–378
21. Cochrane BN, Steward AJ, Ginzler JA, Cauce AM. Challenges faced by homeless sexual minorities. *Am J Public Health.* 2002;92(5):773–777
22. Parsons JT, Kelly BC, Weiser JD. Initiation into methamphetamine use for young gay and bisexual men. *Drug Alcohol Depend.* 2007;90(2–3):135–144
23. Rosario M, Schrimshaw EW, Hunter J. Predictors of substance use over time among gay, lesbian, and bisexual youths: an examination of three hypotheses. *Addict Behav.* 2004;29(8):1623–1631
24. American Academy of Pediatrics. Recommendations for preventive pediatric health care. 2008. Available at: http://pediatrics.aappublications.org/cgi/data/120/6/1376/DC1/1. Accessed February 4, 2009

25. Benson PA, Hergenroeder AC. Bacterial sexually transmitted infections in gay, lesbian, and bisexual adolescents: medical and public health perspectives. *Semin Pediatr Infect Dis.* 2005; 16(3):181–191
26. Saewyc EM, Bearinger LH, Blum RW, Resnick MD. Sexual intercourse, abuse and pregnancy among adolescent women: does sexual orientation make a difference? *Fam Plann Perspect.* 1999;31(3):127–131
27. Meckler GD, Elliott MN, Kanouse DE, Beals KP, Schuster MA. Nondisclosure of sexual orientation to a physician among a sample of gay, lesbian, and bisexual youth. *Arch Pediatr Adolesc Med.* 2006;160(12):1248–1254
28. Goldenring JM, Rosen DS. Getting into adolescent heads: an essential update. *Contemp Pediatr.* 2004;21(1):64–90
29. Rosario M, Schrimshaw EW, Hunter J. A model of sexual risk behaviors among young gay and bisexual men: longitudinal associations of mental health, substance abuse, sexual abuse, and the coming-out process. *AIDS Educ Prev.* 2006;18(5):444–460
30. Duncan PM, Garcia AC, Frankowski BL, et al. Inspiring healthy adolescent choices: a rationale for and guide to strength promotion in primary care. *J Adolesc Health.* 2007;41(6):525–535
31. Centers for Disease Control and Prevention; Workowski KA, Berman SM. Sexually transmitted diseases treatment guidelines, 2006 [published correction appears in *MMWR Recomm Rep.* 2006;55(36):997]. *MMWR Recomm Rep.* 2006;55(RR-11):1–94
32. Bakotic WL, Willis D, Birdsong G, Tadross TS. Anal cytology in an HIV-positive population: a retrospective analysis. *Acta Cytol.* 2005;49(2):163–168

An Overview of the Use of Dialectical Behavior Therapy With Adolescents for Primary Care Physicians

Christopher Jones, PhD*, Roy Chancey, LCSW, Eamonn Walsh, LCSW, Jamie Bray, LCSW, Emily Potts, LMSW

Hillside, Inc, 690 Courtenay Drive, Atlanta, GA 30306, USA

Primary care physicians are often the first point of contact for adolescents with mental health problems. Mental health problems among children and adolescents are a global public health problem.[1] In the United States, 1 in 5 children and adolescents has a diagnosable mental health disorder. One in 10 children and adolescents experiences a serious mental health disorder that severely affects daily functioning.[2] Many of these youths' conditions go undiagnosed, and they do not receive treatment for their mental health problems. Of those youth who do receive a diagnosis, fewer than 30% receive treatment.[3] Many of these youth who receive treatment are treated by their primary care physicians. Among adolescents who have attempted suicide, only 50% receive follow-up treatment for their mental health problems, and among those who receive treatment, a majority (as much as 77%) fail to attend their appointments or complete treatment.[4] When mental health problems go untreated among children and adolescents, these youth are at increased risk of suicide, juvenile delinquency, school dropout, and substance abuse.[5]

Dialectical behavior therapy (DBT) is a psychotherapeutic treatment developed to treat individuals with a history of chronic suicide attempts, parasuicidal acts, intentional self-harm, and borderline personality disorder (BPD). DBT is currently the only mental health treatment that has been found to be effective at reducing attempts at suicide and self-injurious behavior in more than 1 clinical trial. On the basis of DBT's effectiveness with adults, the treatment has been adapted for treatment of adolescents who have comorbid mental health problems and are suicidal.[4] Because primary care physicians are often the first point of contact for these youth and are left with the task of identifying the most

---

*Corresponding author.
E-mail address: cjones@hside.org (C. Jones).

Copyright © 2009 American Academy of Pediatrics. All rights reserved. ISSN 1934-4287

appropriate treatment for these youth and their families, the following is an overview of DBT, its effectiveness with adolescents, and its application to work with adolescents.

WHAT IS DBT?

DBT is an empirically researched psychotherapeutic treatment developed by Marsha Linehan, PhD, Professor of Psychology at the University of Washington. This therapy employs cognitive and behavioral principles and is rapidly becoming a standard for treating patients with BPD. The essential functions of DBT are "improving client motivation to change; enhancing client capabilities; generalization of new behaviors; structuring the environment; and enhancing therapist capability and motivation."[4]

Dr Linehan's biosocial theory provides the theoretical framework for DBT and views an individual's behaviors as resulting from both biological and environmental factors. Biological factors are described as a persistent dysfunction in an individual's emotion-regulation system. This emotional dysregulation is characterized by heightened sensitivity to emotion, increased emotional intensity, and a slow return to emotional baseline. An individual's initial vulnerability to emotional dysregulation is theorized as stemming from biological factors such as genetics, prenatal conditions, brain development, and nervous system development. Behaviors and emotional experiences commonly associated with BPD theoretically result from the expression of this biological dysfunction in combination with environmental factors.[6]

The environmental factors of biosocial theory stem from a social environment that the individual experiences as invalidating. An invalidating environment is characterized by the individual's behaviors and communications being rejected and ignored, any emotional displays and painful behaviors being met with punishment that is erratically administered and intermittently reinforced, and oversimplification of how problems are solved or needs are met. Most individuals are able to manage an invalidating environment by changing their behavior to meet expectations, changing the environment so that it is no longer invalidating, or simply leaving the environment. For individuals with BPD or borderline features, this invalidating environment intensifies their vulnerability to emotion dysregulation.[6]

Another important component of DBT is the concept of dialectical dilemmas, the ongoing synthesis of opposing ideas. The primary dialectic that defines the core treatment strategies in DBT is acknowledging the balance between acceptance of the individual and the expectation that he or she needs to change.[7] Acceptance strategies, drawn from Zen practice, involve emotional, behavioral, and cognitive validation, as well as teaching the patient personal strategies for validation.[6] One example of a validation strategy would be recognizing how self-mutilation can be an individual's attempt at being adaptive or regulating his emotions.[8]

The antithesis of acceptance is the expectation of change. This expectation is embodied in behavioral therapy with its emphasis on problem solving, rationality, logic, and gaining knowledge by testing beliefs. Strategies for promoting change include problem solving, contingency procedures, skills training, exposure, and cognitive modification.[9] An example of a problem-solving procedure is the use of a "behavior chain analysis" to diminish cutting (self-mutilation) behaviors. A chain analysis reviews the environmental and personal antecedents and consequences of the cutting behavior in great detail. An important goal of this procedure is to identify points during the chain of events when the patient has an opportunity to implement effective change. This sets the stage for the patient to avoid the problematic behavior in the future.[4]

COMPONENTS OF TREATMENT

DBT treatment is organized along a 4-stage hierarchy. Treatment emphasis is placed initially on the pretreatment targets of commitment to therapy and orientation. The next stage of treatment focuses on achieving competence and mastery by targeting areas on the basis of their degree of importance.[6] The most important target area involves decreasing suicidal and parasuicidal behaviors.[6,8] This is followed by decreasing behaviors that interfere with therapy, addressing behaviors that interfere with quality of life, and increasing behavioral skills. The other stages, which target posttraumatic stress, increasing self-respect, and achieving individual goals, are not formally addressed with an adolescent population.[6,8,9]

DBT emphasizes 5 problem areas that involve emotional, interpersonal, self, cognitive, and behavioral dysregulation along with 5 corresponding skills modules that include mindfulness, distress tolerance, emotional regulation, interpersonal effectiveness, and middle path. These modules are presented in a didactic format through a skills-training group. The goals of skills training are to change behavioral, emotional, and thinking patterns that cause personal misery and interpersonal distress. Specific goals include reducing dysregulation while increasing adaptive (eg, more regulated) behaviors. Patients are taught to attend to the moment without judgment or impulsivity, a quality described as "core mindfulness." Newly learned skills enable patients to improve their emotional, cognitive, and interpersonal functioning.[6,7]

The primary components of DBT include individual psychotherapy once per week, a weekly skills-training group, and telephone consultations with the individual therapist as needed. Skills training is slightly modified to accommodate the adolescent's family. Parents are included in the skills-training group to learn and reinforce skills within the home. An additional skills module, "middle path," was developed specifically for families. This skills module addresses parent-child conflicts.[10]

TREATMENT EFFECTIVENESS

There are many advantages to using DBT within a treatment framework. DBT effectively addresses noncompliance and focuses on continual reengagement of the patient in the treatment process. Furthermore, the problem areas addressed in DBT are specific to the developmental stages of adolescents in particular. The nonjudgmental approach used within DBT facilitates and promotes empathy toward the patient. There are also empirical data that support the efficacy of DBT in reducing parasuicidal behavior, therapy dropout, and inpatient hospitalization compared with standard treatment interventions.[8,9]

Linehan et al conducted[8,11] a clinical trial and subsequent replication trials to assess the effectiveness of DBT among adult women who were suicidal and met criteria for BPD. DBT was compared with treatment as usual (TAU), typically consisting of psychopharmacologic treatment and intermittent supportive psychotherapy. When compared with TAU, subjects assigned to receive DBT had significantly fewer and less-severe parasuicidal behaviors during the treatment year. These results were obtained although DBT was no better than TAU at improving self-reports of hopelessness, suicide ideation, or reasons for living. DBT was also dramatically more effective than TAU in limiting treatment dropout, the most serious behavior interfering with therapy. At the end of 1 year, only 16.4% of patients who were receiving DBT had left treatment. In contrast, ~50% of patients receiving TAU had dropped out. Another important finding was that subjects assigned to receive DBT had a tendency to enter psychiatric inpatient units less often and had fewer inpatient psychiatric days. Those receiving DBT had an average of 8.46 inpatient days over the year compared with 38.86 inpatient days for those who were receiving TAU. This finding suggests that DBT is cost-effective. Finally, subjects receiving DBT rated themselves as more successful at changing their emotions and improving general emotional control. They also had significantly lower scores on self-reported measures of anger and anxious rumination.[8,11,12]

DBT's effectiveness with adults has lead to successful modification for adolescents who also suffer from emotional dysregulation. These structural changes have been made for DBT to accommodate the adolescent and family. Adolescents served within DBT programs typically have symptoms that mirror those of adult patients with BPD, with adolescents having stronger identifiable characteristics involving affective instability and uncontrolled anger.

DBT has been extended from its original scope of treating adults with BPD to use with adolescents with various behavioral and emotional problems and to other target populations beyond the scope of this review. The initial extension for teenagers was to provide DBT to adolescents with suicidal and parasuicidal behaviors, maintaining the same behavioral targets as DBT for adults and modifying the treatment to better speak to an adolescent population. The primary modifications of DBT to treat adolescents were length of treatment (shortening the initial treatment phase from 1 year to 12–16 weeks), changing the handouts to be more developmentally appropriate, and including the family as a critical part of the treatment (creating a family DBT skills group and including the family in some sessions with the individual therapist).[4] In addition to being extended to treating adolescents with suicidal and parasuicidal behaviors, DBT has also begun to be extended to treat adolescents outside the original BPD population for which it was developed. DBT has been used to treat adolescents with both substance abuse and suicidal behavior; incarcerated juvenile offenders; adolescents with bipolar disorder; and adolescents with binge-eating disorder.[13–16] Finally, as it has been in the adult population, DBT has been extended for use with adolescents in both inpatient and outpatient settings.[17]

Miller et al[13] provided the initial research on adapting DBT to suicidal adolescents on an outpatient basis. Subsequent publications[4,18] by these same authors made adaptations to the length of treatment and included parents/guardians in the treatment. In addition, to address the dialectical dilemmas common in parent-teenager relationships, Miller et al added a training module called the middle path.[4]

A preliminary study by Washington State's Juvenile Rehabilitation Administration found that youth who received DBT in residential care had lower felony recidivism rates after 1 year than youth who lived in the program before the implementation of DBT.[14] Miller et al[13] found that suicidal teenagers in outpatient treatment receiving DBT were more likely to complete treatment and have fewer psychiatric hospitalizations than youth who did not receive DBT in outpatient treatment.

Trupin et al[16] extended DBT to incarcerated female juvenile offenders. Noting that this population has similarities in emotional problems to those with BPD, they tested offenders with mental health issues, offenders from the general population, and a general population control group. Female youth offenders on the mental health unit demonstrated a significant decrease in behavior problems such as suicidal acts, aggression, and class disruption when compared via records to the same unit in the previous year. Youth in the general population did not demonstrate a significant difference in behavior problems after treatment, although they started out with less suicidal and self-injurious behavior.

A single case study performed by Safer et al[15] provided preliminary support for adapting DBT to adolescent populations with binge-eating disorder. Adaptations described included the use of family sessions.

Adolescents with bipolar disorder and treated in a pediatric bipolar specialty outpatient clinic were studied by Goldstein et al.[17] They received DBT through individual therapy and family skills groups for a 1-year period. Results indicated that patients stayed in the treatment to completion and that treatment satisfaction was high. Pretreatment/posttreatment results showed significant decreases in suicidality, nonsuicidal self-injurious behavior, emotional dysregulation, and depressive symptoms. It should be noted that the subject group was small and, therefore, not generalizable.

Although DBT has been extended to adolescents, families, and other target populations, the effectiveness of such extensions has not been researched rigorously. In essence, the research is in its infancy and contains problems with generalization, validity, and methodology. These studies are important in terms of exploring DBT for various populations yet, clearly, can only be interpreted narrowly.

OVERVIEW OF SKILLS TRAINING

Skills training is one of the key change procedures used in DBT to help the individual learn the skills, strengthen his or her ability to use the skills, and generalize use of the skills through direct application. The 5 skills modules taught through skills training include mindfulness, distress tolerance, emotional regulation, interpersonal effectiveness, and middle path. Each module consists of a set of skills that target the related problem areas of emotional, interpersonal, self, cognitive, and behavioral dysregulation. Skills training is taught in a structured format and aimed at teaching skills that assist the individual in changing dysfunctional behavioral, emotional, and thought patterns. Each of the 5 modules consists of a set of skills designed to actively engage the individual in identifying alternative solutions to the identified problem and then practicing the skills.[4,6,7]

The mindfulness skills are referred to as the "core" skills and were designed to teach individuals awareness of their environment and self (thoughts, emotions, and behaviors). One concept taught in this module is the 3 states of mind: the emotional mind; the reasonable mind; and the wise mind. When someone is in the emotional mind, he or she is thinking and acting impulsively according to his or her current emotional state. The reasonable mind is looking at a situation intellectually through analyzing data and facts. If someone is primarily in reasonable mind, there is a danger he or she will overanalyze a situation and not take action. One moves from the reasonable mind to the wise mind once he or she has taken into account his or her feelings and intellect and has a plan to put into action. The skills taught in this module are aimed at helping an individual move to the wise mind. For example, the "what" skills taught in this module include: "observe" the experience, thoughts, behaviors, and feelings; "describe" the experience by applying a verbal label (eg, "I feel sad right now"); and "participate" fully by being one with the experience without being self-conscious.[4,6,7]

Hillside, Inc is a private not-for-profit agency in Atlanta, Georgia, that treats children and adolescents aged 7 to 17 years with a wide range of severe emotional and behavioral problems. Hillside has incorporated DBT into its psychiatric residential treatment program, community intervention program, and therapeutic foster care. At Hillside, each skills-training group session begins with a mindfulness practice exercise. These practice exercises are used to coach the patients in developing their awareness of self and their environment. For example, the "what" skill described above is taught by asking patients to sit quietly for 5 minutes and focus on their breathing. Patients are encouraged to "observe" their thoughts, feelings, and behaviors during the exercise. The group leaders coach the patients in noticing distractions and returning their focus to their breathing. After the exercise is over, we practice "describe" by each patient telling the group about the thoughts, feelings, and behaviors they experienced during the exercise.

The distress-tolerance module consists of skills for coping with painful events and emotions. This module helps the individual accept that pain and suffering are a part of life and provides him or her with skills to cope with this reality. The skills taught in this module include crisis-survival and acceptance skills. One of the 4 crisis-survival strategies taught in this module is to "self-soothe" by using the 5 senses.[4,6,7] An adolescent who experiences distress when visiting his or her primary care physician could, for example, use a stress ball to focus attention on the sense of touch and to distract him or her from worrying thoughts about the visit.

John, a 12-year-old boy in Hillside's residential program, provides us with another example of this same skill. He learned to use self-soothing skills to manage his emotion dysregulation when he is not able to reach his family members on the telephone. When John attempted to contact his family members and was not able to reach them, he experienced intense feelings of "loneliness" and thoughts of "no one likes me." When John became emotionally dysregulated, he often responded aggressively by throwing the telephone or hitting the wall with his hand. John learned to use the self-soothe skill by rubbing hand lotion on his hands and focusing on the smell of the lotion and sensation of the lotion on his skin if he was not able to reach his family members on the telephone. Using this skill shifted his attention from his intense emotions and worry thoughts and allowed him to regain control of his thoughts, feelings, and behaviors.

The emotional regulation module provides individuals with skills to regulate their affective levels. The skills in this module focus on identifying and labeling emotions, identifying the functions and reinforcers of emotional behaviors, reducing vulnerability to emotional reactivity, increasing positive emotions through positive experiences and events, increasing awareness of current emotions without judgment or inhibition, and applying distress-tolerance skills to tolerate negative emotions. One specific set of skills taught in this module is the "ABC" skills. These skills teach individuals to "A, accumulate positive experiences" by finding pleasant experiences to produce positive emotions (eg, physical exercise, listening to music, setting long- and short-term goals). The "B" represents "build mastery" by scheduling activities that are pleasurable every day that will foster a sense of accomplishment (eg, taking up a new hobby). Finally, the "C" stands for "coping ahead" by anticipating stressful situations and developing an individualized plan to deal with the situation.[4,6,7]

For example, Sally is a 15-year-old girl who lives with her mother and stepfather and spends every other weekend with her father. While Sally was in Hillside's residential program, she learned to use the DBT skill of coping ahead to manage her anxiety in "going back and forth" between her parents' homes. In joint family therapy sessions with her mother, stepfather, and father, Sally was able to identify that a factor increasing her anxiety during these transitions was the "different rules" at each home. The family used "cope ahead" to establish consistent behavior expectations between both homes and strategies to help the parents communicate about Sally's behavior progress. Despite their differences in parenting styles, Sally's parents were able to agree on expectations for schoolwork, curfew, telephone privileges, and peer groups. The family continued to use this skill by her parents speaking over the telephone about her behavior progress over the past week before each visit to her father's home. Sally also made telephone calls to her father before each visit to review any changes in her behavior expectations and any scheduled events.

The interpersonal effectiveness module teaches skills needed for effectiveness in social settings. These skills teach individuals how to identify their goal for social interaction and the skills required to accomplish that goal. The skills taught address the goals of asking for something effectively, saying "no" effectively, keeping a good relationship with the other person, and keeping self-respect. The module uses specific interpersonal response patterns to achieve these goals by targeting both the individual's belief patterns that inhibit effective communication and the individual's affective responses.[4,6,7] For example, the module teaches individuals to change worry thoughts (eg, "I will never be able to do it") by replacing these thoughts with "cheerleading statements" (eg, "I won't know if I don't try . . . let me give it my best shot").

The following is an example of using this skill. Bill is a 14-year-old boy who experienced severe abuse and neglect in his birth home and who was adopted at 8 years of age. Bill displayed a pattern of denying responsibility for his behavior with his adoptive parents when receiving a consequence for his behavior. While in Hillside's residential program, Bill was able to practice using cheerleading statements to change his worry thoughts of how his parents will respond. Because of Bill's experience with abuse and neglect, he often had worry thoughts that his adoptive parents would respond with the same pattern of abuse he experienced in his birth home. To manage these worry thoughts Bill began saying to himself, "my parents are not going to yell at me, they just want me to take responsibility for my behavior."

The fifth module, middle path, was developed in response to the unique family dilemmas experienced by suicidal adolescents and their families. This module emphasizes the concept of dialectics and that there is more than one way to see a problem and more than one way to solve it. The skills taught in the module focus on a willingness to hear other points of view and have an open mind without absolutes and polarized thinking. For example, the skill of "validation" taught in this module helps the individual understand someone else's feelings and emotions in a given situation through active listening, awareness of verbal and nonverbal communication, and reflecting back without judgment.[4] The vignette above about Sally developing the coping-ahead plan with her mother, stepfather, and father also illustrated the use of "validation." During family therapy, Sally's mother and father were able to validate Sally's concerns about the differences in rules between their homes by actively listening to Sally's explanation of feeling "anxious" about "not knowing what to expect" when going between her families' homes. Initially, the families maintained that their style of parenting was the "better" style to assist Sally. However, through family therapy, her parents were able to hear Sally's concern and recognize the need to work together to establish consistent expectations for Sally at each home.

DISCUSSION

As can be seen through the examples provided, skills training is an important component of the problem-solving strategies for DBT. However, DBT is not limited to problem-solving strategies. The concept of dialectic also allows for DBT to incorporate validation strategies to assist the individual with both acceptance and change. Focus on only acceptance offers little hope to an individual who experiences life as painful, whereas an overemphasis on change can be experienced as invalidating to emotionally dysregulated individuals. Individuals with BPD or features of BPD require treatment that balances validation of their experiences and perception with engagement in active problem solving.

Although existing research on the use of DBT with adolescents is limited, the current findings provide a positive outlook on the use of this treatment model with adolescents who have comorbid mental health problems and are suicidal. Research on DBT with adolescents is ongoing, and additional research is needed. The knowledge of the application of this empirically based treatment model can be beneficial for primary care providers, who oftentimes have the first contact with these adolescents. Identification and assessment of these troubled youth, along with appropriate referrals to DBT treatment providers, can help reduce the large number of youth whose conditions go undiagnosed or who do not receive effective treatment for their mental health problems.

REFERENCES

1. World Health Organization. *Caring for Children and Adolescents With Mental Disorders: Setting WHO Directions.* Geneva, Switzerland: World Health Organization; 2003

2. US Department of Health and Human Services. *Report of the Surgeon General's Conference on Children's Mental Health: A National Action Agenda.* Washington, DC: US Department of Health and Human Services; 2000
3. Platt R, Fothergill K, Wissow S. Talking with adolescents and their families about emotional and behavioral concerns. *Adolesc Med.* 2008;19(1):41–53
4. Miller AL, Rathus JH, Linehan MM. *Dialectical Behavior Therapy With Suicidal Adolescents.* New York, NY: Guilford Press; 2007
5. Centers for Disease Control and Prevention. Healthy youth! Health topics: mental health. Available at: www.cdc.gov/HealthyYouth/mentalhealth. Accessed August 13, 2008
6. Linehan MM. *Cognitive-Behavioral Treatment of Borderline Personality Disorder.* New York, NY: Guilford Press; 1993
7. Linehan MM. *Skills Training Manual for Treating Borderline Personality Disorder.* New York, NY: Guilford Press; 1993
8. Linehan MM, Armstrong HE, Suarez A, Allman D, Heard HL. Cognitive-behavioral treatment of chronically parasuicidal borderline patients. *Arch Gen Psychiatry.* 1991;48(12):1060–1064
9. Shearin EN, Linehan MM. Dialectical behavioral therapy for borderline personality disorder: theoretical and empirical foundations. *Acta Psychiatr Scand.* 1994;89(suppl 379):61–68
10. D'Amico Guthrie DM. *Adolescent Borderline Personality Disorder and Dialectical Behavior Therapy: Praxis.* Chicago, IL: Loyola University Press; 2006
11. Linehan MM, Heard HL, Armstrong HE. Naturalistic follow-up of a behavioral treatment for chronically parasuicidal borderline patients. *Arch Gen Psychiatry.* 1993;50(12):971–974
12. Linehan MM, Comtois KA, Murry AM, et al. Two-year randomized controlled trial and follow-up of dialectical behavior therapy vs therapy by experts for suicidal behaviors and borderline personality disorder [published correction appears in *Arch Gen Psychiatry.* 2007; 64(12):1401]. *Arch Gen Psychiatry.* 2006;63(7):757–766
13. Miller AL, Rathus JH, Linehan MM, Wetzler S, Leigh E. Dialectical behavior therapy adapted for suicidal adolescents. *J Pract Psychiatry Behav Health.* 1997;3(1):78–86
14. Washington State Institute for Public Policy. *Preliminary Findings for the Juvenile Rehabilitation Administration's Dialectical Behavior Therapy Program.* Olympia, WA: Washington State Institute for Public Policy; 2002
15. Safer DL, Lock J, Couturier JL. Dialectical behavior therapy modified for adolescent binge eating disorder: a case report. *Cogn Behav Pract.* 2007;14(2):157–167
16. Trupin EW, Stewart DG, Beach B, Boesky L. Effectiveness of a dialectical behaviour therapy program for incarcerated female juvenile offenders. *Child Adolesc Mental Health.* 2002;7(3): 121–127
17. Goldstein TR, Axelson DA, Birmaher B, Brent DA. Dialectical behavior therapy for adolescents with bipolar disorder: a 1-year open trial. *J Am Acad Child Adolesc Psychiatry.* 2007;46(7): 820–830
18. Miller AL. Dialectical behavior therapy: A new treatment approach for suicidal adolescents. *Am J Psychother.* 1999;53(3):413–417

A

Adenosine deaminase (ADA) deficiency, 130, 142
Adolescent contraceptive care for the practicing pediatrician, **168–187**
Alcohol use
 adolescent brain development and, 85–86, 85–87
 by adolescents with ADHD, 206
 screening for, in the office setting, 9–20
Americans With Disabilities Act (ADA), 212
Amygdala, 78, 87, 88
Antidepressants, 83
Anxiety
 diagnosis and treatment, 188–193
 test anxiety, 155–156
Anxiety and anxiety-related disorders in the adolescent population: an overview of diagnosis and treatment, **188–202**
Anxiolytic agents. see Tranquilizers
An approach to obesity management in primary care: yes, we can make a difference, **91–108**
Armed Forces qualifying test, 214
Athletes, management of adolescent concussion victims, 41–55
Attention-deficit/hyperactivity disorder
 grade failures, 156
 helping adolescents transition toward adulthood, 203–218
 prescription stimulants, abuse of, 4–6, 206
 promoting strengths of adolescents, 30
Autoimmune polyendocrinopathy candidiasis ectodermal dystrophy (APECED) syndrome, 131

B

Behavioral interventions
 anxiety and anxiety-related disorders, 188–201
 dialectical behavior therapy, 243–251
Belonging, promoting as adolescent strength, 26, 27–28, 30
Benzodiazepines, treatment of anxiety, 190–191, 193
Binge-eating disorder, 247
Bipolar disorder, 82, 83, 247–248
Bisexual youth, office-based care, 223–240
Blogs, 57, 58
Boarding school interventions, in obesity management, 93
Body mass index
 data from CDC growth curves, 97
 definitions of obesity and overweight, 91, 111
 management options, 117
 recording, for tracking obesity, 97–98, 118
Borderline personality disorder (BPD), 243, 244, 246, 247, 251
Brain, human, diagram of, 75
Brain development, adolescent
 effects of alcohol and drugs, 10–11, 84–87
 understanding, implications for the clinician, 73–89
Brain injuries, management of concussion victims, 41–55
Bullying. see Cyberbullying

C

Cardiovascular disease
 metabolic syndrome and, 110, 119
 obesity and, 91
Career planning, adolescents with ADHD, 207
Cell phones, 58, 67
Cellular or combined immunodeficiencies, treatment of, 140
Central obesity, 110, 113
Change plans, written, 36, 37

Chat rooms, 57, 58, 61, 66
Chronic granulomatous disease (CGD), 124, 128, 142
Chronic mucocutaneous candidiasis (CMC), 131
Circle of Courage, 24, 25, 26, 27–29, 36, 38
Colleges
  disability-support services, 215
  testing and admissions, 212–213
Common variable immunodeficiency (CVID), 123, 124, 125, 126, 137, 140, 142
Community colleges, students with ADHD, 215
Complement deficiency, treatment of, 141
Computers
  filtering, blocking, and monitoring software, 66–67, 68
  interventions, in obesity management, 93–94
Concussion
  criteria, 43
  definition/location, 42–43
  evaluation/assessment, 44–49
  initial management, 51–52
  neurometabolic cascade, 44
  parent's checklist, 48
  prevention, 53–54
  prognosis/clinical course, 49–51
  return to playing sports after, 52–53
  signs and symptoms, 43
Confidentiality
  adolescents with ADHD, 208
  in contraceptive care, 169
Congenital neutropenia, 124
Consent for care, 169
Contraceptive care, 168–182, 239
Corpus callosum, 80–81, 87
Cortex, changes during adolescence, 74–76
Cortisol, 78
CRAFFT screening tool, 17–18, 33
Cutting, 66, 245
Cyberbullying, 67
Cyclic neutropenia, 128

D

Depo-Provera (DMPA), 170, 177–180
Depression, adolescent brain development and, 82–83
Developmental approach, screening for substance abuse in the office setting, 9–20
Developmental delay, promoting strengths of adolescents, 30
Diabetes mellitus, type 2, 91, 100, 110, 119
Diagnosis
  anxiety and anxiety-related disorders, 188–201
  metabolic syndrome, 111–112
  primary immunodeficiency diseases, 132–137, 142
Dialectical behavior therapy, overview of use with adolescents for primary care physicians, 243–251
DiGeorge syndrome/22q11.2 deletion syndrome, 124, 129
Disabled students, 153–157, 210–212
Driving, adolescents with ADHD, 205–206
Drop-out crisis impacting America: can we turn it around?, **149–167**
Drug use
  adolescent brain development and, 84–87
  by adolescents with ADHD, 206
  nonmedical use of prescription drugs, 1–7
  screening for, in the office setting, 9–20
Dyslipidemia, 91, 100, 114, 116, 118

E

Eating disorders
  binge-eating disorder, 247
  in gay and bisexual men, 230
  Web sites promoting, 66, 69
Education. see also Schools
  drop-out crisis, 149–164
  students with ADHD, 210–215
Elementary school, screening for alcohol and drug use, 15–16
E-mail, 57, 58, 67, 68
Emergency contraception, 170–171, 239
Emotional dysregulation, 244, 246, 248, 251
Emotional reactivity, brain structures involved in, 76–78
Epidemiology, of metabolic syndrome, 111–112
Exercise

F

Facebook, 58, 59, 64, 65, 217
Fatty liver, 92
Foster care, promoting strengths of adolescents, 30, 31–32
Friendship formation, adolescents with ADHD, 207
Frontal lobes, changes during adolescence, 74–76, 77, 80, 81, 82, 88–89

G

Gammaglobulin products, comparison of, 139
Gay youth
  office-based care, 223–240
  risk of sexual victimization, 69
Gender-neutral terms, 235–236
Generosity, promoting as adolescent strength, 26, 28, 30
Genetic counseling, patients with PIDDs, 142, 143
Genetic factors, predisposition to drug and alcohol problems, 12–13, 14, 15, 16, 18
Glucose tolerance, impaired, 91–92
Glycemic index, 94, 96
Goal setting, in obesity management, 93, 99
Graduate Record Examination, 214
Gray-matter volume, changes during adolescence, 74–76, 78, 80

H

HEADSSS interview format, 24, 25, 236
Helping adolescents with attention-deficit/hyperactivity disorder transition toward adulthood, **203–222**
High school
  drop-out crisis, 149–164
  screening for alcohol and drug use, 16–17
HIGM types 2, 3, and 4, 124, 127, 137, 140
Hippocampus, 76, 78, 86
Homosexual orientation, office-based care for youth, 223–240
Human immunodeficiency virus (HIV), 130, 158, 223, 228, 234

in obesity management, 99
use of written change plans, 36, 37

Humoral immune defects, treatment of, 137, 140
Hyper-IgE syndrome, 128–129
Hypertension
  metabolic syndrome and, 114, 116, 117, 118
  obesity and, 91, 104
Hyperventilation syndrome, 193–195
Hypogammaglobulinemia, 123
Hypothalamic-pituitary-adrenal (HPA) axis, 78
Hypothalamus, 78

I

IgA deficiency, 124, 125–126, 137, 140, 142
IgG subclass deficiency, 124, 126, 142
Immune dysregulation, polyendocrinopathy, enteropathy, X-linked (IPEX) syndrome, 124, 130, 142
Immunodeficiencies. see also Human immunodeficiency virus
  primary, presenting in adolescence, 121–143
Implantable contraception, 182
Incarcerated juvenile offenders, 247
Independence, promoting as adolescent strength, 26, 28, 30
Individual Education Plans (IEPs), 210–211, 214
Infections, recurrent, primary immunodeficiencies and, 121–143
Injectable contraception, 170, 177–180
Instant messaging, 57, 58, 66, 67
Insulin resistance, 92, 109–115, 117, 119
Insurance coverage, adolescents with ADHD, 208–210
Interferon γ receptor/interleukin 12 receptor deficiency (IFNγR), 124, 130
Internet
  interventions, in obesity management, 93–94
  online social networking, 57–70, 217–218
Interviewing
  motivational interviewing, 31, 34, 98
  strength-based interviewing, 22–39

Intimacy development, adolescents with ADHD, 207
Intrauterine contraception, 180–182

J

Junior high school, screening for alcohol and drug use, 16–17

L

Laboratory testing
  evaluation of suspected PIDDs, 133–137
  screening of obese adolescents, 100–106
Learning disabilities, students with, 153–154, 210–212
Legal issues. see Confidentiality; Consent for care
Lesbian youth, office-based care, 223–240
Leukocyte adhesion deficiency type 1 (LAD1), 124, 128, 142
Lipid levels, abnormal, 102, 104. see also Dyslipidemia

M

Management of the adolescent concussion victim, **41–56**
Mastery, promoting as adolescent strength, 26, 27, 30
Medications and medication issues
  adolescent brain and, 83–84
  nonmedical use of prescription drugs, 1–7, 206
  traveling with medication, 214
  treatment of anxiety, 190–193
  weight loss in adolescents, 94–95, 103, 106, 116
Mental health issues. see also Attention-deficit/hyperactivity disorder
  anxiety and anxiety-related disorders, 188–201
  dialectical behavior therapy, 243–251
  emergence during adolescent brain development, 82–83
  gay, lesbian, bisexual, and questioning youth, 229–231
Message boards, 57, 58
Metabolic syndrome
  clinical assessment, 113–15
  definitions, 101, 110–111
  diagnostic criteria, 111–112
  epidemiology, 111–112
  management, 115–117
  pathogenesis, 112–113
  prevention, 117–118, 119
  reimbursement, 118

The metabolic syndrome in childhood and adolescents: a clinician's guide, **109–120**
Metformin, 96, 103, 116
Mild traumatic brain injury. see Concussion
Military testing, 214
Motivational interviewing, 31, 34, 98
MySpace, 58–59, 61, 63–65, 67, 68

N

National Education Association (NEA), action plan for reducing school dropout rate, 162–163
Neurometabolic cascade, of concussion, 44
Neuron, depiction of, 79
Nonalcoholic fatty liver disease (NAFLD), 91, 100, 102
The nonmedical use of prescription drugs, **1–8**
Nuclear factor κB essential modulator defects (NEMO), 124, 131, 137, 140, 142
Nucleus accumbens, 77, 88
Nutrition
  goals in obesity management, 99–100
  written change plans, 36, 37

O

Obesity
  definitions, 91, 111
  management, primary care approach, 91–106
  medications for weight loss, 94–95, 103, 106, 116
  metabolic syndrome, 109–119
  prevention, AAP guidelines, 118
  promoting strengths of adolescents, 30
Obsessive compulsive disorder (OCD), 188, 200–201
Obstructive sleep apnea, 91, 105
Occipital lobes, changes during adolescence, 76
Office-based care for gay, lesbian, bisexual, and questioning youth, **223–242**
Office setting, screening for substance abuse, developmental approach, 9–20
Opioids, prescription, abuse of, 2–4
Oral contraceptive pills, 171–175

Orlistat, 94–95, 103
An overview of the use of dialectical behavior therapy with adolescents for primary care physicians, **243–252**
Overweight, definition of, 91

P

Panic disorder, 188, 199–200
Parasuicidal behaviors, 243, 246, 247
Parents
    checklist for concussion, 48
    children's alcohol and drug use issues, 18–20
    protecting kids against Internet hazards, 68–70
    teaching strength-based approaches, 27–29
Parietal lobes, changes during adolescence, 76
Pediatricians, practicing, adolescent contraceptive care for, 168–182, 239
Phagocyte defects, treatment of, 141
Pharmacotherapy
    anxiety, 190–193
    weight loss, 94–95, 103, 106, 116
Polycystic ovary syndrome, 104–105
Post-concussion Scale, 46, 49
Pregnancies, teenage, adolescent contraceptive care, 168–182
Prescription drugs, nonmedical use, 1–7, 206
Primary care
    approach to obesity management, 91–106
    use of dialectical behavior therapy, 243–251
Primary immunodeficiencies presenting in adolescence, **121–148**
Primary immunodeficiency diseases (PIDDs)
    algorithm for testing, 135
    B cell defects, 123, 124, 125–127
    cellular immune defects, 129–131
    clinical presentation, 122–123, 124
    clinical signs, 133
    combined defects, 124, 131–132
    complement defects, 124, 127, 136
    diagnosis, 132–137, 142
    immune reconstitution, 141–142
    laboratory evaluation, 133–137
    phagocytic defects, 124, 128–129
    relative frequency of different types, 122
    T cell defects, 124
    therapy, 137–141
    warning signs, 134
Progestins, 177–180, 182
Psychological development, during adolescence, 78–81
Psychological disorders. see Mental health issues

R

"READY for Life" framework, 25–27, 36, 38
Rehabilitation Act of 1973, Section 504, 211–212, 214
Residential programs, 93, 247, 249
Reward system, adolescent brain development, 78, 84–85
Risk behaviors
    brain structures involved in, 76–78
    underage drinking, 11–14

S

Scholarship aid, students with ADHD, 215
Schools. see also Colleges
    drop-out crisis, 149–164
    Internet safety lessons, 68
    obesity management interventions, 92–93
Screening for substance abuse in the office setting: a developmental approach, **9–21**
Screening tools, substance abuse, 15–17, 33
Sedatives, prescription, abuse of, 6–7
Selective antibody deficiency (SAD), 124, 126, 137, 140, 142
Selective serotonin reuptake inhibitors (SSRIs)
    black-box warning, 191, 201
    treatment of anxiety, 191–192
    treatment of OCD, 201
Self-harm behaviors, 66, 69, 243, 244, 245, 247, 248
Self-management skills, adolescents with ADHD, 215–218

Sexual and reproductive health care
contraceptive care, 168–182, 239
gay, lesbian, bisexual, and questioning youth, 232–234
Sexually transmitted infections (STIs), 158, 223, 226, 234, 240
Sexual orientation, office-based care for gay, lesbian, bisexual, and questioning youth, 223–240
Sexual predators, online social networking, 61–63, 66
Sibutramine, 95–96, 103
Sleep disorders, 91, 105, 188, 196–199
Sleeping pills, prescription, abuse of, 6
Smoking
adolescents with ADHD, 206
nicotine and adolescent brain development, 84, 85
Social networking and adolescents, **57–72**
Social networking web sites, 57–70, 217–218
Socioeconomic factors, in drop-out crisis, 157–159
Sport Concussion Assessment Tool (SCAT), 45, 47
Sports, management of adolescent concussion victims, 41–55
Standardized Assessment of Concussion (SAC), 45, 46
Statins, 103
Stimulants, prescription, abuse of, 4–6, 206
Strength-based interviewing, **22–40**
Stress response, exaggerated, 78
Stroop test, 76, 83
Substance abuse
adolescent brain development and, 84–87
by adolescents with ADHD, 206
dialectical behavior therapy, 247
gay, lesbian, bisexual, and questioning youth, 231–232
nonmedical use of prescription drugs, 1–7
screening for, in the office setting, 9–20
Suicidal behavior, 229–230, 243, 246, 247
Suicide risk
adolescents who take antidepressants, 83–84
SSRI black-box warning, 191, 201
Syncope, 188, 195–196

T

Temporal lobes, changes during adolescence, 76
Test anxiety, 155–156
Text messaging, 67
Time-management tools, adolescents with ADHD, 216
Tobacco use. see Smoking
Tranquilizers, prescription, abuse of, 6–7
Transdermal patch, 175–176
Transgendered youth, 224, 225
Traumatic brain injury. see Concussion
Traveling abroad with medications, 214

U

Understanding adolescent brain development and its implications for the clinician, **73–90**
Uracil-DNA glycosylase deficiency, 124, 127

V

Vaginal contraceptive ring, 176–177
Velocardiofacial syndrome, 129
Vermont Child Health Improvement Program (VCHIP), 38

W

Web logs. see Blogs
Web sites
ADHD resources, 216, 217
social networking, 57–70, 217–218
Weight management
in metabolic syndrome, 115–118
primary care approach, 91–106
White-matter volumes, changes during adolescence, 78–81
Wiskott-Aldrich syndrome (WAS), 124, 132, 140, 142
Workplace issues, adolescents with ADHD, 212

X

X-linked agammaglobulinemia (XLA), 123, 124, 137, 140, 142

X-linked hyper-IgM syndrome (XHIGM), 123

X-linked lymphoproliferative disease (XLP), 131–132, 142